Nutrition Across Reproductive, Maternal, Neonatal, Child, and Adolescent Health Care

Zohra S. Lassi • Rehana A. Salam
Editors

Nutrition Across Reproductive, Maternal, Neonatal, Child, and Adolescent Health Care

Focus on Low and Middle Income Countries

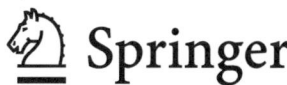# # Springer

Editors
Zohra S. Lassi
School of Public Health
University of Adelaide
Adelaide, SA, Australia

Robinson Research Institute,
Adelaide Medical School
The University of Adelaide
Adelaide, SA, Australia

Rehana A. Salam
The Daffodil Centre, The University
of Sydney, a joint venture with Cancer
Council NSW
Sydney, NSW, Australia

ISBN 978-3-031-95720-8   ISBN 978-3-031-95721-5   (eBook)
https://doi.org/10.1007/978-3-031-95721-5

© The Editor(s) (if applicable) and The Author(s), under exclusive license to Springer Nature Switzerland AG 2025

This work is subject to copyright. All rights are solely and exclusively licensed by the Publisher, whether the whole or part of the material is concerned, specifically the rights of translation, reprinting, reuse of illustrations, recitation, broadcasting, reproduction on microfilms or in any other physical way, and transmission or information storage and retrieval, electronic adaptation, computer software, or by similar or dissimilar methodology now known or hereafter developed.
The use of general descriptive names, registered names, trademarks, service marks, etc. in this publication does not imply, even in the absence of a specific statement, that such names are exempt from the relevant protective laws and regulations and therefore free for general use.
The publisher, the authors and the editors are safe to assume that the advice and information in this book are believed to be true and accurate at the date of publication. Neither the publisher nor the authors or the editors give a warranty, expressed or implied, with respect to the material contained herein or for any errors or omissions that may have been made. The publisher remains neutral with regard to jurisdictional claims in published maps and institutional affiliations.

This Springer imprint is published by the registered company Springer Nature Switzerland AG
The registered company address is: Gewerbestrasse 11, 6330 Cham, Switzerland

If disposing of this product, please recycle the paper.

Contents

Continuum of Care for RMNCAH and Role of Nutrition

Nutrition's Role in Strengthening the RMNCAH Continuum of Care 3
Zohra S. Lassi and Rehana A. Salam

Global Epidemiology and Risk Factors

Preconception Health and Nutrition 11
Patience Castleton, Sohail Lakhani, and Zahra Ali Padhani

Maternal and Child Nutrition in LMICs 27
Blessing Jaka Akombi-Inyang

Nutritional Health of Children Under the Age of Five 49
Bhavita Kumari, Ayesha Arshad Ali, and Jai K. Das

Social Determinants of Health and Nutrition Among School-Age Children and Adolescents 63
Gizachew A. Tessema, Tesfaye S. Mengistu, Adyya Gupta, Amanuel T. Gebremedhin, Eleanor Dunlop, Molla M. Wassie, and Gavin Pereira

Nutritional Challenges and Issues Relevant to Adolescents 79
Emily C. Keats, Maya Kshatriya, Christopher Lee, and Zulfiqar A. Bhutta

Health Sector Interventions

Family Planning 101
Fatima Haider, Mishaal Zulfiqar, and Zahid Ali Memon

Nutrition Intervention During Pregnancy and Lactation 119
Komal Abdul Rahim, Zahra Ali Padhani, and Zohra S. Lassi

Newborn Nutrition 137
Shabina Ariff, Sajid Soofi, Unzela Ghulam, and Aqsa Ishaq

**Nutritional Intervention Among Children Under Five,
School-Age Children, and Adolescents to Overcome Undernutrition** 155
Aamer Imdad, Areeba Fatima, and Uzma Rani

**Nutritional Interventions Among Children and Adolescents
to Prevent/Treat Overweight/Obesity** 177
Doris González-Fernández, Paulo Augusto Neves,
and Zulfiqar A. Bhutta

Non-health Sectoral Interventions

**Educational Settings and Nutrition Promotion:
Practices and Policy** 199
Shelina Bhamani, Zahra Ladhani, Zaibunissa Karim,
and Sameeta Chunara

**The Complementary Role of Social Protection Programs
in Tackling Malnutrition** 209
Wafa Aftab

Food Security and Agriculture.................................. 221
Narjis Fatima Hussain, Hamna Amir Naseem, and Jai K. Das

**Nutritional Empowerment Through Food Fortification
and Biofortification**... 241
Maha Azhar, Rahima Yasin, and Jai K. Das

Anthelminthics and WASH Interventions: Evidence and Gaps......... 261
Rehana A. Salam and Zohra S. Lassi

Women's Empowerment and Nutritional Status..................... 273
Salima Meherali, Mariam Ahmad, Sobia Idrees,
and Amyna Ismail Rehmani

**The Political Economy of Multi-sectoral Programming
of Adolescent Nutrition: Global Discourse
and Emerging Lessons from Pakistan**.............................. 289
Shehla Zaidi

Emerging Challenges

Nutrition in Conflict and Humanitarian Settings 305
Nadia Akseer, Hana Tasic, Sama El Baz, and Shelley Walton

Climate Change and Nutrition 333
Amira M. Khan and Zulfiqar A. Bhutta

**Role of Technologies in Nutritional Advances Along
the RMNCAH Continuum of Care** 353
Samra Naz, Asma Zulfiqar, and Ammarah Kanwal

Conclusion and the Way Forward

Conclusion and Way Forward 369
Rehana A. Salam, Zahra Ali Padhani, and Zohra S. Lassi

Continuum of Care for RMNCAH and Role of Nutrition

Nutrition's Role in Strengthening the RMNCAH Continuum of Care

Zohra S. Lassi and Rehana A. Salam

Malnutrition, encompassing both undernutrition and overnutrition, remains a persistent and multifaceted public health challenge in low- and middle-income countries (LMICs) [1]. Undernutrition, manifesting as stunting, wasting and micronutrient deficiencies, continues to disproportionately impact vulnerable groups, particularly women, children, and adolescents. Concurrently, overnutrition, characterised by overweight and obesity, is escalating at an alarming pace, driven by rapid urbanisation, dietary shifts towards energy-dense and nutrient-poor foods, and increasingly sedentary lifestyles [2]. These dual burdens of malnutrition not only compromise individual health outcomes but also impede socio-economic progress and the overall trajectory of sustainable human development [3, 4].

Despite notable advancements in global health, including improvements in healthcare delivery, food security, and education, malnutrition persists as a significant barrier to achieving equitable and sustainable development [5] (Fig. 1). It reinforces cycles of poverty and ill health, undermines economic productivity, and exacerbates inequalities both within and across communities. This challenge is especially critical within the continuum of reproductive, maternal, neonatal, child, and adolescent health (RMNCAH), where nutritional inadequacies at any stage can perpetuate intergenerational cycles of poor health and compromised developmental outcomes [1].

Z. S. Lassi (✉)
School of Public Health, University of Adelaide, Adelaide, SA, Australia

Robinson Research Institute, Adelaide Medical School, The University of Adelaide, Adelaide, SA, Australia
e-mail: zohra.lassi@adelaide.edu.au

R. A. Salam
The Daffodil Centre, The University of Sydney, a joint venture with Cancer Council NSW, Sydney, NSW, Australia
e-mail: rehana.abdussalam@sydney.edu.au

© The Author(s), under exclusive license to Springer Nature Switzerland AG 2025
Z. S. Lassi, R. A. Salam (eds.), *Nutrition Across Reproductive, Maternal, Neonatal, Child, and Adolescent Health Care*,
https://doi.org/10.1007/978-3-031-95721-5_1

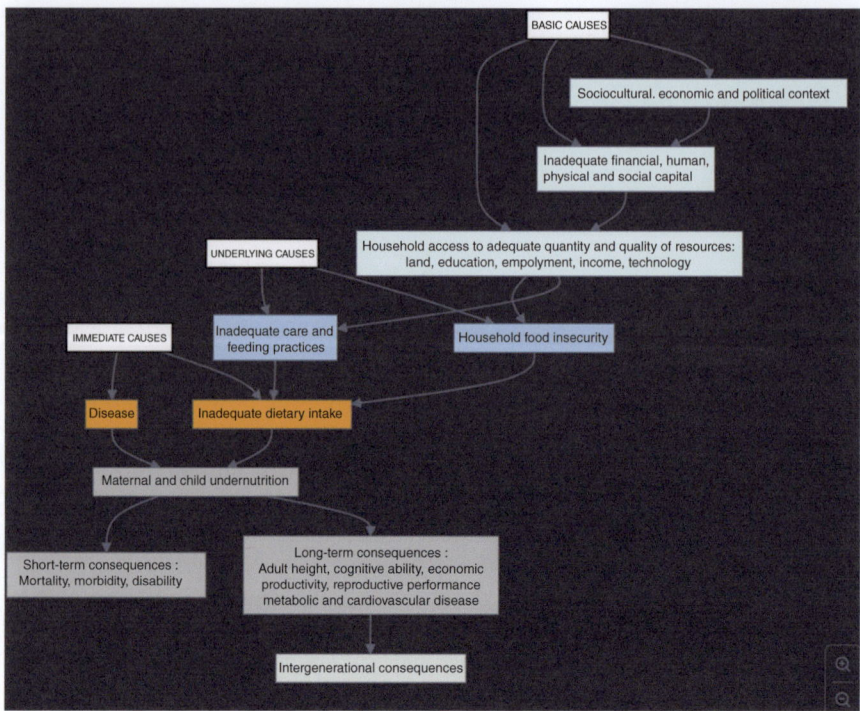

Fig. 1 Conceptual framework of malnutrition. (Adapted UNICEF framework on maternal and child undernutrition 2013 [6]; https://data.unicef.org/resources/improving-child-nutrition-the-achievable-imperative-for-global-progress/)

Malnutrition is not solely a clinical issue but a complex, multifactorial challenge driven by the intersection of social, economic, environmental, and political determinants [7]. Structural inequities, including poverty, food insecurity, inadequate access to quality healthcare, and gender inequality, play a central role in its persistence [8]. Environmental challenges such as climate change, natural disasters, and resource depletion further destabilise food systems and exacerbate vulnerabilities, particularly in LMICs [9]. Additionally, political instability and weak governance often compound these issues, hindering the development and implementation of effective nutrition policies and programmes [10].

1 The Burden of Malnutrition

Malnutrition, a global health crisis, is a significant contributor to morbidity and mortality, particularly among vulnerable populations. It is estimated that nearly half of all deaths among children under 5 years of age are attributable to malnutrition, with undernutrition weakening immune systems and increasing susceptibility to preventable illnesses such as pneumonia and diarrhoea [11]. Among women of reproductive age, malnutrition is a leading cause of adverse pregnancy outcomes, including intrauterine growth restriction, preterm birth, and low birth weight, which significantly elevate neonatal mortality risks [12]. Furthermore, children who survive malnutrition face lifelong consequences, including stunted growth, impaired cognitive development, and diminished economic productivity [13].

Adding complexity to this issue is the growing prevalence of the double burden of malnutrition, particularly in low- and middle-income countries (LMICs). In these settings, undernutrition coexists with overnutrition and obesity, driven by rapid urbanisation, dietary transitions, and the proliferation of ultra-processed, calorie-dense, nutrient-poor foods [14]. This paradoxical coexistence creates a dual challenge for health systems, as both conditions often stem from common socio-economic and environmental determinants, such as poverty, limited access to nutritious food, and inadequate healthcare services.

Micronutrient deficiencies, often termed "hidden hunger", further exacerbate the burden of malnutrition, affecting billions of individuals worldwide. Deficiencies in critical nutrients such as iron, iodine, vitamin A, and zinc impair physical growth, compromise immune function, and hinder cognitive development [15]. In pregnant women, these deficiencies increase the risk of complications during childbirth, anaemia, and preeclampsia, while in children, they contribute to learning difficulties and reduced school performance [16]. Hidden hunger not only diminishes individual potential but also perpetuates intergenerational cycles of poverty and ill-health, as malnourished mothers are more likely to give birth to malnourished infants, reinforcing the cycle.

The long-term consequences of malnutrition extend beyond immediate health impacts. Malnourished children are at increased risk of developing noncommunicable diseases (NCDs) such as diabetes, hypertension, and cardiovascular diseases later in life [17]. This phenomenon, often explained by the "developmental origins of health and disease" hypothesis, underscores the importance of optimal nutrition during critical periods of growth and development to prevent long-term health complications.

In LMICs, where malnutrition is most prevalent, the economic burden is staggering. Productivity losses due to stunting, wasting, and micronutrient deficiencies cost national economies billions of dollars annually, impeding progress towards achieving sustainable development goals. These challenges highlight the need for comprehensive, context-specific strategies to address malnutrition in all its forms.

This complex and multifaceted burden underscores the urgency of integrating targeted interventions across the continuum of reproductive, maternal, neonatal, child, and adolescent health (RMNCAH) (Fig. 2). Addressing malnutrition at every life stage, while considering the social, economic, and environmental factors that drive it, is essential to breaking the cycle of poor health and poverty and ensuring the well-being of current and future generations.

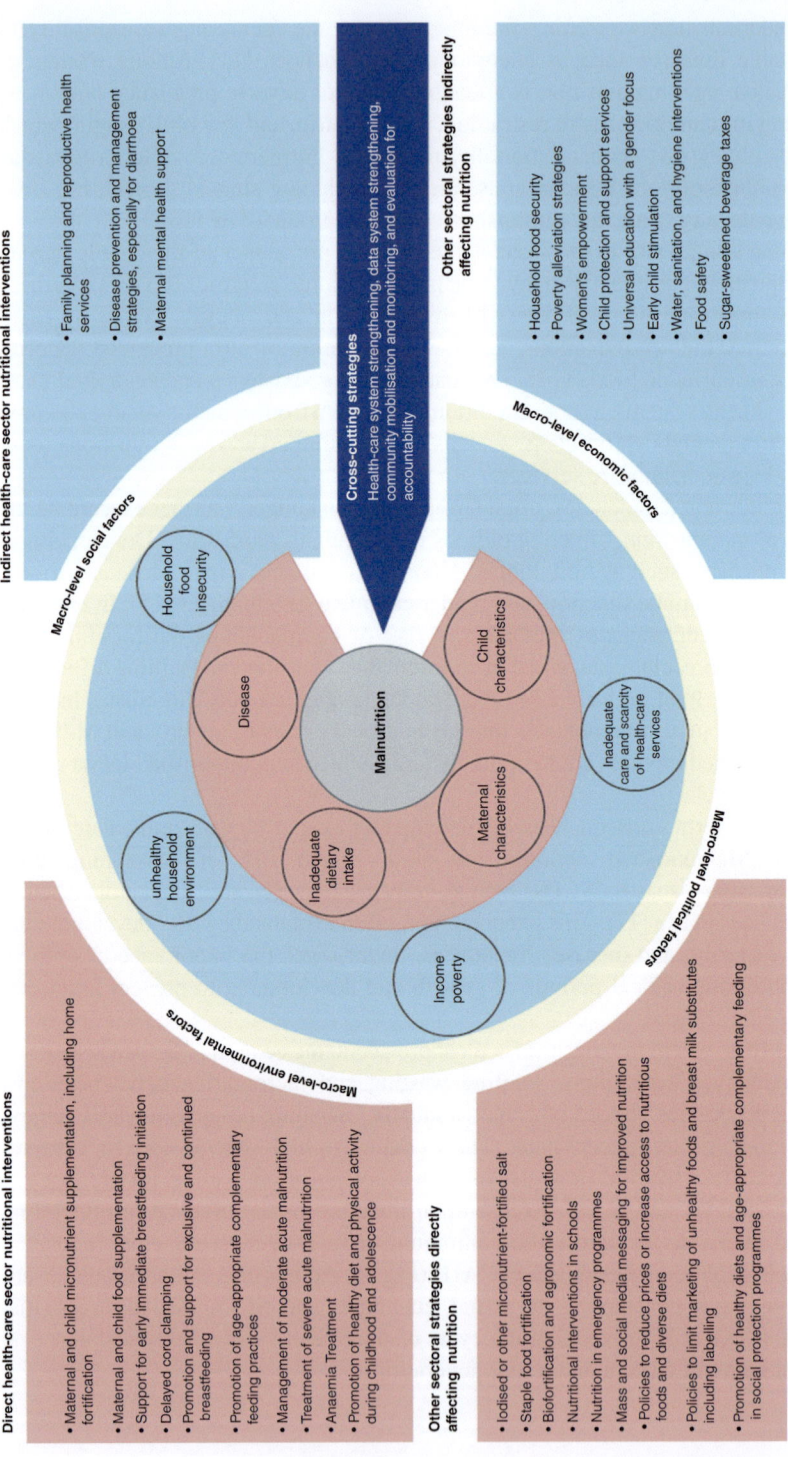

Fig. 2 Nutrition interventions for RMNCAH. (Reprinted from: The Lancet Child & Adolescent Health, 5/5, Emily C Keats et al., Effective interventions to address maternal and child malnutrition: an update of the evidence, 367–384, Copyright (2021), with permission from Elsevier)

2 A Continuum of Care Approach

The RMNCAH continuum of care framework is a cornerstone of global health, recognising the critical interconnections between health and nutrition across different stages of life. This holistic framework acknowledges that health outcomes in one stage, such as maternal nutrition during pregnancy, profoundly influence the subsequent stages, from neonatal survival to adolescent development. By focusing on the continuum, it emphasises that health and nutrition are not isolated events but part of a lifelong trajectory where interventions at key life stages can have transformative and enduring effects.

Central to this framework is the identification of "critical windows of opportunity" during preconception, pregnancy, infancy, early childhood, and adolescence. These periods are pivotal for growth and development and present the greatest potential for impactful interventions. For instance, adequate maternal nutrition before and during pregnancy is essential to prevent adverse outcomes such as low birth weight and preterm birth, while exclusive breastfeeding and optimal complementary feeding practices during infancy can significantly reduce the risk of malnutrition and promote cognitive development. Similarly, adolescence represents a crucial period for breaking intergenerational cycles of poor nutrition, as it is a time of rapid growth and the formation of lifelong health behaviours.

The continuum of care approach also underscores the importance of integrating services across health systems to address the multifaceted nature of malnutrition. This includes bridging gaps between preventive and curative services, ensuring continuity of care across life stages, and fostering collaboration between health and non-health sectors. For example, addressing health disparities requires not only strengthening healthcare systems but also tackling the underlying social determinants of health, such as poverty, education, food security, and gender inequality. Equitable access to quality nutrition interventions is central to this approach, particularly in LMICs, where systemic inequities often hinder progress.

This book delves into the vital role of nutrition across the RMNCAH continuum, highlighting how both health-specific and broader sectoral interventions can combat malnutrition at its root. It provides an in-depth exploration of nutrition's impact on health outcomes at each stage of the continuum, from preconception care to adolescent health, drawing on robust evidence and case studies from diverse settings.

Each section builds a comprehensive understanding of malnutrition, its drivers, and potential solutions, aimed at empowering policymakers, researchers, and practitioners to design and implement effective, context-specific interventions. By adopting this continuum of care perspective, the book aims to inspire a paradigm shift in how malnutrition is addressed, moving beyond siloed approaches to integrated, equity-focused strategies that prioritise the health and well-being of women, children, and adolescents.

References

1. Escher NA, et al. The effect of nutrition-specific and nutrition-sensitive interventions on the double burden of malnutrition in low-income and middle-income countries: a systematic review. Lancet Glob Health. 2024;12(3):e419–32.
2. Le TH. An analysis of changing dietary trends and the implications for global health. Bournemouth University; 2021.
3. Kiosia A, et al. The double burden of malnutrition in individuals: identifying key challenges and re-thinking research focus. Nutr Bull. 2024;49:132.
4. Takhelchangbam ND, et al. Epidemiology of double burden of malnutrition: causes and consequences. Prev Med Res Rev. 2024;1(6):305–9.
5. Sowards DB, McCauley SM, Munoz N. Impacting malnutrition, food insecurity, and health equity: an overview of academy of nutrition and dietetics priorities and future opportunities. J Acad Nutr Diet. 2022;122(10):S7–S11.
6. UNICEF. Improving child nutrition: the achievable imperative for global progress. New York: UNICEF; 2013.
7. Delisle HF. Poverty: the double burden of malnutrition in mothers and the intergenerational impact. Ann N Y Acad Sci. 2008;1136(1):172–84.
8. Bowen S, Elliott S, Hardison-Moody A. The structural roots of food insecurity: how racism is a fundamental cause of food insecurity. Sociol Compass. 2021;15(7):e12846.
9. Swinburn BA, et al. The global syndemic of obesity, undernutrition, and climate change: the Lancet Commission report. Lancet. 2019;393(10173):791–846.
10. Ogunniyi AI, et al. Governance quality, remittances and their implications for food and nutrition security in Sub-Saharan Africa. World Dev. 2020;127:104752.
11. Morales F, et al. Effects of malnutrition on the immune system and infection and the role of nutritional strategies regarding improvements in children's health status: a literature review. Nutrients. 2023;16(1):1.
12. Keats EC, et al. Effective interventions to address maternal and child malnutrition: an update of the evidence. Lancet Child Adolesc Health. 2021;5(5):367–84.
13. Okolo CV, Okolo BO, Anika NN. Nutrition for pre-school children in Africa and Asia: a review analysis on the economic impact of children's malnutrition. Economy. 2021;8(1):10–5.
14. Popkin BM, Corvalan C, Grummer-Strawn LM. Dynamics of the double burden of malnutrition and the changing nutrition reality. Lancet. 2020;395(10217):65–74.
15. Benton D, ILSI Europe a.i.s.b.l. Micronutrient status, cognition and behavioral problems in childhood. Eur J Nutr. 2008;47:38–50.
16. Lassi ZS, et al. Essential pre-pregnancy and pregnancy interventions for improved maternal, newborn and child health. Reprod Health. 2014;11:1–19.
17. Grey K, et al. Severe malnutrition or famine exposure in childhood and cardiometabolic noncommunicable disease later in life: a systematic review. BMJ Glob Health. 2021;6(3):e003161.

Global Epidemiology and Risk Factors

Preconception Health and Nutrition

Patience Castleton, Sohail Lakhani, and Zahra Ali Padhani

1 What Is Preconception?

The preconception period is one of the most sensitive phases in human development that not only affects pregnancy outcomes but also carries long-term implications for both the mother and her child [1]. The preconception period is categorised into two phases: the proximal period, which refers to the time immediately before pregnancy (up to 2 years before conception), and the distal preconception period, which encompasses the mother's early years, adolescence, and the 2-plus years preceding a pregnancy (not necessarily the first pregnancy) [2].

The 2018 Lancet series on preconception health introduced three perspectives for conceptualising the preconception period. These include the individual perspective, which involves a deliberate intention to conceive, usually taking place weeks to months before pregnancy; the biological perspective, which concentrates on the days to weeks leading up to embryo development; and the public health perspective, which spans months to years to address preconception risk factors. These definitions serve as the basis for a variety of individual and community health initiatives targeted at enhancing preconception health outcomes. They also offer a helpful, empirically supported framework for identifying critical preconception intervals [3, 4].

P. Castleton · Z. A. Padhani (✉)
School of Public Health, University of Adelaide, Adelaide, SA, Australia

Robinson Research Institute, University of Adelaide, Adelaide, SA, Australia
e-mail: patience.castleton@adelaide.edu.au; zahraali.padhani@adelaide.edu.au

S. Lakhani
Community Health Sciences, Aga Khan University, Karachi, Pakistan
e-mail: sohail.lakhani2@aku.edu

© The Author(s), under exclusive license to Springer Nature Switzerland AG 2025
Z. S. Lassi, R. A. Salam (eds.), *Nutrition Across Reproductive, Maternal, Neonatal, Child, and Adolescent Health Care*,
https://doi.org/10.1007/978-3-031-95721-5_2

2   Why Is Preconception Health Important?

Women bear a disproportionate burden of challenges related to reproductive health, including teenage or unintended pregnancies, domestic or intimate partner violence, and sexually transmitted diseases (STIs) [5]. Maternal mortality, particularly during labour, childbirth, or immediately postpartum, remains a significant concern despite progress towards achieving Sustainable Development Goal (SDG) 3.1 by 2030 [6, 7]. In 2020, the World Health Organization (WHO) reported an alarming figure that an estimated 800 women lost their lives daily due to preventable causes, translating to around 287,000 deaths among women of reproductive age (WRA) that year [8]. The majority of these tragic incidents occurred in low-income settings (430 per 100,000 live births) compared to high-income settings, where the rate was substantially lower (12 per 100,000 live births) [8].

The year 2021 witnessed a concerning trend as newborns faced a heightened risk of mortality within the first month of birth, with a rate of 18 deaths per 1000 live births [9]. Many of these neonatal deaths resulted from factors like premature birth, low birth weight (LBW), asphyxia, and severe infections. Optimising women's health before pregnancy, as well as across the maternal continuum of care, could potentially improve the health outcomes for mothers and newborns [4, 6, 10, 11]. The persistent high burden of adverse maternal, pregnancy, and neonatal health outcomes underscores the urgency of targeting this crucial phase in the continuum of care.

3   Preconception Health Risk Factors

The well-being of both prospective parents at preconception and during pregnancy plays a vital role in fostering a healthy pregnancy and optimal foetal growth and development [12]. Various factors, including health behaviours, exposures, and risks such as comorbidities, poor mental health, use of alcohol and substances, malnutrition, environment, and infections, have been identified as contributors to maternal and child morbidity and mortality [13]. Given the unpredictability of the time of conception and the understanding that the health of both partners contributes to a successful pregnancy, the importance of preconception care cannot be overstated [4]. It is recommended that preconception care be extended to all individuals of reproductive age. Providing such care and recognizing the significance of preconception care can help minimise the health risks and create an environment conducive to a healthy conception and pregnancy [13].

The preconception period is a critical time during which a woman's physical condition can have significant impacts on her future pregnancy and the health of both herself and her child [14]. It is recommended that women start pregnancy at an optimal weight, with a healthy diet and low-stress levels [15–17]. Maintaining a healthy lifestyle is vital for both parents in ensuring a successful and healthy pregnancy and a child of full physical and mental health. These recommendations are even stronger for women with a history of mental and/or physical health conditions, including diabetes, anaemia, and depression. Extensive research shows that successful and healthy pregnancies are significantly more likely amongst women who have a healthy lifestyle before pregnancy, with some studies also showing that rectifying these poor habits (including diet, inadequate exercise, and alcohol exposure) during pregnancy does not positively impact the child's health status [4].

Nutrition is one of the key preconception health determinants that has been extensively studied and correlated with poor pregnancy and child outcomes. Preconception nutrition exerts a distinct impact on birth outcomes in comparison to maternal nutrition during pregnancy. Research shows that the nutritional status of mothers before conception significantly impacts the linear growth of their children during the initial 1000 (from conception to 6 months) days of life [18]. Throughout the first half of this crucial period, the mother plays the indispensable role of being the sole provider of nutrition for the developing child. This essential nourishment begins during pregnancy while the child is in the womb and continues during the initial 6 months of life, during which exclusive breastfeeding is highly encouraged [19]. The nutritional well-being of a mother significantly influences her baby's nutritional status, as essential micronutrients are passed from the mother to the foetus through the placental barrier [2]. The degree of transfer of micronutrients across the placental barrier depends on the specific mechanism utilised by each micronutrient, making it unique for each nutrient. During the early stages of gestation, when organogenesis takes place, various biological pathways involve micronutrients. For instance, iron, iodine, zinc, and long-chain n-3 polyunsaturated fatty acids are crucial for the development of the brain and nervous system. Inadequate levels of vitamins A, B6, B12, and folate during embryogenesis may result in foetal malformations and pregnancy loss [20]. The immediate effects of micronutrient deficiencies during pregnancy and preconception on both the mother and infant are reasonably well-known, but the long-term implications of these inadequacies have not been entirely clarified. Although some evidence from animal studies and observational research in humans indicates a connection between intrauterine micronutrient status and the potential risk of chronic diseases, the comprehension of the molecular mechanisms underlying these effects for many micronutrients is limited [21]. Studies, from both high-income countries (HIC) and low- and middle-income countries (LMIC), have indicated that dietary habits within the 3 years leading up to pregnancy, marked by a high consumption of fruits, vegetables, legumes, nuts, and fish, coupled with a low intake of red and processed meat, are linked to a decreased likelihood of experiencing gestational diabetes mellitus [22], hypertensive disorders during pregnancy [23], and preterm birth [24]. Poor nutrition choices are an ever-increasing epidemic worldwide, with urbanisation increasing consumption of junk foods and decreasing activity levels. It is a key area for improvement and one that can be taught and managed by all people. A UK-based study revealed that a significant number of women in their reproductive years lack adequate nutritional preparation for pregnancy, even when considering lower reference nutrient intake levels [4, 25]. This was particularly notable among young women, especially in terms of mineral intake, with 77% of women aged 18–25 reporting dietary intakes below the daily recommended nutrient intake (RNI) for iodine [25]. Further, 96% of women in this age range also had inadequate levels of iron and folate for a healthy pregnancy, indicating they would be at increased risk of adverse outcomes if they were to enter pregnancy. The strong correlation between preconception nutrition and maternal and child health outcomes, including chronic diseases and mental health, highlights the critical need for relevant and accurate preconception care services and information.

Research highlights some association between preconception eating disorders, including anorexia nervosa, binge eating disorder, and/or bulimia nervosa, and negative pregnancy and child outcomes [26, 27]. Whilst severe eating disorders can result in infertility and lifelong difficulties in conceiving [28], mothers who suffer from binge-eating disorder and/or bulimia nervosa prior to conception face an increased risk of miscarriage [27]. A recent meta-analysis reported a mean decrease of 0.19 kg in childbirth weight amongst mothers with a history of anorexia nervosa, as compared to mothers with no history of an eating disorder [29]. In a study of over 1000 young mothers, the risk of LBW was twice as high amongst mothers who had previously been hospitalised for an eating disorder when compared to mothers who had never suffered an eating disorder [26]. This same study also showed a 70% increased risk of preterm delivery and an 80% increase in small-for-gestational age (SGA) delivery for women who had previously suffered from an eating disorder [26]. Studies have also found a significant association between preconception and pregnancy eating disorders and postnatal depression [30–32], with most mothers continuing to suffer from their eating disorder throughout and after pregnancy [32]. However, the research in this domain is scarce, and a large gap in our understanding surrounds eating disorders in preconception care.

Apart from malnutrition and eating disorders, maternal smoking either before or during pregnancy has a detrimental impact on health, leading to loss of pregnancy, intrauterine growth restriction (IUGR), LBW, and behavioural, physical, and learning difficulties in a child [4, 33, 34]. There is no available evidence on the impact of smoking prevention before pregnancy. However, smoke-free legislation has shown a significant reduction in preterm births (-10.4%, 95% confidence interval (CI): $-18.8, -2.0$; from four cohort studies; $n = 1,366,862$ pregnancies) [4, 35]. Further, government bodies worldwide recommend alcohol abstinence for women who are planning a pregnancy or who are already pregnant due to the risk of foetal alcohol syndrome (FAS). FAS occurs when alcohol passes through the mother's umbilical cord to the child, thus exposing them to alcohol, resulting in central nervous system problems, intellectual disabilities, and/or birth defects [36]. Whilst the literature is scarce with human trials, studies on mice and rats have shown that alcohol consumption 2 weeks prior to pregnancy significantly increased the risk of abnormal foetal development and placed the mother at greater risk of macrosomia [37]. Alcohol exposure before and during pregnancy is an increasing risk factor for poor maternal and child health worldwide, with one study showing almost 23% of African participants continuing to consume alcohol once pregnant [38]. A recent cohort study even showed that paternal smoking increases the risk of child behavioural problems, including depression, anxiety, and sleep problems at up to 6 years of age. It is important to be cautious of alcohol consumption as women can be pregnant for up to 6 weeks without knowing, thus exposing their child to alcohol long before getting the opportunity to stop. Further, it is recommended that fathers also decrease their alcohol exposure prior to, and during, pregnancy, in support of their partners. According to Stephen et al., public health actions such as smoke-free legislation and the pricing of alcohol have contributed to reducing risky behaviours [4].

High blood sugar levels at the time of conception have been known to increase the risk of stillbirth, birth defects, and preterm birth [39]. Preconception diabetes has been found to significantly increase the risk of miscarriage, macrosomia, [40] and stillbirth [41], as well as intrauterine growth and developmental abnormalities [42], contributing to child morbidity and early mortality. Women with pre-existing diabetes mellitus (type 1 and 2) are recommended to obtain exhaustive preconception care to discuss treatments, health-related risks, and management. To reduce type 2 diabetes and gestational diabetes mellitus (GDM), studies and government bodies urge at-risk mothers to maintain a healthy body mass index (BMI), eat nutritious foods, and exercise regularly [43]. Studies have also revealed that women living in low socio-economic regions are unlikely to seek medical preconception care and/or treatments, even when struggling with health conditions such as diabetes [44].

4 Impact of Malnutrition During Preconception on Maternal and Child Health and Nutrition Outcomes

4.1 Overweight/Obesity

Maternal and child health outcomes are significantly compromised by high preconception maternal BMI. With approximately 40% of women worldwide entering pregnancy overweight or obese, [45] appropriate preconception care needs to directly address these challenges are crucial. A meta-analysis found that high-income countries (HIC) constituted 35% of the burden of overweight and obese pregnancies, and low- and middle-income countries (LMIC) constituted 39.1% of the burden [46], thus depicting its global impact. Further, a recent meta-analysis supported this idea, showing that 20.5% of women in LMIC/LICs were overweight or obese prior to pregnancy [47]. Increases in urbanisation in both HIC and LMIC in recent years have been predicted to be contributing factors to the increasing overweight/obesity epidemic, with the availability of different foods and sedentary lifestyles all negatively impacting healthy lifestyles worldwide [46].

Women who enter pregnancy overweight are at a greatly increased risk of excessive gestational weight gain and the associated consequences of this, including pre-eclampsia and hypertension [45]. Recent data has indicated that women who enter pregnancy obese gain significantly more weight than recommended during their pregnancy [48]. Further in a recent meta-analysis of studies conducted in LMIC and LIC, excess gestational weight gain was associated with an increased risk of preterm birth (adjusted RR: 1.22, 95% CI: 1.13–1.31), large for gestational age (adjusted RR: 1.44, 95% CI: 1.33–1.57), and macrosomia (adjusted RR: 1.52, 95% CI: 1.33–1.73) [47]. This meta-analysis concluded that these child outcomes were modified by the mothers' BMI prior to pregnancy, thus further supporting the important role that preconception health plays in child outcomes. In a Canada-based population study involving 226,958 singleton pregnancies, it was observed that a preconception weight loss of 10%, whilst remaining in the healthy BMI range, correlated with a substantial and clinically significant reduction in the risk of preeclampsia, gestational diabetes mellitus, preterm delivery, macrosomia, and stillbirth [49]. Further, a study amongst African women showed that the risk of preeclampsia increased with an increase in the mothers' BMI, being up to 1.8 times more likely to experience it when compared to mothers in the healthy BMI range before conception [50].

Maternal obesity is also associated with an increased risk of labour complications, including delivery haemorrhage, caesarean section delivery, and infections [51–53], as well as short gestation periods, and in one American study, neonatal death [54]. Elevated BMI at conception and excessive gestational weight gain have also been associated with excessive childhood weight gain during infant years, as well as early childhood [55], which have previously been linked to lifelong obesity and high BMI [56]. Furthermore, children born to mothers who are overweight or obese during early pregnancy are at a significantly increased risk of suffering from hypertension, asthma, and coronary heart disease later in life, greatly inhibiting their quality of life, often resulting in early mortality [57–59]. Childhood stunting has also been seen to be increased twofold in mothers who are overweight or obese [60], which can greatly inhibit the child's learning capacity and development, as well as increase their risk of non-communicable diseases and infections [61]. Moreover, women who enter pregnancy overweight or obese are significantly more likely to experience GDM and are also more likely to gain excessive weight during pregnancy, compared to mothers who do not experience GDM [62], placing both the mother and child at increased risk of adverse health outcomes.

Research has shown that insufficient knowledge and understanding of the optimal diet and physical activity levels in the preconception period are significant barriers for overweight women to make appropriate lifestyle changes before conception [63]. As changes to body composition are not fast or easy for an individual to make, it is essential for women to understand the negative repercussions of preconception obesity before trying to get pregnant [63]. Further, early interventions must be sought for women who unintentionally conceive whilst at an increased BMI to minimise risks to both mothers and their children.

4.2 Underweight

Women who lack key macronutrients and are undernourished are commonly underweight, with approximately 7.3% of women of reproductive age in low- and middle-income countries recording BMIs under those recommended by the WHO [64]. However, a recent meta-analysis of 53 studies (118, 207 participants) found that 15.6% of women in LMIC/LICs were underweight before pregnancy [47]. Underweight women at preconception are at significantly increased risk of poor birth outcomes, including a three-fold increase in the chance of preterm birth and LBW [65, 66].

Research has also indicated an association between underweight mothers and poor child mental and physical development [67], with findings relating to underweight mothers and subsequent underweight children showing increased signs of food-related anxiety and refusal behaviours as well as moodiness and anger [68]. Further, women who enter pregnancy underweight are also more likely to have insufficient gestational weight gain, increasing their risk of negative pregnancy outcomes [69]; notably, they face a 2.3 times increased risk of small-for-gestational age (SGA) birth [69]. This was further supported in a recent meta-analysis of evidence from LMICs and LICs which found inadequate gestational weight gain significantly increases the risk of SGA (adjusted RR: 1.44, 95% CI: 1.36–1.54), microcephaly (adjusted RR: 1.57, 95% CI: 1.31–1.88), and LBW (adjusted RR: 1.62, 95% CI: 1.51–1.72) babies [47]. Women with a pre-pregnancy body mass index (BMI) below the "healthy range" of 17.5, or 18 kg/m^2, face an elevated risk of having a child with stunted growth at the age of two; an elevation of one standard deviation in preconception weight has been linked to a 283 g increase in birth weight (95% confidence interval (CI): 279 to 286) in Vietnam [70]. Women with a preconception weight below 43 kg (and under the "healthy" BMI range) are almost three times more likely to deliver an infant with SGA [71] or LBW [72]. Low birth weight has been previously linked to difficulties with cognitive function and verbal comprehension in later childhood [73, 74]. A recent study also found no association between preconception underweight mothers who showed average gestational weight gain and improvements in the intellectual development of their children, compared to mothers who had below-average gestational weight gain [73].

4.3 Micronutrient Deficiencies

Micronutrients are found in dietary foods and supplements and are essential for all humans for many biological processes. Micronutrients must be supplied externally to the body, thus resulting in many men and women suffering from deficiencies. Deficiencies during pregnancy can result in many adverse maternal outcomes, including preeclampsia, as well as negative child outcomes, including preterm birth, LBW, and neural tube defects [75]. Further, studies have shown that women suffering from certain micronutrient deficiencies, such as vitamin B12, have lower fertility levels and are significantly less likely to conceive compared to women with adequate micronutrient levels [76]. Further, women living in low-income countries are at heightened risk of micronutrient deficiencies due to their poor diet, which places their children at an equally high risk of micronutrient deficiencies throughout their lives [77]. Additionally, women who enter pregnancy with a micronutrient deficiency are significantly more likely to retain this deficiency during their pregnancy due to the increased nutritional requirements of the growing foetus [78, 79].

Research on micronutrient supplementation during the preconception, and pregnancy, period shows largely inconclusive data on improving maternal and child health and nutrition outcomes. However, a recent randomised controlled trial saw that micronutrient supplementation at least 6 months prior to conception was able to improve nutrient stores during pregnancy. The study also concluded that children born to mothers with increased levels of folic acid, iron, and multiple micronutrients from external supplementations had improved cognitive functions at up to 7 years of age [80, 81]. Up-to-date research on other key micronutrients is currently limited, however, insufficient vitamin D has previously been linked to preeclampsia and perinatal mortality [82] and deficiencies in calcium have been associated with increased blood pressure during pregnancy [83, 84].

4.4 Iron Deficiency Anaemia

Low haemoglobin levels (<110 g/L), or anaemia, are attributed to low consumption and/or absorption of iron in the diet (commonly attributed to iron deficiency) and are a highly prevalent condition that impacts approximately 29% of non-pregnant women, and 28% of pregnant women globally (Stevens 2013). Without appropriate dietary supplementation, anaemia can significantly increase the risk of preeclampsia, placenta previa, and caesarean delivery [85], thus risking further pregnancy and labour complications and adverse child health.

Studies have further shown associations between maternal anaemia and preterm birth, small-for-gestational-age births, and perinatal mortality [85] as well as childhood anaemia [65, 86]. Women with suboptimal nutritional status prior to conception are at increased risk of developing and sustaining anaemia during pregnancy; adolescents, women with low socio-economic status, and women with unplanned pregnancies are at greatly increased risk of anaemia [87]. A meta-analysis found that almost 43% of pregnant women in low- and middle-income countries suffered anaemia, with this attributing to 12% of LBW children, 18% of perinatal mortality, and 19% of preterm births [88]. A recent study conducted in Vietnam also found significant associations between preconception anaemia and decreased motor and language skills at 12 months, however, the low home environments of the mother and child could have had a confounding impact on this data [65]. Therefore, women in low- and middle-income countries are negatively, disproportionately affected by anaemia [86]. It is important to evaluate their unique and high-risk needs during preconception care.

4.5 Folic Acid Deficiency

In low- and middle-income countries, the largest contributing factor to LBW children is intrauterine growth restriction [89], a complication that is well-known to be reduced in the presence of sufficient folic acid [89]. Intrauterine growth restriction can also result in major birth defects, including spina bifida and anencephaly, greatly compromising a child's development and quality of life [90], all of which have been proven to be decreased in the presence of folic acid supplementation [90, 91]. The Centres for Disease Prevention and Control (CDC) recommends that women of reproductive age consume 400 mcg folic acid at least 1 month before getting pregnant and throughout the first 3 months of conception; however, only 30% of women worldwide take a folate supplement before conception [92]. Substantial research spanning many years has shown strong associations between reductions in neural birth defects and sufficient folate acid intake [92]. This unequivocal evidence has prompted more than 75 countries to implement fortification programmes, promoting the benefits of adequate folate acid and ensuring women's folic acid intake is sufficient before, and after, conception [92]. However, global research has shown that women living in low- and middle-income countries have poor retention of daily folic acid supplementation [67], thus placing them at higher risk of negative pregnancy and child outcomes, indicating a greater need for research into food fortification in these countries.

5 Preconception Care

Preconception care refers to a series of interventions designed to identify and address biomedical, behavioural, and social risks that may impact a woman's health and/or pregnancy outcome. The primary goal of preconception care is to prevent and manage these risks holistically, considering the mother's physical, emotional, and social needs. This involves implementing initiatives that extend beyond nutrition, such as promoting women's education and empowerment. Preconception care also involves specific health interventions, including vaccinations and the use of vitamin and mineral supplements.

This type of care is also referred to as pre-pregnancy care, interpregnancy care, or periconceptional medicine [93]. Healthcare professionals and researchers highlight that numerous effective interventions for preconception care could yield improved outcomes if initiated during the preconception period [2].

5.1 Preconception Health Interventions to Improve Nutrition

The preconception health of women has received the limelight since the release of the WHO guidelines in 2013 [94], followed by a series of reviews by Dean et al. and Lassi et al. in 2014 [6, 95–97] and the Lancet series in 2018 [4, 10, 98]. These guidelines and reviews have highlighted preconception health as a critical period for shaping the health outcomes of both mothers and their children.

There is a lack of interventional trials aiming to improve health and nutrition among both men and women in their reproductive years, especially adolescents [10, 25, 99]. Most of the trials aim to improve the health of mothers, usually involving women during pregnancy, due to short follow-up time and an easy recruitment process [10]. There are a variety of interventions to improve nutrition and micronutrient deficiencies among women [100]. These interventions are broadly classified as nutrition-specific and nutrition-sensitive interventions. Nutrition-specific interventions are those interventions that target the immediate determinants of foetal and child development and nutrition [101]. Nutrition-specific interventions related to preconception health involve dietary and micronutrient supplementation, food fortification and biofortification, disease prevention, dietary modification, and nutrition in emergency settings, while nutrition-sensitive interventions address the underlying determinants of foetal and child development and nutrition [101]. Nutrition-sensitive interventions related to preconception health include food security and agriculture, social support or social safety nets, women's empowerment, family planning services, improving mental health, and water, sanitation, and

Table 1 Preconception health interventions to improve nutrition outcomes among women and their children

Domain	Interventions
Improving nutrition and preventing micronutrient deficiencies and eating disorders	Nutrition education Lifestyle modification Physical activity Diet modification Food fortification and biofortification Multiple micronutrient supplementation Iron folic acid supplementation Screening Weight control and management Improve access to water, sanitation, and hygiene Deworming
Poverty alleviation	School education programmes Social protection programmes such as conditional and unconditional cash transfers, food and cash vouchers, food baskets, and rations
Maternal age and pregnancy prevention	Family planning education Birth spacing or interpregnancy intervals Contraceptive use or distribution Abortion care
Prevention of female genital mutilation and intimate partner violence	Women empowerment Community support groups Counselling services Social support
Prevention of sexually transmitted infections	Sex education Contraceptive use or distribution Counselling services Provision of treatment and access to medications Immunisation
Prevention of infections	Immunisation Deworming
Prevention of chronic diseases, e.g. phenylketonuria	Timely screening, diagnosis, and management of diseases Counselling services Lifestyle modification
Prevent alcohol, tobacco, and substance use	Taxation Law enforcement Counselling services
Improving oral health	Health promotion Dental checkups

Sources: Dean et al. [95], Snyder et al. [100], World Health Organization [102], Moos et al. [103]

hygiene (WASH) [101]. Dean et al. [95], Padhani et al. [99], and the WHO [34] suggests and discusses preconception health interventions which could help contribute to the health of mothers and their children (see Table 1).

6 Conclusion and Future Implications

As demonstrated through this chapter, women and their children are at high risk of poor health outcomes due to inadequate nutrient intake, micronutrient deficiencies, and poor lifestyle behaviours. Recently, there has been more focus on the preconception health of women, but there is very limited research on the preconception health and nutrition of men, adolescents, and young adults. To improve the health of women and their children, the chapter suggests:

- Robust trials targeting both men and women in their reproductive years to study the impact of preconception nutrition interventions on lifelong health outcomes.
- Prevent and target all the health and nutritional risk factors at an early stage of life (i.e. adolescence).
- Trials and reviews that evaluate the effectiveness, impact, and cost of different preconception nutrition interventions for men and women in LMIC/LICs.
- More research into the role that paternal preconception nutrition has on pregnancy and child outcomes, with a particular focus on paternal diabetes, obesity, and micronutrient deficiencies. This recommendation further extends to randomised controlled trial (RCT) interventions involving men in improving preconception care and nutrition.
- Further research on the impact that paternal eating disorders, restricted and binge eating types, have on pregnancy and child outcomes, as there is a significant gap in this research extending to men.
- Further studies on the impact that different diets, low carb, intermittent fasting, etc. during preconception periods have on pregnancy and child health outcomes.

References

1. Mumford SL, et al. Preconception care: it's never too early. Reprod Health. 2014;11(1):73.
2. Hanson MA, et al. The International Federation of Gynecology and Obstetrics (FIGO) recommendations on adolescent, preconception, and maternal nutrition: "Think Nutrition First". Int J Gynaecol Obstet. 2015;131(Suppl 4):S213–53.
3. Preconception health | Lancet Series. 2018; Available from: https://www.thelancet.com/series/preconception-health.
4. Stephenson J, et al. Before the beginning: nutrition and lifestyle in the preconception period and its importance for future health. Lancet. 2018;391(10132):1830–41.
5. WHO. Preconception care report of a regional expert group consultation 6–8 August 2013. New Delhi: World Health Organization; 2014.
6. Dean SV, et al. Preconception care: nutritional risks and interventions. Reprod Health. 2014;11(3):1–15.

7. Institute for Health Metrics and Evaluation (IHME). Findings from the Global Burden of Disease Study 2017. Seattle: IHME; 2018.
8. WHO. Trends in maternal mortality 2000 to 2020: estimates by WHO, UNICEF, UNFPA, World Bank Group and UNDESA/Population Division. Geneva: World Health Organization; 2023. Licence: CC BY-NC-SA 3.0 IGO.
9. UNICEF. Levels and trends in child mortality United Nations Inter-Agency Group For Child Mortality Estimation (UN IGME): Report 2020: Estimates developed by the UN inter-agency Group for Child Mortality Estimation. New York: ONU. p. 2023.
10. Barker M, et al. Intervention strategies to improve nutrition and health behaviours before conception. Lancet. 2018;391(10132):1853–64.
11. Mason E, et al. Preconception care: advancing from 'important to do and can be done' to 'is being done and is making a difference'. Reprod Health. 2014;11:1–9.
12. Moss JL, Harris KM. Impact of maternal and paternal preconception health on birth outcomes using prospective couples' data in add health. Arch Gynecol Obstet. 2015;291:287–98.
13. Dean SV, et al. Preconception care: closing the gap in the continuum of care to accelerate improvements in maternal, newborn and child health. Reprod Health. 2014;11(3):1–8.
14. Caulfield, Laura E., Victoria Elliot, Program in Human Nutrition, the Johns Hopkins Bloomberg School of Public Health, for SPRING. Nutrition of Adolescent Girls and Women of Reproductive Age in Low- and Middle-Income Countries: Current Context and Scientific Basis for Moving Forward. Arlington: Strengthening Partnerships, Results, and Innovations in Nutrition Globally (SPRING) project; 2015.
15. Lang AY, et al. Optimizing preconception health in women of reproductive age. Minerva Ginecol. 2017;70(1):99–119.
16. Frayne DJ, et al. Health care system measures to advance preconception wellness: consensus recommendations of the clinical workgroup of the National Preconception Health and Health Care Initiative. Obstet Gynecol. 2016;127(5):863–72.
17. National Institute for Health and Care Excellence. Fertility problems: assessment and treatment: National Institute for Health and Care Excellence. 2016 [cited 2023 01/03/2023]; Available from: https://www.nice.org.uk/guidance/cg156/chapter/Recommendations.
18. 1000 days. Nutrition in the first 1000 days: A foundation for brain development and learning. 2023 [cited 2024 August 6]; Available from: Available from: https://thousanddays.org/wp-content/uploads/1000Days-Nutrition_Brief_Brain-Think_Babies_FINAL.pdf.
19. Mason JB, et al. The first 500 days of life: policies to support maternal nutrition. Glob Health Action. 2014;7:23623.
20. Ramakrishnan U, et al. Effect of women's nutrition before and during early pregnancy on maternal and infant outcomes: a systematic review. Paediatr Perinat Epidemiol. 2012;26(Suppl 1):285–301.
21. Christian P, Stewart CP. Maternal micronutrient deficiency, fetal development, and the risk of chronic disease. J Nutr. 2010;140(3):437–45.
22. Bao W, et al. Prepregnancy low-carbohydrate dietary pattern and risk of gestational diabetes mellitus: a prospective cohort study. Am J Clin Nutr. 2014;99(6):1378–84.
23. Schoenaker DA, Soedamah-Muthu SS, Mishra GD. The association between dietary factors and gestational hypertension and pre-eclampsia: a systematic review and meta-analysis of observational studies. BMC Med. 2014;12:157.
24. Grieger JA, Grzeskowiak LE, Clifton VL. Preconception dietary patterns in human pregnancies are associated with preterm delivery. J Nutr. 2014;144(7):1075–80.
25. Cuskelly GJ, McNulty H, Scott JM. Effect of increasing dietary folate on red-cell folate: implications for prevention of neural tube defects. Lancet. 1996;347(9002):657–9.
26. Sollid CP, et al. Eating disorder that was diagnosed before pregnancy and pregnancy outcome. Am J Obstet Gynecol. 2004;190(1):206–10.
27. Kimmel MC, et al. Obstetric and gynecologic problems associated with eating disorders. Int J Eat Disord. 2016;49(3):260–75.

28. Easter A, Treasure J, Micali N. Fertility and prenatal attitudes towards pregnancy in women with eating disorders: results from the Avon Longitudinal Study of Parents and Children. BJOG. 2011;118(12):1491–8.
29. Solmi F, et al. Low birth weight in the offspring of women with anorexia nervosa. Epidemiol Rev. 2014;36(1):49–56.
30. Meltzer-Brody S, et al. Eating disorders and trauma history in women with perinatal depression. J Womens Health (Larchmt). 2011;20(6):863–70.
31. Morgan JF, Lacey JH, Chung E. Risk of postnatal depression, miscarriage, and preterm birth in bulimia nervosa: retrospective controlled study. Psychosom Med. 2006;68(3):487.
32. Knoph Berg C, et al. Factors associated with binge eating disorder in pregnancy. Int J Eat Disord. 2011;44(2):124–33.
33. Courtney, R., The Health Consequences of Smoking—50 Years of Progress: A Report of the Surgeon General, 2014 Us Department of Health and Human Services Atlanta, GA: Department of Health and Human Services, Centers for Disease Control and Prevention, National Center for Chronic Disease Prevention and Health Promotion, Office on Smoking and Health, 2014 1081 pp. Online (grey literature): http://www.surgeongeneral.gov/library/reports/50-years-of-progress. 2015, Wiley Online Library.
34. Reeves S, Bernstein I. Effects of maternal tobacco-smoke exposure on fetal growth and neonatal size. Expert Rev Obstet Gynecol. 2008;3(6):719–30.
35. Been JV, et al. Effect of smoke-free legislation on perinatal and child health: a systematic review and meta-analysis. Lancet. 2014;383(9928):1549–60.
36. Prevention, C.f.D.C.a., Fetal Alcohol Spectrum Disorders (FASDs). 2023.
37. Lee YJ, et al. Alcohol consumption before pregnancy causes detrimental fetal development and maternal metabolic disorders. Sci Rep. 2020;10(1):10054.
38. Mulat B, Alemnew W, Shitu K. Alcohol use during pregnancy and associated factors among pregnant women in Sub-Saharan Africa: further analysis of the recent demographic and health survey data. BMC Pregnancy Childbirth. 2022;22(1):361.
39. Mackin ST, et al. Factors associated with stillbirth in women with diabetes. Diabetologia. 2019;62(10):1938–47.
40. Zhang S, et al. Hypertensive disorders of pregnancy in women with gestational diabetes mellitus on overweight status of their children. J Hum Hypertens. 2017;31(11):731–6.
41. Lauenborg J, et al. Audit on stillbirths in women with Pregestational type 1 diabetes. Diabetes Care. 2003;26(5):1385–9.
42. Diabetes in pregnancy: management from preconception to the postnatal period. Dec 16 2020: London: National Institute for Health and Care Excellence (NICE).
43. Prevention, C.f.D.C.a. Diabetes During Pregnancy. 2018; Available from: https://www.cdc.gov/reproductivehealth/maternalinfanthealth/diabetes-during-pregnancy.htm#:~:text=Diabetes%20during%20pregnancy%E2%80%94including%20type,%2C%20stillbirth%2C%20and%20preterm%20birth.
44. Ukoha WC, Mtshali NG, Adepeju L. Current state of preconception care in sub-Saharan Africa: a systematic scoping review. Afr J Prim Health Care Fam Med. 2022;14(1):e1–e11.
45. Goldstein RF, et al. Association of gestational weight gain with maternal and infant outcomes: a systematic review and meta-analysis. JAMA. 2017;317(21):2207–25.
46. Chen C, Xu X, Yan Y. Estimated global overweight and obesity burden in pregnant women based on panel data model. PLoS One. 2018;13(8):e0202183.
47. Perumal N, et al. Suboptimal gestational weight gain and neonatal outcomes in low and middle income countries: individual participant data meta-analysis. BMJ. 2023;382:e072249.
48. Institute of, M. and I.O.M.P.W.G. National Research Council Committee to Reexamine, The National Academies Collection: Reports funded by National Institutes of Health, in Weight Gain During Pregnancy: Reexamining the Guidelines, K.M. Rasmussen and A.L. Yaktine, Editors. 2009, National Academies Press (US) Copyright © 2009, National Academy of Sciences: Washington, DC.

49. Schummers L, et al. Risk of adverse pregnancy outcomes by prepregnancy body mass index: a population-based study to inform prepregnancy weight loss counseling. Obstet Gynecol. 2015;125(1):133–43.
50. Mrema D, et al. The association between pre pregnancy body mass index and risk of preeclampsia: a registry based study from Tanzania. BMC Pregnancy Childbirth. 2018;18(1):56.
51. Aviram A, Hod M, Yogev Y. Maternal obesity: implications for pregnancy outcome and long-term risks-a link to maternal nutrition. Int J Gynaecol Obstet. 2011;115(Suppl 1):S6–10.
52. Denison FC, et al. Obesity, pregnancy, inflammation, and vascular function. Reproduction. 2010;140(3):373–85.
53. Arrowsmith S, Wray S, Quenby S. Maternal obesity and labour complications following induction of labour in prolonged pregnancy. BJOG. 2011;118(5):578–88.
54. Chen A, et al. Maternal obesity and the risk of infant death in the United States. Epidemiology. 2009;20(1):74–81.
55. Lau EY, et al. Maternal weight gain in pregnancy and risk of obesity among offspring: a systematic review. J Obes. 2014;2014:524939.
56. Singh AS, et al. Tracking of childhood overweight into adulthood: a systematic review of the literature. Obes Rev. 2008;9(5):474–88.
57. Ziyab AH, et al. Developmental trajectories of body mass index from infancy to 18 years of age: prenatal determinants and health consequences. J Epidemiol Community Health. 2014;68(10):934–41.
58. Burgess JA, et al. Childhood adiposity predicts adult-onset current asthma in females: a 25-yr prospective study. Eur Respir J. 2007;29(4):668–75.
59. Bjørge T, et al. Body mass index in adolescence in relation to cause-specific mortality: a follow-up of 230,000 Norwegian adolescents. Am J Epidemiol. 2008;168(1):30–7.
60. Félix-Beltrán L, Macinko J, Kuhn R. Maternal height and double-burden of malnutrition households in Mexico: stunted children with overweight or obese mothers. Public Health Nutr. 2021;24(1):106–16.
61. De Sanctis V, et al. Early and Long-term consequences of nutritional stunting: from childhood to adulthood. Acta Biomed. 2021;92(1):e2021168.
62. MayoClinic. Gestational Diabetes. [2022 October 18 2023]; Available from: https://www.mayoclinic.org/diseases-conditions/gestational-diabetes/symptoms-causes/syc-20355339.
63. Lim S, et al. Addressing obesity in preconception, pregnancy, and postpartum: a review of the literature. Curr Obes Rep. 2022;11(4):405–14.
64. Reyes Matos U, Mesenburg MA, Victora CG. Socioeconomic inequalities in the prevalence of underweight, overweight, and obesity among women aged 20-49 in low- and middle-income countries. Int J Obes. 2020;44(3):609–16.
65. Young MF, et al. Long-term association between maternal preconception hemoglobin concentration, anemia, and child health and development in Vietnam. J Nutr. 2023;153(5):1597–606.
66. El Rafei R, et al. Association of pre-pregnancy body mass index and gestational weight gain with preterm births and fetal size: an observational study from Lebanon. Paediatr Perinat Epidemiol. 2016;30(1):38–45.
67. Black RE, et al. Maternal and child undernutrition and overweight in low-income and middle-income countries. Lancet. 2013;382(9890):427–51.
68. Ammaniti M, et al. Malnutrition and dysfunctional mother-child feeding interactions: clinical assessment and research implications. J Am Coll Nutr. 2004;23(3):259–71.
69. Montvignier Monnet A, et al. In underweight women, insufficient gestational weight gain is associated with adverse obstetric outcomes. Nutrients. 2022;15(1)
70. Young MF, et al. Role of maternal preconception nutrition on offspring growth and risk of stunting across the first 1000 days in Vietnam: a prospective cohort study. PLoS One. 2018;13(8):e0203201.
71. Young MF, et al. The relative influence of maternal nutritional status before and during pregnancy on birth outcomes in Vietnam. Eur J Obstet Gynecol Reprod Biol. 2015;194:223–7.
72. Tshotetsi L, et al. Maternal factors contributing to low birth weight deliveries in Tshwane District, South Africa. PLoS One. 2019;14(3):e0213058.

73. Li C, et al. Effect of maternal pre-pregnancy underweight and average gestational weight gain on physical growth and intellectual development of early school-aged children. Sci Rep. 2018;8(1):12014.
74. Li C, et al. Effect of prenatal and postnatal malnutrition on intellectual functioning in early school-aged children in rural western China. Medicine (Baltimore). 2016;95(31):e4161.
75. Schaefer E, Nock D. The impact of Preconceptional multiple-micronutrient supplementation on female fertility. Clin Med Insights Womens Health. 2019;12:1179562x19843868.
76. Hosseini B, Eslamian G. Association of Micronutrient Intakes with female infertility: review of recent evidence. Thrita. 2015;4(1):e25586.
77. Gernand AD, et al. Micronutrient deficiencies in pregnancy worldwide: health effects and prevention. Nat Rev Endocrinol. 2016;12(5):274–89.
78. Parisi F, et al. Micronutrient supplementation in pregnancy: who, what and how much? Obstet Med. 2019;12(1):5–13.
79. Darnton-Hill I, Mkparu UC. Micronutrients in pregnancy in low- and middle-income countries. Nutrients. 2015;7(3):1744–68.
80. Veena SR, et al. Association between maternal nutritional status in pregnancy and offspring cognitive function during childhood and adolescence; a systematic review. BMC Pregnancy Childbirth. 2016;16(1):220.
81. Prado EL, et al. Maternal multiple micronutrient supplementation and other biomedical and socioenvironmental influences on children's cognition at age 9–12 years in Indonesia: follow-up of the SUMMIT randomised trial. Lancet Glob Health. 2017;5(2):e217–28.
82. Palacios C, Kostiuk LK, Peña-Rosas JP. Vitamin D supplementation for women during pregnancy. Cochrane Database Syst Rev. 2019;7(7):Cd008873.
83. Imdad A, Jabeen A, Bhutta ZA. Role of calcium supplementation during pregnancy in reducing risk of developing gestational hypertensive disorders: a meta-analysis of studies from developing countries. BMC Public Health. 2011;11(3):S18.
84. Hofmeyr GJ, et al. Calcium supplementation during pregnancy for preventing hypertensive disorders and related problems. Cochrane Database Syst Rev. 2018;10
85. Smith C, et al. Maternal and perinatal morbidity and mortality associated with anemia in pregnancy. Obstet Gynecol. 2019;134(6):1234–44.
86. Balarajan Y, et al. Anaemia in low-income and middle-income countries. Lancet. 2011;378(9809):2123–35.
87. Iseyemi A, et al. Socioeconomic status as a risk factor for unintended pregnancy in the contraceptive CHOICE project. Obstet Gynecol. 2017;130(3):609–15.
88. Rahman MM, et al. Maternal anemia and risk of adverse birth and health outcomes in low- and middle-income countries: systematic review and meta-analysis. Am J Clin Nutr. 2016;103(2):495–504.
89. Jonker H, et al. Maternal folic acid supplementation and infant birthweight in low- and middle-income countries: a systematic review. Matern Child Nutr. 2020;16(1):e12895.
90. Imbard A, Benoist JF, Blom HJ. Neural tube defects, folic acid and methylation. Int J Environ Res Public Health. 2013;10(9):4352–89.
91. Wald NJ. Folic acid and neural tube defects: discovery, debate and the need for policy change. J Med Screen. 2022;29(3):138–46.
92. Bailey RL, West KP Jr, Black RE. The epidemiology of global micronutrient deficiencies. Ann Nutr Metab. 2015;66(Suppl. 2):22–33.
93. Berghella V, et al. Preconception care. Obstet Gynecol Surv. 2010;65(2):119–31.
94. World Health Organization. Meeting to develop a global consensus on preconception care to reduce maternal and childhood mortality and morbidity. Geneva: World Health Organization; 2013.
95. Dean SV, et al. Systematic review of preconception risks and interventions. Pakistan: Division of Women and Child Health, Aga Khan University; 2013.
96. Lassi ZS, et al. Preconception care: caffeine, smoking, alcohol, drugs and other environmental chemical/radiation exposure. Reprod Health. 2014;11(3):1–12.

97. Lassi ZS, et al. Effects of preconception care and periconception interventions on maternal nutritional status and birth outcomes in low-and middle-income countries: a systematic review. Nutrients. 2020;12(3):606.
98. Fleming TP, et al. Origins of lifetime health around the time of conception: causes and consequences. Lancet. 2018;391(10132):1842–52.
99. Padhani ZA, et al. Exploring preconception health in adolescents and young adults: identifying risk factors and interventions to prevent adverse maternal, perinatal, and child health outcomes–a scoping review. PLoS One. 2024;19(4):e0300177.
100. Snyder TM, et al. A role for preconception nutrition. In: The biology of the first 1,000 days. CRC Press; 2017. p. 423–38.
101. Ruel MT, Alderman H. Nutrition-sensitive interventions and programmes: how can they help to accelerate progress in improving maternal and child nutrition? Lancet. 2013;382(9891):536–51.
102. World Health Organization. Global technical strategy for malaria 2016–2030. World Health Organization; 2015.
103. Moos MK, Dunlop AL, Jack BW, Nelson L, Coonrod DV, Long R, Boggess K, Gardiner PM. Healthier women, healthier reproductive outcomes: recommendations for the routine care of all women of reproductive age. Am J Obstet Gynecol. 2008;199(6):S280–9.

Maternal and Child Nutrition in LMICs

Blessing Jaka Akombi-Inyang

1 Background

The nutritional health of mothers and their children holds a pivotal role in assessing and predicting the overall health of a population, as it plays a significant role in shaping the foundation of the next generation's health. By focusing on the nutritional needs of pregnant women and young children, societies can effectively safeguard positive health outcomes across a range of domains, encompassing physical, mental, and long-term well-being. Prioritizing the nutritional needs of these individuals is not only a means of ensuring their immediate health but also an investment in the long-term vitality and resilience of society [1].

The relationship between maternal and child nutrition (MCN) is intricate and interdependent. During pregnancy, a mother's nutritional intake directly impacts the development of the foetus [2]. Insufficient or imbalanced nutrition during this crucial period can lead to stunted growth, cognitive impairments, and even developmental abnormalities in the child [3]. Moreover, maternal nutrition affects pregnancy outcomes, influencing the likelihood of preterm births and low birth weight [4]. These factors, in turn, contribute to the child's immediate and future health prospects [1].

Proper maternal nutrition ensures that the growing foetus receives essential nutrients necessary for healthy development [5]. Adequate intake of nutrients like protein, vitamins, and minerals is vital for the formation of organs, tissues, and bones. A well-nourished foetus has a higher likelihood of achieving optimal birth weight and size, reducing the risk of complications during childbirth, and increasing the infant's resilience to infections and illnesses [6, 7].

B. J. Akombi-Inyang (✉)
School of Population Health, University of New South Wales, Sydney, NSW, Australia
e-mail: b.akombi@unsw.edu.au

© The Author(s), under exclusive license to Springer Nature Switzerland AG 2025
Z. S. Lassi, R. A. Salam (eds.), *Nutrition Across Reproductive, Maternal, Neonatal, Child, and Adolescent Health Care*,
https://doi.org/10.1007/978-3-031-95721-5_3

Nutrition is intricately linked to brain development. Nutrient deficiencies during critical developmental stages can lead to cognitive impairments, affecting a child's learning abilities, memory, and overall cognitive functioning [8, 9]. Proper nutrition, on the other hand, supports healthy brain development, enhancing a child's potential for intellectual growth and emotional well-being [8, 9].

Early life nutrition has a lasting impact on long-term health outcomes [10]. Malnutrition during childhood, especially in the form of undernutrition, can predispose individuals to chronic diseases such as diabetes [11], cardiovascular disease [12], and obesity later in life [13]. By prioritizing maternal and child nutrition, societies can potentially mitigate the risk of such diseases and promote healthier aging.

Emphasizing maternal and child nutrition is crucial for breaking the cycle of intergenerational malnutrition [14, 15]. Poor maternal nutrition can lead to undernourished children, perpetuating a cycle of malnutrition and poor health across generations [15]. By ensuring that mothers receive adequate nutrition before, during, and after pregnancy, this cycle can be disrupted, leading to better health outcomes for both mothers and their children.

2 Issues in Maternal and Child Nutrition

Good nutrition is essential in reducing maternal and child mortality and in achieving the Sustainable Development Goals (SDGs) on child health. Maternal and child malnutrition, including undernutrition (underweight, wasting, and stunting), overnutrition (overweight and obesity), and micronutrient deficiencies, represents one of the most urgent global challenges. Malnutrition has profound implications for survival, its long-term association with chronic diseases, and its influence on economic development and productivity, both at the individual and societal levels, make it a significant public health challenge. Furthermore, factors related to infant and young child feeding (IYCF), water, sanitation, and hygiene (WASH), and family planning also play a significant role in shaping maternal and child nutrition on an individual basis.

2.1 Undernutrition

Maternal undernutrition presents a significant health concern in most developing nations. The nutritional status of a mother before conception, during pregnancy, and following childbirth exerts multifaceted effects on a child's development. It not only elevates the risks of maternal and child mortality but also imparts lasting impacts on the child's well-being. One particularly noteworthy consequence is stunting. Inadequate nutrition adversely affects cognitive functions, leading to enduring consequences such as reduced learning capabilities in both childhood and adulthood, resulting in diminished earnings and heightened susceptibility to diseases. Stunting that occurs during the early years of life tends to be largely irreversible and contributes to an intergenerational cycle of poor growth and development. The underlying mechanism for these long-term effects can be attributed to insufficient growth and tissue restructuring during critical developmental phases due to inadequate nutritional resources [16]. Foetal growth unfolds in a sequential manner, and any deficiency in nutrition during any phase can lead to maldevelopment. This can be explained by genetic alterations and subsequent epigenetic changes. These epigenetic modifications transpire during the embryo's formation and are highly sensitive to the nutritional provisions made available to the foetus by the mother. Consequently, these abnormalities can be prevented through proper maternal nutrition practices [16].

Child undernutrition contributes significantly to the global disease burden. It stems primarily from causes including foetal growth restrictions, stunting, wasting, micronutrient deficiencies, and suboptimal breastfeeding practices [17]. Undernutrition directly impacts child health by compromising immune function as a result of exposure to pathogens in the environment thus increasing susceptibility to infectious diseases, and accelerating the onset, severity, and duration of illnesses. Additionally, it is often a consequence of poor health, as infectious diseases like diarrhea, acute respiratory infections, tuberculosis, and HIV raise energy requirements while reducing appetite and nutrient absorption, as depicted in Fig. 1.

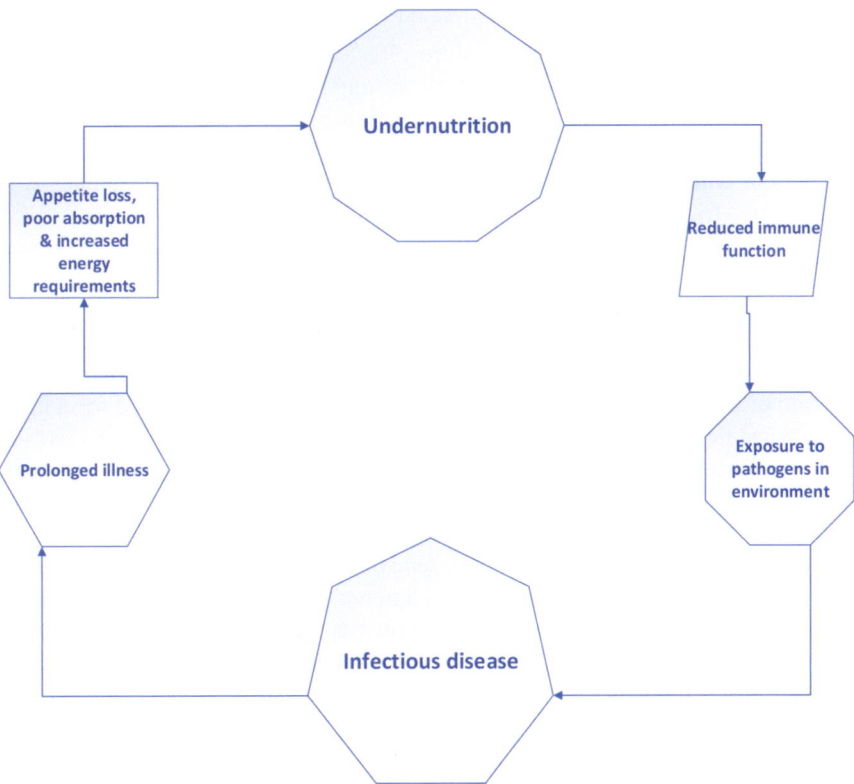

Fig. 1 The cycle of undernutrition and disease

The synergistic and interactive consequences of undernutrition and disease are frequently masked by the proximate factors contributing to child mortality. Nonetheless, it is imperative to acknowledge that undernutrition persists as a significant underlying determinant of child mortality [18]. Therefore, implementing timely nutrition interventions to address undernutrition at crucial stages of the life cycle can reduce child mortality rates in high-burden countries. For instance, focusing on nutrition interventions for children during the critical "1,000-day window of opportunity" from conception to 2 years of age has the potential to substantially decrease the prevalence of childhood stunting [19].

A significant number of women worldwide grapple with undernutrition, micronutrient deficiencies, and overweight concerns [20]. Among women aged 15–49, about 30% are affected by anemia, 10% are underweight, and 35% are overweight, with 13% falling into the category of obesity [20]. Furthermore, micronutrient deficiencies, particularly those involving vitamin A, zinc, iodine, and iron, cast a shadow over the well-being of more than two billion individuals on a global scale. These deficiencies have dire consequences, ranging from premature mortality and deteriorating health to impaired vision, stunted growth, compromised cognitive development, and diminished productivity [20]. In 2022, approximately 148.1 million children under the age of 5 years, accounting for 22.3% of the global population in that age group, were reported to be stunted [21]. In addition, about 45 million children under 5, equivalent to 6.8%, were affected by wasting, with a subset of 13.6 million (2.1%) suffering from severe wasting [21]. The prevalence of stunting is disproportionately concentrated in two regions: Asia, where 52% of cases are found, and Africa, where 43% of cases are prevalent [21]. Likewise, over three-quarters of children afflicted by severe wasting reside in Asia, with another 22% residing in Africa.

2.2 Micronutrient Deficiencies

Micronutrients are crucial for numerous physiological processes, including the production of enzymes, hormones, and other essential compounds needed for normal growth and development [22]. Deficiencies in these nutrients pose serious risks to child development, leading to a range of adverse outcomes such as physical stunting, developmental delays, cognitive impairments, increased susceptibility to infections, higher illness and mortality rates, and reduced productivity later in life [22].

Globally, micronutrient deficiencies remain widespread, with recent estimates showing that 56% of preschool-aged children and 69% of women of reproductive age are deficient in at least one vital micronutrient, including iron, vitamin A, zinc, or folate [23, 24]. The highest rates of deficiency are found in South Asia and Sub-Saharan Africa, though even high-income countries are affected; for example, about 50% of women in the UK and 33% in the USA have at least one micronutrient deficiency [24]. Among these, iron, iodine, and vitamin A deficiencies are the most common, particularly affecting children and pregnant women due to their increased nutritional needs.

Research has shown that iron deficiency anemia in infancy and early childhood has been linked to suboptimal motor development and irreversible cognitive deficits, which hinder learning and reduce educational achievements [25]. Childhood iodine deficiency has also been identified as a risk factor for developmental delays [25], while vitamin A deficiency raises the risk of blindness in children and susceptibility to common ailments like diarrhea and measles, which can be life-threatening [26].

Additionally, zinc deficiency has been associated with impaired growth and compromised immune function, resulting in conditions such as stunting, wasting, and more severe infections. Micronutrient supplementation involves the provision of single or multiple micronutrients (including iodine, iron, folic acid, vitamin A, vitamin B12, vitamin D, and zinc) in the form of capsules, tablets, drops, or syrup to children. Micronutrient supplementation is one of the simplest and most cost-effective public health interventions available [27]. For instance, vitamin A supplementation has demonstrated a reduction in overall mortality and deaths related to diarrhea in children aged 6–59 months [28], while zinc supplementation has lowered the incidence of diarrhea [29].

2.3 Inadequate Infant and Young Child Feeding (IYCF) Practices

Practicing appropriate feeding techniques for infants and young children, including early and exclusive breastfeeding, and providing complementary foods after thorough handwashing with soap, has been demonstrated to enhance child health significantly [30]. Breast milk is a vital source of energy and essential nutrients for children aged 6–23 months. It can supply over half of a child's energy requirements between the ages of 6 and 12 months, and about one-third of energy needs from 12 to 24 months. Furthermore, breast milk plays a crucial role in providing energy and nutrients during periods of illness, reducing mortality among malnourished children [31].

Initiating breastfeeding within the first hour after birth shields newborns from infections and lowers newborn mortality rates [32]. Infants who are either partially breastfed or not breastfed at all face an elevated risk of mortality due to conditions like diarrhea and other infections. Exclusive breastfeeding for the first 6 months offers numerous benefits for both the infant and the mother. Infants who are not exclusively breastfed are at a higher risk of succumbing to infections, including pneumonia and diarrhea, not only in developing but also in industrialized countries [33].

Children and adolescents who were breastfed during infancy are less prone to becoming overweight or obese. Additionally, they tend to perform better on intelligence assessments and exhibit higher school attendance rates [34]. Breastfeeding has also been correlated with increased income in adulthood, thereby fostering child development and diminishing healthcare expenses, which ultimately translates into economic advantages for both individual families and at the national level.

Data on IYCF indicators indicate that globally, approximately 44% of infants under 6 months are exclusively breastfed [35]. However, this figure is significantly lower in some LMIC regions, especially in South Asia and Sub-Saharan Africa, where various socioeconomic and cultural barriers impact breastfeeding rates [35]. In LMICs, early initiation of breastfeeding within the first hour of life varies widely, with rates as low as 50% in certain regions.

Additionally, the percentage of children receiving adequate dietary diversity, which is essential for meeting nutritional needs, remains low across LMICs. Less than 30% of children aged 6–23 months receive the minimum dietary diversity needed to support healthy growth and development [35].

According to the World Health Organization (WHO), children aged 6–23 months should receive a variety of foods to ensure their nutritional needs are met. Diversifying food groups has been associated with improved linear growth in young children. A lack of dietary diversity can heighten the risk of micronutrient deficiencies, which can negatively impact children's physical and cognitive development [36].

In addition to ensuring dietary diversity, the frequency of providing complementary foods to a child is crucial. Breastfed infants aged 6–8 months should receive complementary foods 2–3 times per day, while breastfed children aged 9–23 months should be given complementary foods 3–4 times daily, along with additional nutritious snacks offered 1–2 times a day. Providing meals and snacks less frequently than recommended can compromise the overall intake of energy and micronutrients, potentially leading to growth faltering, stunting, and micronutrient deficiencies [19].

2.4 Water, Sanitation, and Hygiene (WASH)

Inadequate sanitation and poor hygiene practices contribute to the presence of fecal pathogens in the environment. When these pathogens are ingested through contaminated food and water sources, they can lead to various diseases. The provision of safe drinking water, proper sanitation facilities, and good hygiene practices is of paramount importance for human health and overall well-being. Access to safe water, sanitation, and hygiene (WASH) not only serves as a fundamental requirement for health but also has a positive impact on livelihoods, school attendance, and human dignity. It plays a crucial role in fostering resilient communities that live in healthy environments.

Recent data on water, sanitation, and hygiene (WASH) indicators for low- and middle-income countries (LMICs) highlight ongoing challenges, particularly regarding access to safe drinking water and sanitation. According to the World Health Organization (WHO), about 50% of the global population still lacks adequate access to safe drinking water and sanitation services, a shortfall that could prevent an estimated 1.4 million deaths and 74 million disability-adjusted life years annually. LMICs bear the brunt of these deficiencies, with Sub-Saharan Africa and South Asia showing the highest burden, where diarrheal diseases, primarily caused by unsafe water and poor sanitation, are a leading cause of child mortality [37].

Maintaining appropriate levels of sanitation, practicing good hygiene, and ensuring access to safe drinking water can significantly reduce the prevalence of childhood mortality, malnutrition, and stunting. This reduction occurs by preventing conditions like diarrhea, parasitic diseases, and environmental enteropathy, which can negatively affect the body's capacity to absorb nutrients and hinder normal growth and cognitive development.

For infants under the age of 6 months, diarrhea can cause irreversible damage to intestinal development, impairing their ability to absorb essential nutrients. Diarrhea ranks as the second-leading cause of death among children under the age of 5 years worldwide [38, 39]. Children suffering from persistent diarrhea are at a significantly elevated risk of malnutrition and exhibit reduced resistance to infections, making them more susceptible to fatal infectious diseases [39, 40]. Implementing water, sanitation, and hygiene interventions to reduce the incidence of diarrheal diseases can prevent nearly two million deaths attributable to undernutrition annually [38, 39, 41].

2.5 Overnutrition

Overnutrition in MCN is a multifaceted issue with significant implications for public health. While undernutrition has traditionally been the focus of global health efforts, overnutrition has emerged as a growing concern globally, particularly in LMICs, due to increasing urbanization and dietary shifts toward high-calorie, ultra-processed foods [42–45]. A 2023 report on food security and nutrition reported that around 12.6% of the global population is affected by obesity, with LMICs experiencing notable increases in childhood obesity and adult overweight. Specifically, LMICs report a combined overweight and obesity prevalence of about 8.4% in children under 5, with variations across regions [46].

Maternal overnutrition can also lead to foetal overgrowth, resulting in macrosomia (high birth weight). This increases the risk of birth complications for both the mother and the baby, such as shoulder dystocia and birth injuries [47, 48]. Furthermore, maternal overnutrition can have long-term consequences for the offspring, predisposing them to obesity, metabolic syndrome, and other chronic diseases later in life through mechanisms such as epigenetic modifications [49].

Recent data highlight the rising global and LMIC rates of maternal overnutrition, with significant implications for maternal and child health outcomes. The 2023 Global Nutrition Report estimates that globally, 40% of women aged 20 years and older are overweight or obese, with rates highest in middle-income countries, where 62% of adult women face overnutrition risks [50]. In LMICs specifically, maternal overnutrition is escalating, particularly in urban areas with increased access to calorie-dense, nutrient-poor foods. Studies show higher rates in regions like Latin America, the Caribbean, and parts of Africa, where urbanization and shifts in diet have contributed to obesity prevalence among women of reproductive age, often surpassing 30% in some countries [17, 50].

Excessive weight gain during pregnancy is an increasing concern worldwide, especially in LMICs, where it has been linked to adverse outcomes for both mothers and infants. These include gestational diabetes, hypertension, preeclampsia, and an increased risk of caesarean delivery [51, 52]. While data varies, recent studies estimate that nearly 20% of pregnancies in LMICs involve excessive gestational weight gain [53, 54].

Early childhood is a critical period for growth and development, and overnutrition during this time can have lasting effects on health. Excessive calorie intake, often from energy-dense and nutrient-poor foods, contributes to childhood obesity, which has reached epidemic proportions globally [55].

Childhood obesity is associated with a myriad of health problems, including type 2 diabetes, cardiovascular disease, fatty liver disease, and psychological issues such as low self-esteem and depression [55]. Overnutrition in infancy, such as overfeeding or early introduction of high-calorie solid foods, can disrupt the establishment of healthy eating habits and metabolic regulation, setting the stage for lifelong health challenges [55].

Recent data on childhood obesity reveals alarming trends both globally and in LMICs. According to the World Obesity Federation's *World Obesity Atlas 2023*, more than 39 million children aged under 5 years are affected by overweight or obesity worldwide, representing nearly 6% of children in this age group. LMICs continue to report an increase in childhood obesity from 5% to 14% in girls, and from 6% to 16% in boys for the period 2020–2035 [55].

Several factors contribute to overnutrition in MCN, including changes in food environments, cultural norms, socioeconomic status, and marketing practices [56–60]. For instance, in many societies, there is a cultural preference for larger body sizes, which can influence perceptions of health and contribute to the normalization of overnutrition. Likewise, socioeconomic disparities play a significant role, with lower-income populations often having limited access to nutritious foods and relying on cheaper, calorie-dense options that contribute to overnutrition and obesity. The availability and affordability of highly processed and energy-dense foods, coupled with sedentary lifestyles, promote overconsumption and weight gain [61–67].

Addressing overnutrition requires a comprehensive approach that encompasses policy, environmental, and behavioral strategies. Policies aimed at promoting healthy eating environments, such as taxation on sugary beverages, restrictions on unhealthy food marketing to children, and subsidies for fruits and vegetables, can help shift consumption patterns toward healthier options [55]. In addition, nutrition education and counselling for expectant mothers and caregivers are crucial for raising awareness about the importance of balanced diets, appropriate portion sizes, and responsive feeding practices. Creating supportive environments that facilitate physical activity and promote breastfeeding as the optimal source of nutrition for infants can also help prevent overnutrition and its associated health consequences.

3 Determinants of Maternal and Child Nutrition

The determinants of maternal and child nutrition are diverse yet interconnected and influence maternal health and child growth at various levels. The socioeconomic, political, and cultural context in which a child is born can shape their access to food, health status, and overall well-being. For example, a woman who is poor and malnourished is more likely to have a low birth weight baby, which can increase the risk of chronic health problems for the child later in life. The daily living conditions of a child, such as their access to clean water and sanitation, can also play a role in their nutritional status. Improving maternal and child nutrition requires addressing all the determinants of malnutrition. This includes interventions targeting the socioeconomic, political, cultural, and individual health-related factors that influence nutritional status.

The *socioeconomic determinants* of maternal and child nutrition include factors such as income, education, and employment. These factors can affect the ability of mothers to access nutritious food, as well as their nutrition knowledge. The *political determinants* of maternal and child nutrition include factors such as government policies on food security, agriculture, and health care. These policies can affect the availability and affordability of food, as well as the quality of healthcare services. The *cultural determinants* of maternal and child nutrition include factors such as beliefs about food, feeding practices, and gender roles. These factors can influence the choices that mothers and children make about food, as well as the way that they are cared for. The *individual health-related determinants* of maternal and child nutrition include factors such as genetics, health status, age, and gender. These factors can affect the body's ability to absorb and use nutrients, as well as the risk of developing certain diseases, as shown in Fig. 2. For example, a child who is born with a genetic disorder that affects their absorption of nutrients may be more likely to experience malnutrition.

These determinants could also be broadly classified into three levels as highlighted in the UNICEF conceptual framework [68]. This framework provides a comprehensive understanding of the various factors that influence MCN outcomes and emphasizes a multi-sectoral approach that considers the immediate, underlying, and enabling determinants of nutrition.

3.1 Immediate Determinants

As shown in Fig. 3, these are the direct factors that influence the food and nutrient intake of mothers and children. These determinants directly impact MCN outcomes.

(i) *Dietary Intake:*
- Dietary intake refers to the quality and quantity of food consumed by mothers and children. Adequate dietary intake is essential for meeting nutrient requirements and supporting optimal growth, development, and health.

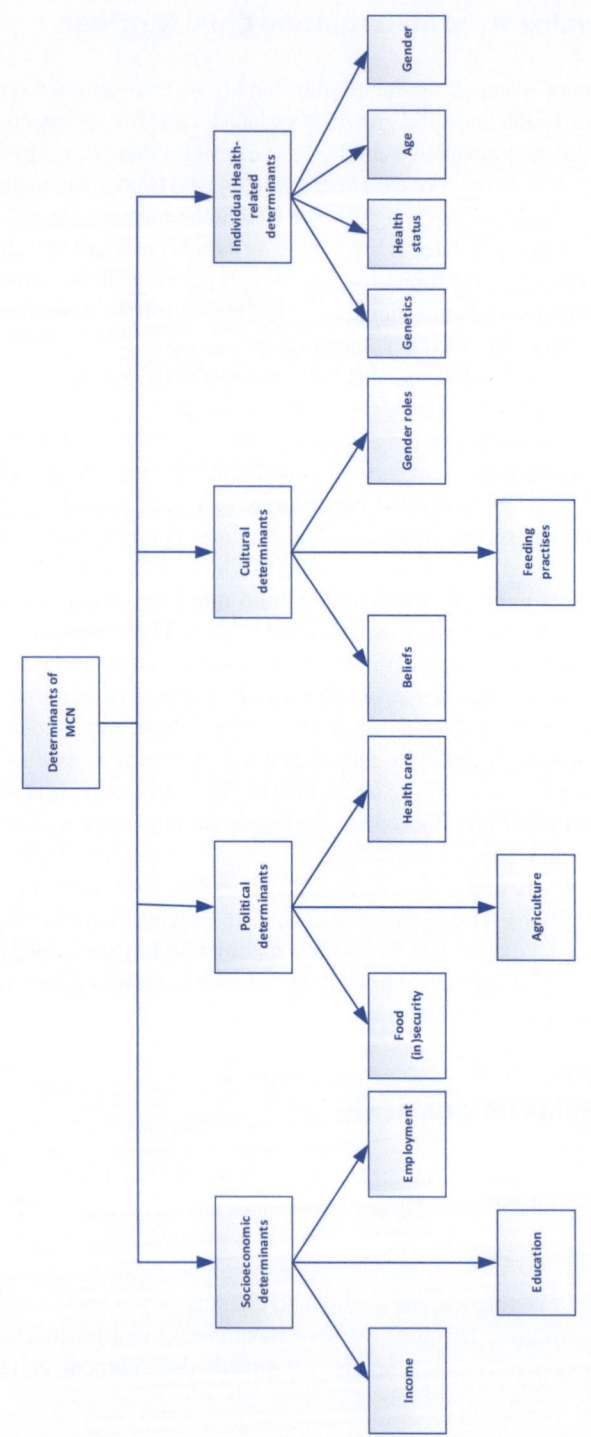

Fig. 2 Determinants of maternal and child nutrition

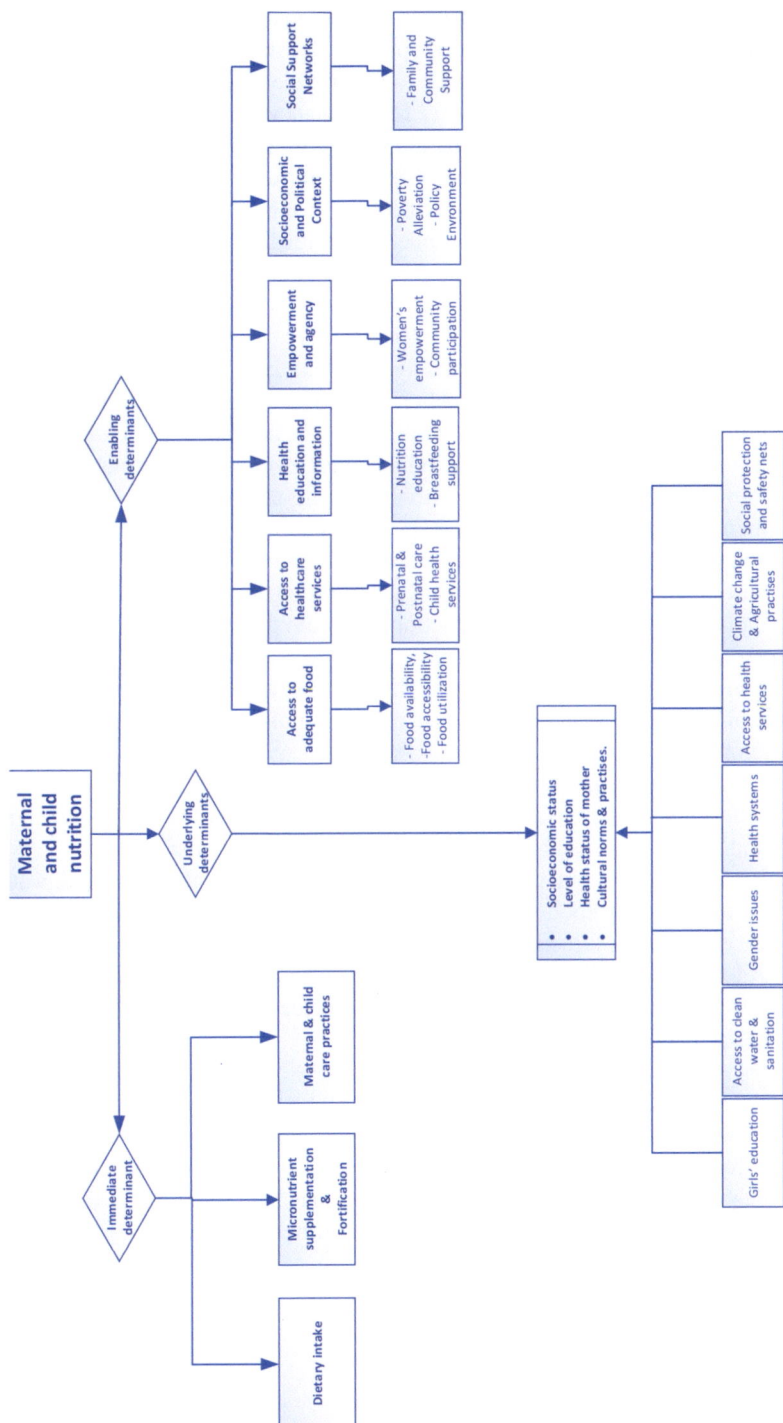

Fig. 3 Determinants of maternal and child nutrition

- For pregnant and lactating women, proper nutrition is crucial to support maternal health and foetal development. Consuming a balanced diet that includes a variety of nutrient-rich foods provides essential vitamins, minerals, and macronutrients necessary for pregnancy and breastfeeding.
- For infants and young children, appropriate infant and young child feeding (IYCF) practices are critical for meeting their nutritional needs. Exclusive breastfeeding for the first 6 months of life, followed by the introduction of complementary foods and continued breastfeeding up to 2 years of age or beyond, provides essential nutrients and promotes healthy growth and development.

(ii) *Micronutrient Supplementation and Fortification:*
- Micronutrients, such as vitamins and minerals, play vital roles in maternal and child health and nutrition. Micronutrient supplementation and fortification programs aim to address deficiencies in key micronutrients, such as iron, folic acid, vitamin A, and iodine, among vulnerable populations.
- Prenatal supplements, such as iron and folic acid, are commonly recommended for pregnant women to prevent anemia and neural tube defects. Vitamin A supplementation helps reduce the risk of maternal and child mortality and morbidity. Iodized salt and fortified foods contribute to iodine intake, essential for thyroid function and brain development.

(iii) *Maternal and Childcare Practices:*

Maternal and childcare practices directly impact MCN outcomes and are critical for preventing infections and promoting optimal growth and development.
- Responsive feeding involves recognizing and responding to hunger and satiety cues in infants and young children. It encourages feeding on demand and supports the establishment of healthy eating patterns.
- Proper hygiene practices, including handwashing with soap and water before handling food and after using the toilet, help prevent diarrheal diseases and other infections that can compromise nutritional status.
- Adequate sanitation facilities, such as improved toilets and access to clean water, contribute to better hygiene and reduce the risk of waterborne diseases that can impact nutritional status.

By addressing these immediate determinants of maternal and child nutrition, policymakers, healthcare providers, and caregivers can promote optimal nutrition outcomes for mothers and children. Ensuring access to nutritious foods, promoting appropriate feeding practices, and improving hygiene and sanitation conditions are essential components of interventions aimed at improving MCN.

3.2 Underlying Determinants

These are the broader contextual factors that influence the immediate determinants of MCN. These factors are embedded within the household and community levels and contribute to the occurrence of undernutrition.

(i) *Socioeconomic Status:* The socioeconomic status of the family is a crucial determinant of MCN. Poverty and economic disparities impact access to nutritious foods, healthcare services, and resources necessary for optimal nutrition. Families with lower socioeconomic status may face challenges in affording nutritious foods, accessing health care, and practicing healthy behaviors.

(ii) *Level of Education:* Education plays a significant role in shaping MCN outcomes. Higher levels of education, particularly for women, are associated with improved nutrition knowledge, healthier dietary practices, better healthcare-seeking behaviors, and increased empowerment. Education empowers individuals to make informed decisions regarding nutrition and health for themselves and their families.

(iii) *Health Status of the Mother:* The health status of the mother directly affects MCN outcomes. Maternal health conditions, such as malnutrition, anemia, and chronic diseases, can impact pregnancy outcomes and the health of the foetus or newborn. Addressing maternal health issues through access to healthcare services and appropriate interventions is essential for improving MCN.

(iv) *Cultural Norms and Practices:* Cultural norms and practices related to food and feeding behaviors influence MCN. These include traditional dietary patterns, breastfeeding practices, weaning practices, food taboos, and beliefs about food and health. Understanding and respecting cultural practices are essential for designing culturally sensitive nutrition interventions.

These underlying determinants are further influenced by additional factors:

- *Access to Health Services:* Limited access to healthcare services, including prenatal care, postnatal care, and child health services, can hinder efforts to improve MCN outcomes. Improving access to quality healthcare services, especially in rural and underserved areas, is crucial for addressing the underlying determinants of undernutrition.
- *Climate Change and Agricultural Practices:* Climate change and agricultural practices impact food production, availability, and access to nutritious foods. Climate-related events, such as droughts, floods, and extreme weather, can disrupt food systems, leading to food insecurity and undernutrition. Sustainable agricultural practices and climate-resilient food systems are essential for ensuring food security and nutrition.

- *Social Protection and Safety Nets:* Social protection programs, such as cash transfers, food assistance, and nutrition programs, play a vital role in reducing poverty and improving access to nutritious foods and healthcare services among vulnerable populations. Social safety nets provide a cushion against economic shocks and help protect families from food insecurity and malnutrition.
- *Girls' Education:* Investing in girls' education has multiple benefits for MCN. Educated girls are more likely to delay marriage and childbearing, have smaller family sizes, and make informed decisions about health and nutrition for themselves and their families, contributing to improved MCN outcomes.
- *Access to Clean Water and Sanitation:* Lack of access to clean water and sanitation facilities increases the risk of waterborne diseases and malnutrition. Poor sanitation and hygiene practices contribute to diarrheal diseases, which can lead to malnutrition, especially among young children. Improving access to clean water and sanitation is essential for preventing undernutrition.
- *Gender Issues:* Gender inequalities, including unequal access to resources, decision-making power, and opportunities, affect MCN outcomes. Women and girls often face barriers to accessing nutritious foods, healthcare services, and education, which can perpetuate cycles of undernutrition and poverty.
- *Health Systems:* Weak health systems, including limited infrastructure, human resources, and funding, pose challenges to addressing MCN. Strengthening health systems, including primary healthcare services, nutrition programs, and community-based interventions, is essential for improving MCN outcomes.

The underlying determinants of MCN are complex and multifaceted. Therefore, addressing these requires multi-sectoral approaches, policy interventions, and investments in health, education, social protection, and agriculture to create enabling environments that promote optimal maternal and child nutrition outcomes.

3.3 Enabling Determinants

These are various factors and conditions that facilitate or hinder access to essential resources, services, and knowledge necessary for optimal nutrition during pregnancy, lactation, and early childhood. Understanding these determinants is critical for improving MCN outcomes.

(i) *Access to Adequate Food:*
- *Food Availability:* Availability of a diverse range of nutritious foods within communities and households is essential for meeting the dietary needs of pregnant and lactating women, as well as infants and young children. Factors influencing food availability include agricultural productivity, food production systems, market infrastructure, and trade policies.
- *Food Accessibility:* Economic factors, such as household income, food prices, and access to markets and food distribution channels, determine the ability of families to obtain nutritious foods. Socioeconomic disparities can

lead to unequal access to food, exacerbating malnutrition among vulnerable populations.
- *Food Utilization:* Knowledge, skills, and practices related to food preparation, storage, and utilization influence food utilization within households. Nutrition education programs can promote healthy cooking methods, dietary diversity, and optimal feeding practices for mothers and children.

(ii) *Access to Healthcare Services:*
- *Prenatal and Postnatal Care:* Access to quality prenatal and postnatal care services is essential for promoting maternal nutrition, monitoring foetal growth, and addressing maternal health issues. Antenatal care visits offer opportunities for nutritional counselling, supplementation, and screening for conditions that may affect maternal and foetal well-being.
- *Child Health Services:* Routine well-child visits, immunizations, growth monitoring, and nutritional supplementation programs are crucial components of child health services. Access to these services ensures early detection and management of malnutrition and other health conditions in children.

(iii) *Health Education and Information:*
- *Nutrition Education:* Providing accurate and culturally appropriate nutrition education empowers mothers and caregivers to make informed decisions about dietary choices, breastfeeding, and complementary feeding practices. Health education interventions delivered through various channels, including healthcare facilities, community health workers, and media campaigns, promote healthy nutrition behaviors.
- *Breastfeeding Support:* Access to lactation support services and counselling encourages and enables mothers to initiate and sustain breastfeeding. Breastfeeding promotion programs provide information on the benefits of breastfeeding, overcoming breastfeeding challenges, and proper breastfeeding techniques.

(iv) *Empowerment and Agency:*
- *Women's Empowerment:* Gender equality, women's education, and economic empowerment are critical for improving maternal and child nutrition outcomes. Empowered women have greater control over household resources, decision-making processes, and access to healthcare services, leading to better nutrition outcomes for themselves and their children.
- *Community Participation:* Engaging communities in nutrition-related interventions fosters community ownership, participation, and sustainability. Community-based approaches, such as women's groups, community health workers, and participatory nutrition education programs, empower communities to identify local nutrition challenges and implement context-specific solutions.

(v) *Socioeconomic and Political Context:*
- *Poverty Alleviation:* Addressing poverty and socioeconomic disparities is fundamental for improving maternal and child nutrition. Poverty under-

mines access to food, healthcare, education, and other essential resources, contributing to malnutrition and poor health outcomes among mothers and children.
- *Policy Environment:* Supportive policy frameworks, investments in nutrition-sensitive sectors (such as agriculture, education, and social protection), and political commitment are essential for advancing maternal and child nutrition agendas. Policies that promote food security, breastfeeding support, micronutrient supplementation, and nutrition education contribute to improved nutrition outcomes.

(vi) *Social Support Networks:*
- *Family and Community Support:* Social support from family members, peers, and community networks provides emotional, practical, and social support to mothers and caregivers. Strong social support networks can help alleviate stress, provide childcare assistance, and reinforce positive nutrition behaviors.

By addressing these enabling determinants of MCN, policymakers, healthcare providers, and community stakeholders can create an enabling environment that promotes equitable access to nutritious food, healthcare services, and resources. Empowering mothers and caregivers with knowledge, skills, and support networks strengthens their ability to provide optimal nutrition for themselves and their children, leading to improved MCN outcomes.

4 Maternal and Child Nutrition and the SDGs

The impact of maternal and child nutrition on the Sustainable Development Goals (SDGs) is profound and far-reaching, intertwining with various dimensions of global development. The SDGs, adopted by the United Nations in 2015, provide a comprehensive framework for addressing the most pressing challenges faced by our world, ranging from poverty eradication to environmental sustainability. Maternal and child nutrition, as integral components of health and well-being, are intricately linked to several of these goals, thereby contributing to the overall achievement of the SDG agenda.

Starting with SDG 2—Zero Hunger, maternal and child nutrition stands as a cornerstone for addressing food security and ending all forms of malnutrition. Adequate maternal nutrition is essential not only for the well-being of mothers but also for the development of healthy infants. Similarly, focusing on the nutritional needs of children ensures that they have the best possible start in life, enhancing their physical and cognitive development and paving the way for a productive future.

In terms of SDG 3—Good Health and Well-Being, maternal and child nutrition play a pivotal role in reducing child mortality and improving maternal health. Proper nutrition during pregnancy reduces the risk of complications and enhances the chances of safe childbirth. Furthermore, addressing malnutrition in children reduces the prevalence of stunting, wasting, and underweight, leading to healthier populations and decreased child mortality rates.

SDG 4—Quality Education is also intricately linked to maternal and child nutrition. Malnourished children often face cognitive impairments that hinder their ability to learn and excel in school. Adequate nutrition is a prerequisite for effective learning and the realization of educational goals.

Additionally, SDG 5—Gender Equality is influenced by maternal and child nutrition. Women's well-being and nutrition have direct implications for their empowerment and participation in society. When women have access to proper nutrition and health care, they are more likely to engage in economic activities and contribute to their families and communities.

Furthermore, maternal and child nutrition intersect with SDG 6—Clean Water and Sanitation, as clean water and sanitation facilities are crucial for maintaining hygiene and preventing infections that could impact nutrition.

The impact of maternal and child nutrition on the SDGs is substantial and multifaceted. Improving maternal and child nutrition aligns with numerous SDGs, contributing to the eradication of hunger, the enhancement of health and well-being, the promotion of gender equality, the advancement of education, and the overall improvement of human development. Recognizing the interconnectedness of these goals underscores the need for integrated and comprehensive efforts to ensure that maternal and child nutrition is prioritized as a fundamental component of sustainable development.

5 Conclusion

Maternal and child nutrition is essential to global health and development. It transcends mere sustenance, instead represents an investment in the well-being of individuals, families, and societies at large. The journey from conception to early childhood is a pivotal window of opportunity, one that can shape not only the physical growth but also the cognitive and emotional development of the next generation.

The strides made in understanding the multifaceted determinants of maternal and child nutrition, coupled with innovative interventions, hold the potential to reshape the trajectory of millions of lives. From advocating for improved water and sanitation to ensuring access to essential health services, from leveraging microfinance to harnessing the power of food fortification, each approach contributes to the overarching goal of breaking the cycle of malnutrition and poverty in LMICs.

Maternal and child nutrition is a complex issue that is influenced by a variety of factors. Therefore, it is important to take a collaborative approach to addressing this issue, involving governments, nongovernmental organizations, healthcare providers, communities, and individuals in a shared commitment to the well-being of mothers and their children.

References

1. The first 1,000 days of a child's life are the most important to their development – and our economic success. [Sep; 2022]. 2017. Available at https://www.weforum.org/agenda/2017/01/the-first-1-000-days-of-a-childs-life-are-the-most-important-to-their-development-and-our-economic-success/. Accessed 21 Nov 2023.
2. Marshall NE, Abrams B, Barbour LA, Catalano P, Christian P, Friedman JE, Hay WW Jr, Hernandez TL, Krebs NF, Oken E, Purnell JQ, Roberts JM, Soltani H, Wallace J, Thornburg KL. The importance of nutrition in pregnancy and lactation: lifelong consequences. Am J Obstet Gynecol. 2022;226(5):607–32. https://doi.org/10.1016/j.ajog.2021.12.035. Epub 2021 Dec 27. PMID: 34968458; PMCID: PMC9182711.
3. Roberts M, Tolar-Peterson T, Reynolds A, Wall C, Reeder N, Rico Mendez G. The effects of nutritional interventions on the cognitive development of preschool-age children: a systematic review. Nutrients. 2022;14(3):532. https://doi.org/10.3390/nu14030532. PMID: 35276891; PMCID: PMC8839299.
4. Gete DG, Waller M, Mishra GD. Effects of maternal diets on preterm birth and low birth weight: a systematic review. Br J Nutr. 2020;123(4):446–61. https://doi.org/10.1017/S0007114519002897. Epub 2019 Nov 12
5. Lowensohn RI, Stadler DD, Naze C. Current concepts of maternal nutrition. Obstet Gynecol Surv. 2016;71(7):413–26. https://doi.org/10.1097/OGX.0000000000000329. PMID: 27436176; PMCID: PMC4949006.
6. Abu-Saad K, Fraser D. Maternal nutrition and birth outcomes. Epidemiol Rev. 2010;32(1):5–25. https://doi.org/10.1093/epirev/mxq001.
7. Woldeamanuel GG, Geta TG, Mohammed TP, Shuba MB, Bafa TA. Effect of nutritional status of pregnant women on birth weight of newborns at Butajira Referral Hospital, Butajira, Ethiopia. SAGE Open Med. 2019;7:2050312119827096. https://doi.org/10.1177/2050312119827096. PMID: 30728970; PMCID: PMC6351719.
8. Likhar A, Patil MS. Importance of maternal nutrition in the first 1,000 days of life and its effects on child development: a narrative review. Cureus. 2022;14(10):e30083. https://doi.org/10.7759/cureus.30083. PMID: 36381799; PMCID: PMC9640361.
9. Cusick SE, Georgieff MK. The role of nutrition in brain development: the Golden opportunity of the "first 1000 days". J Pediatr. 2016;175:16–21. https://doi.org/10.1016/j.jpeds.2016.05.013. Epub 2016 Jun 3. PMID: 27266965; PMCID: PMC4981537
10. He S, Stein AD. Early-life nutrition interventions and associated long-term Cardiometabolic outcomes: a systematic review and meta-analysis of randomized controlled trials. Adv Nutr. 2021;12(2):461–89. https://doi.org/10.1093/advances/nmaa107. PMID: 33786595; PMCID: PMC8009753.
11. Rajamanickam A, Munisankar S, Dolla CK, Thiruvengadam K, Babu S. Impact of malnutrition on systemic immune and metabolic profiles in type 2 diabetes. BMC Endocr Disord. 2020;20:1–3.
12. Eroğlu AG. Malnutrition and the heart. Turk Pediatr Ars. 2019;54(3):139–40. https://doi.org/10.14744/TurkPediatriArs.2019.03764. PMID: 31619924; PMCID: PMC6776449.
13. Kobylińska M, Antosik K, Decyk A, Kurowska K. Malnutrition in obesity: is it possible? Obes Facts. 2022;15(1):19–25. https://doi.org/10.1159/000519503. Epub 2021 Nov 8. PMID: 34749356; PMCID: PMC8820192.
14. Arlinghaus KR, Truong C, Johnston CA, Hernandez DC. An intergenerational approach to break the cycle of malnutrition. Curr Nutr Rep. 2018;7:259–67.
15. Siddiqui F, Salam RA, Lassi ZS, Das JK. The intertwined relationship between malnutrition and poverty. Front Public Health. 2020;8:453.
16. Fall CH. Fetal malnutrition and long-term outcomes. In: Maternal and child nutrition: the first 1,000 days, vol. 74. Karger Publishers; 2013. p. 11–25.

17. United Nations Children's Fund (UNICEF). Improving maternal nutrition: an acceleration plan to prevent malnutrition and anaemia during pregnancy (2024–2025). New York: UNICEF; 2024.
18. Bhutta ZA, Berkley JA, Bandsma RH, Kerac M, Trehan I, Briend A. Severe childhood malnutrition. Nat Rev Dis Primers. 2017;3(1):1–8.
19. UNICEF. Infant and young child feeding. Available at https://data.unicef.org/topic/nutrition/infant-and-young-child-feeding/. Accessed 23 Oct 2023.
20. WHO, UNICEF & International Bank for Reconstruction and Development/The World Bank. Maternal nutrition. https://www.unicef.org/nutrition/maternal#. Accessed 23 Oct 2023.
21. World Health Organization. Levels and trends in child malnutrition: UNICEF/WHO/World Bank Group joint child malnutrition estimates: key findings of the 2023 edition. https://www.who.int/publications/i/item/9789240073791. Accessed 23 Oct 2023.
22. World Health Organization. Micronutrients. Available at https://www.who.int/health-topics/micronutrients#tab=tab_1. Accessed 23 Oct 2023.
23. UNICEF. Undernourished and overlooked, a global nutrition crisis in adolescent girls and women. UNICEF; 2023.
24. Stevens GA, Beal T, Mbuya MN, Luo H, Neufeld LM, Addo OY, Adu-Afarwuah S, Alayón S, Bhutta Z, Brown KH, Jefferds ME. Micronutrient deficiencies among preschool-aged children and women of reproductive age worldwide: a pooled analysis of individual-level data from population-representative surveys. Lancet Glob Health. 2022;10(11):e1590–9.
25. East P, Doom JR, Blanco E, Burrows R, Lozoff B, Gahagan S. Iron deficiency in infancy and neurocognitive and educational outcomes in young adulthood. Dev Psychol. 2021;57(6):962.
26. Institute of Medicine (US) Committee on Micronutrient Deficiencies. In: Howson CP, Kennedy ET, Horwitz A, editors. Prevention of micronutrient deficiencies: tools for policymakers and public health workers. Washington, DC: National Academies Press (US); 1998. 4, Prevention of Vitamin A Deficiency. Available from: https://www.ncbi.nlm.nih.gov/books/NBK230106/.
27. Haridas S, Ramaswamy J, Natarajan T, Nedungadi P. Micronutrient interventions among vulnerable population over a decade: a systematic review on Indian perspective. Health Promot Perspect. 2022;12(2):151–62. https://doi.org/10.34172/hpp.2022.19. PMID: 36276418; PMCID: PMC9508398.
28. Imdad A, Mayo-Wilson E, Haykal MR, Regan A, Sidhu J, Smith A, Bhutta ZA. Vitamin a supplementation for preventing morbidity and mortality in children from six months to five years of age. Cochrane Database Syst Rev. 2022;3(3):CD008524. https://doi.org/10.1002/14651858.CD008524.pub4. PMID: 35294044; PMCID: PMC8925277
29. Khan WU, Sellen DW. Zinc supplementation in the management of diarrhoea. World Health Organization; 2011. p. 4.
30. World Health Organization. Infant and young child feeding. Available at https://www.who.int/data/nutrition/nlis/info/infant-and-young-child-feeding. Accessed 20 Nov 2023.
31. World Health Organization. Breastfeeding. Available at https://www.who.int/health-topics/breastfeeding#tab=tab_1. Accessed 20 Nov 2023.
32. UNICEF. From the first hour of life. https://www.unicef.org/media/49801/file/From-the-first-hour-of-life-ENG.pdf
33. Hossain S, Mihrshahi S. Exclusive breastfeeding and childhood morbidity: a narrative review. Int J Environ Res Public Health. 2022;19(22):14804. https://doi.org/10.3390/ijerph192214804. PMID: 36429518; PMCID: PMC9691199.
34. Victora CG, Horta BL, Loret de Mola C, Quevedo L, Pinheiro RT, Gigante DP, Gonçalves H, Barros FC. Association between breastfeeding and intelligence, educational attainment, and income at 30 years of age: a prospective birth cohort study from Brazil. Lancet Glob Health. 2015;3(4):e199–205. https://doi.org/10.1016/S2214-109X(15)70002-1. PMID: 25794674; PMCID: PMC4365917
35. World Health Organization. Global breastfeeding scorecard 2023: rates of breastfeeding increase around the world through improved protection and support.

36. World Health Organization. Indicators for assessing infant and young child feeding practices: definitions and measurement methods. Geneva: World Health Organization and the United Nations Children's Fund (UNICEF); 2021. Licence: CC BYNC-SA 3.0 IGO; https://creative-commons.org/licenses/by-nc-sa/3.0/igo.
37. World Health Organization. Burden of disease attributable to unsafe drinking-water, sanitation and hygiene, 2019 update. World Health Organization; 2023.
38. Pruss-Ustun A, World Health Organization. Safer water, better health: costs, benefits and sustainability of interventions to protect and promote health. World Health Organization; 2008.
39. World Health Organization. Diarrhoeal disease. Available at https://www.who.int/news-room/fact-sheets/detail/diarrhoeal-disease#:~:text=Diarrhoeal%20disease%20is%20the%20second,and%20adequate%20sanitation%20and%20hygiene. Accessed 20 Nov 2023.
40. Rodríguez L, Cervantes E, Ortiz R. Malnutrition and gastrointestinal and respiratory infections in children: a public health problem. Int J Environ Res Public Health. 2011;8(4):1174–205. https://doi.org/10.3390/ijerph8041174. Epub 2011 Apr 18. PMID: 21695035; PMCID: PMC3118884
41. World Health Organization. Preventing diarrhoea through better water, sanitation and hygiene: exposures and impacts in low-and middle-income countries. In: Preventing diarrhoea through better water, sanitation and hygiene: exposures and impacts in low-and middle-income countries. WHO; 2014.
42. Nnyepi MS, Gwisai N, Lekgoa M, Seru T. Evidence of nutrition transition in southern Africa. Proc Nutr Soc. 2015;74(4):478–86.
43. Popkin BM, Ng SW. The nutrition transition to a stage of high obesity and noncommunicable disease prevalence dominated by ultra-processed foods is not inevitable. Obes Rev. 2022;23(1):e13366.
44. Swinburn BA, Kraak VI, Allender S, Atkins VJ, Baker PI, Bogard JR, et al. The global syndemic of obesity, undernutrition, and climate change: The Lancet Commission report. Lancet. 2019;393(10173):791–846.
45. Popkin BM. Relationship between shifts in food system dynamics and acceleration of the global nutrition transition. Nutr Rev. 2017;75(2):73–82.
46. World Health Organization. The State of Food Security and Nutrition in the World 2023: Urbanization, agrifood systems transformation and healthy diets across the rural–urban continuum. Food & Agriculture Org; 2023.
47. Johnson J, Clifton RG, Roberts JM, Myatt L, Hauth JC, Spong CY, Varner MW, Wapner RJ, Thorp JM Jr, Mercer BM, Peaceman AM. Pregnancy outcomes with weight gain above or below the 2009 Institute of Medicine guidelines. Obstet Gynecol. 2013;121(5):969–75.
48. Rong K, Yu K, Han X, Szeto IM, Qin X, Wang J, Ning Y, Wang P, Ma D. Pre-pregnancy BMI, gestational weight gain and postpartum weight retention: a meta-analysis of observational studies. Public Health Nutr. 2015;18(12):2172–82.
49. Suter MA, Chen A, Burdine MS. Understanding the mechanisms of maternal obesity and the impact on the offspring metabolic and reproductive health. Endocrinology. 2019;160(9):2355–66.
50. Di Cesare M, Ghosh S, Osendarp S, Mozaffarian D. A world free from malnutrition: an assessment of progress towards the global nutrition targets. In: Global nutrition report: the state of global nutrition; 2021. p. 20–34.
51. Kelly B, King L, Jamiyan B, Dittrich J, Chandrasiri J, Sievert K. Protecting children from the harmful effects of food and drink marketing. Nutrients. 2019;11(11):2813.
52. Harris JL, Pomeranz JL, Lobstein T, Brownell KD. A crisis in the marketplace: how food marketing contributes to childhood obesity and what can be done. Annu Rev Public Health. 2009;30:211–25.
53. Perumal N, Wang D, Darling AM, Liu E, Wang M, Ahmed T, Christian P, Dewey KG, Kac G, Kennedy SH, Subramoney V. Suboptimal gestational weight gain and neonatal outcomes in low and middle income countries: individual participant data meta-analysis. BMJ. 2023:382.

54. Kac G, Carrillo T, Rasmussen K, Del Rosso J. What we know about weight gain during pregnancy in low- and middle-income countries, Technical brief. Washington, DC: Alive & Thrive; 2022. https://www.aliveandthrive.org/en/resources/weight-gain-during-pregnancy-in-low-and-middle-income-countries.
55. World Obesity Federation. World Obesity Atlas. 2023. https://data.worldobesity.org/publications/?cat=19.
56. Drewnowski A. The economics of food choice behavior: why poverty and obesity are linked. In: Obesity treatment and prevention: new directions, vol. 73. Karger Publishers; 2012. p. 95–112.
57. Walls HL, Peeters A, Proietto J, McNeil JJ. Public health campaigns and obesity-a critique. BMC Public Health. 2011;11:1–7.
58. Popkin BM, Reardon T. Obesity and the food system transformation in Latin America. Obes Rev. 2018;19(8):1028–64.
59. Monteiro CA, Cannon G, Levy RB, Moubarac JC, Louzada ML, Rauber F, Khandpur N, Cediel G, Neri D, Martinez-Steele E, Baraldi LG. Ultra-processed foods: what they are and how to identify them. Public Health Nutr. 2019;22(5):936–41.
60. Swinburn BA, Kraak VI, Allender S, Atkins VJ, Baker PI, Bogard JR, Brinsden H, Calvillo A, De Schutter O, Devarajan R, Ezzati M. The global syndemic of obesity, undernutrition, and climate change: the Lancet Commission report. Lancet. 2019;393(10173):791–846.
61. Ng M, Fleming T, Robinson M, Thomson B, Graetz N, Margono C, Mullany EC, Biryukov S, Abbafati C, Abera SF, Abraham JP. Global, regional, and national prevalence of overweight and obesity in children and adults during 1980–2013: a systematic analysis for the Global Burden of Disease Study 2013. Lancet. 2014;384(9945):766–81.
62. Montmayeur JP, Le Coutre J. Fat detection: taste, texture, and post ingestive effects. CRC Press; 2009.
63. Hall KD, Ayuketah A, Brychta R, Cai H, Cassimatis T, Chen KY, Chung ST, Costa E, Courville A, Darcey V, Fletcher LA. Ultra-processed diets cause excess calorie intake and weight gain: an inpatient randomized controlled trial of ad libitum food intake. Cell Metab. 2019;30(1):67–77.
64. Vandevijvere S, Chow CC, Hall KD, Umali E, Swinburn BA. Increased food energy supply as a major driver of the obesity epidemic: a global analysis. Bull World Health Organ. 2015;93:446–56.
65. WHO I. Report of the commission on ending childhood obesity. WHO; 2016.
66. Hawkes C, Smith TG, Jewell J, Wardle J, Hammond RA, Friel S, Thow AM, Kain J. Smart food policies for obesity prevention. Lancet. 2015;385(9985):2410–21.
67. Taillie LS, Busey E, Stoltze FM, Dillman Carpenter FR. Governmental policies to reduce unhealthy food marketing to children. Nutr Rev. 2019;77(11):787–816.
68. UNICEF. UNICEF conceptual framework on maternal and child nutrition. UNICEF; 2022. Accessed 18 May 2021.

Nutritional Health of Children Under the Age of Five

Bhavita Kumari, Ayesha Arshad Ali, and Jai K. Das

1   Background

Malnutrition in children under 5 years is a critical global health issue that encompasses a range of nutritional imbalances, including deficiencies, excesses, and imbalances of energy and nutrients. The "triple burden of malnutrition" describes the concurrent presence of undernutrition, micronutrient deficiencies (commonly referred to as "hidden hunger"), and overnutrition (overweight and obesity) [1].

Undernutrition includes wasting, stunting, and being underweight. Wasting, characterized by low weight-for-height, indicates weight loss due to inadequate intake of food and/or an illness such as diarrhea. Low height-for-age is known as stunting and is the result of chronic undernutrition commonly associated with poor maternal health and early childhood nutrition, poor socioeconomic conditions, recurrent illness, and/or inappropriate infant and young child feeding practices. Children who are underweight have low weight-for-age and may be stunted, wasted, or both [2].

Obesity can be classified using body mass index (BMI), which is an index of weight-for-height and is calculated by dividing a person's weight in kilograms by the square of height in meters (kg/m^2). BMI thresholds for overweight and obesity

---

B. Kumari · A. A. Ali
Institute for Global Health and Development, Aga Khan University, Karachi, Pakistan
e-mail: bhavita.kumari2@aku.edu; ayesha.arshad@aku.edu

J. K. Das (✉)
Institute for Global Health and Development, The Aga Khan University, Karachi, Pakistan

Division of Women and Child Health, The Aga Khan University, Karachi, Pakistan
e-mail: jai.das@aku.edu

© The Author(s), under exclusive license to Springer Nature Switzerland AG 2025
Z. S. Lassi, R. A. Salam (eds.), *Nutrition Across Reproductive, Maternal, Neonatal, Child, and Adolescent Health Care*,
https://doi.org/10.1007/978-3-031-95721-5_4

vary by age in children. Overweight and obesity are due to an imbalance between energy consumption and expenditure (too much energy is consumed and too little expended) [2].

Currently, the world faces an unprecedented crisis of the triple burden of malnutrition, which usually coexists within the same population, often in low-income communities [1]. This chapter discusses the nutritional health status of children under the age of 5 years and the associated factors, causes, and consequences of malnutrition in early childhood.

2 Burden of Childhood Malnutrition

2.1 Epidemiology

The global nutrition crisis, present even prior to the onset of COVID-19 [3], has exacerbated significantly, with alarming patterns observed in various forms of malnutrition, ranging from hunger to obesity. According to the United Nations Children's Fund (UNICEF), 45 million children under the age of 5 years were estimated to be wasted, while 37.0 million were living with obesity or were overweight in the year 2022. Overweight and obesity have increased from 33.0 million obese or overweight children in 2000, as global dietary patterns continue to fall short of the minimum standards for healthy and sustainable diets [4], contributing to a rise in obesity and diet-related noncommunicable diseases. The prevalence of stunting among children under 5 years old has decreased from 204.2 million—that is, 33%—in 2000 to 148.1 million, or 22.3%, in 2022 (Fig. 1). However, the global target to reduce stunting to 89 million by 2030 is not likely to be achieved.

Existing policy interventions have not been very effective in reversing these trends, while global conflicts and the unrelenting impacts of climate change persist as key drivers of malnutrition [21]. According to a recent analysis, the potential impact of COVID-19-related economic decline, food insecurity, and disruptions in community-based programs for detecting and managing malnutrition could lead to a 10–50% increase in the prevalence of wasting. This increase could result in an additional 40,000–2,000,000 child deaths [22].

2.2 Disparities and Inequities

Children are most vulnerable to malnutrition in countries that face food insecurity [4]. One in five children under the age of five is experiencing stunted growth overall. Most stunting cases are distributed in two continents—Asia (nearly two out of five children in South Asia were affected) and Africa (two out of five children in Sub-Saharan Africa were affected) [6]. The estimated projection based on the current progress is expected to be 39.6 million affected children, out of which 80% would be expected in Africa [7]. The prevalence of wasting and severe wasting is estimated at 45 million (6.8%) and 13.6 million (2.1%), respectively, in 2022, and the cases

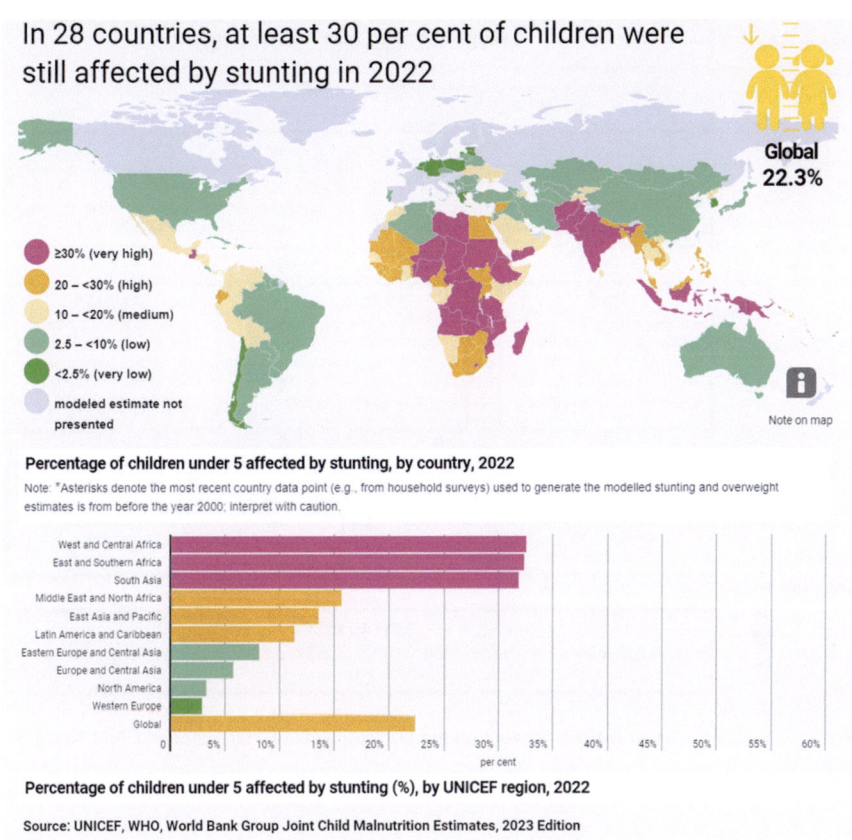

Fig. 1 UNICEF, WHO, and World Bank Group Joint Child Malnutrition Estimates, 2023 [5]. (Published in Open Access under CC BY-NC-SA 3.0 IGO License)

are distributed as 75% in Asia and 22% in Africa [7]. Almost half of deaths among children under the age of five are associated with undernutrition, and these mostly occur in low- to middle-income countries (LMICs) [2]. On the other hand, North Africa and the Middle East had the highest prevalence of overweight children in 2022, with 10.3% affected, followed by the Caribbean and Latin America at 8.6% [6]. The lowest prevalence was seen in South Asia at 2.7% [5].

3 Risk Factors of Childhood Malnutrition

The UNICEF conceptual framework on determinants of maternal and child nutrition highlights the multifaceted causes of malnutrition (Fig. 2). Broadly, these include poverty, leading to limited access to highly nutritious foods; inadequate dietary choices, stemming from a lack of awareness regarding optimal nutrition and a healthy diet; and challenges within the food supply chain, marked by the

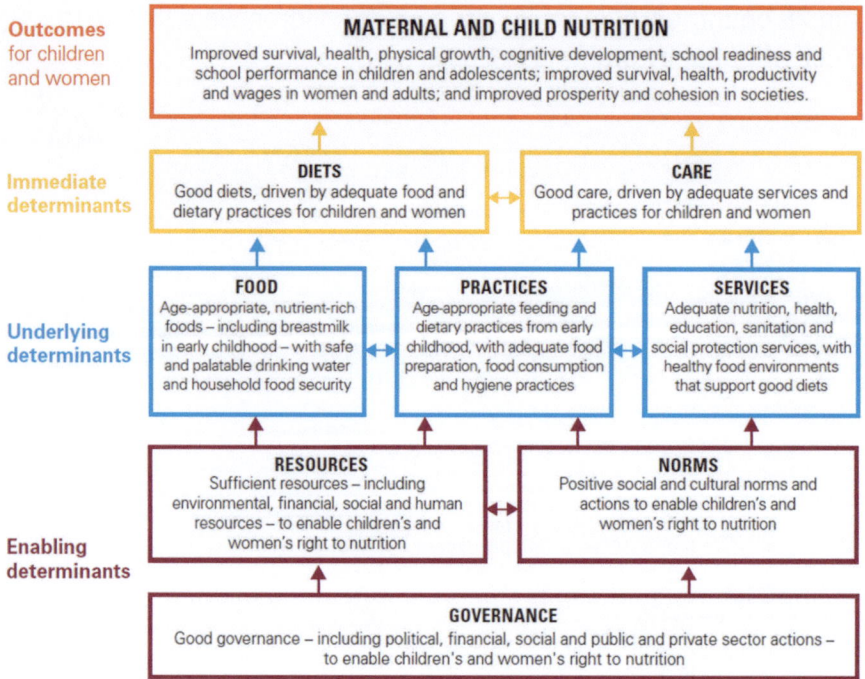

Fig. 2 UNICEF's Conceptual Framework on the Determinants of Maternal and Child Nutrition, 2020 [22]

production and promotion of inexpensive, low-quality foods [1]. Food security, safe handling, and gender disparity disproportionately affect child nutrition in LMICs along with immediate factors like dietary intake and health status, underlying factors such as food security, caregiving resources, and health services, and basic factors including socioeconomic and political contexts. Child malnutrition has also been associated with maternal education, poverty, socioeconomic status and sanitation facilities, child's age, sex, birthweight and birth order, family size, and maternal nutrition [8].

3.1 Immediate Determinants

Dietary factors are directly linked to childhood nutritional outcomes. Adequate quantity and quality of food consumed ensures that children receive the necessary nutrients required for growth, development, and maintaining health. Food insecurity, defined as the lack of reliable access to adequate, affordable, and nutritious food, is a major determinant of malnutrition. Children in food-insecure households are more likely to experience hunger and inadequate nutrient intake, which can have long-term impacts on their growth and development [9].

Diseases and infections can impair a child's ability to absorb nutrients, leading to malnutrition. Diarrheal diseases are a leading cause of malnutrition in children. These include infectious as well as chronic diarrhea, such as environmental enteropathy and inflammatory bowel disease, leading to the loss of fluids and nutrients, which can result in dehydration and nutrient deficiencies. Frequent episodes of diarrhea can impair a child's ability to absorb nutrients from food, leading to chronic malnutrition and growth faltering. Human Immunodeficiency Virus (HIV) or Acquired Immunodeficiency Syndrome (AIDS) and malaria also commonly contribute to poor nutritional status in children. The virus itself can lead to increased nutrient needs, while opportunistic infections associated with HIV/AIDS can impair nutrient absorption and utilization [10]. Additionally, children with HIV/AIDS may experience reduced appetite and increased energy expenditure, further exacerbating malnutrition as indicated by the high prevalence of undernutrition among HIV infected children [11, 12]. Hence, access to quality health services, including prenatal and postnatal care, immunizations, and treatment for illnesses, is essential for maintaining good health.

3.2 Underlying Determinants

Poor infant and young child feeding practices, such as early cessation of breastfeeding, improper introduction of complementary foods, and reliance on nutrient-poor foods, also contribute to malnutrition. Exclusive breastfeeding for the first 6 months of life is crucial for providing essential nutrients and antibodies. The UNICEF Breastfeeding Scorecard (2022) indicates that the global rate of exclusive breastfeeding for infants under 6 months of age is 48%. Globally, 45% of children aged 12–23 months stop breastfeeding before reaching two years of age [13].

Many infants are introduced to solid foods too early or too late, and the foods provided often lack the necessary nutrients, leading to malnutrition [14]. An analysis of the UNICEF global database reported the initiation of complementary feeding in one-third of infants aged 4–5 months [15]. The same study reported that 20% of infants aged 10–11 months had not consumed solid food a day prior to the survey [15].

Children require a balanced diet that includes a variety of nutrients to support their rapid growth and development. Diets that are deficient in key vitamins and minerals, such as iron, vitamin A, and zinc, can lead to specific nutritional deficiencies and overall poor health outcomes.

Environmental factors, particularly those related to water, sanitation, and hygiene (WASH), are critical determinants of childhood nutritional status. Among children under five years of age, there were 297,000 deaths attributable to WASH-related diarrheal diseases, accounting for 5.3% of all fatalities in this age group in 2016 [16]. Evidence indicates that inadequate WASH conditions significantly harm child growth and development, and this is attributable to continuous exposure to enteric pathogens as well as broader social and economic factors [17]. To harness WASH's full potential in reducing stunting, it is essential to intensify efforts to ensure

3.3 Enabling Determinants

Socioeconomic factors play a critical role in childhood nutritional outcomes. Poverty is a significant barrier to accessing adequate nutrition, as families with limited financial resources may struggle to afford nutritious food. This lack of access often results in diets that provide relatively adequate calories but are low in essential nutrients, leading to malnutrition [9]. Furthermore, exposure to indoor air pollution from solid cooking fuel use or indoor smoking, etc., particularly in low-income households, can lead to stunting [18].

Education, particularly maternal education, is another crucial factor [19]. Mothers with higher levels of education are more likely to have knowledge about proper nutrition and health practices, which can lead to better dietary choices for their children. Conversely, lack of education can perpetuate cycles of malnutrition due to poor feeding practices and limited understanding of nutritional needs.

Inadequate healthcare services also contribute to childhood malnutrition. Limited access to healthcare can result in untreated infections and diseases that impair nutrient absorption and utilization. Moreover, a lack of healthcare means fewer opportunities for monitoring and addressing growth and development issues in children, which can lead to chronic malnutrition and stunting. Several reviews have examined the positive impact of improved healthcare services and child nutrition outcomes [20, 21]. Factors such as poverty, limited employment opportunities, inadequate social policies, political instability, and poor governance contribute to malnutrition by restricting access to nutritious food, healthcare, and essential services. Infrastructure development and education, particularly for women and girls, are crucial in improving nutritional outcomes by enabling better access to markets, healthcare, and knowledge about nutrition.

4 Hidden Hunger in Under-Five Children

Hidden hunger, defined as the presence of multiple micronutrient deficiencies in individuals not experiencing an energy deficit, is a common issue [8]. The deficiencies most frequently observed include iron, zinc, iodine, and vitamin A, often resulting from diets rich in calories but poor in essential nutrients [23]. It is estimated that over two billion people worldwide are affected by hidden hunger, with prevalence notably high in LMICs, where diets are often restricted to inexpensive staple foods due to poverty, leading to a lack of dietary diversity [24].

Between 1990 and 2017, there was a 41% reduction in the prevalence of hidden hunger [25]; however, the burden still remains high. A pooled analysis of micronutrient status among preschool children (6–59 months) in 24 countries from 2003 to 2019 revealed that 56%, or 372 million children, had a deficiency in at least one of three micronutrients, that is, iron, zinc, or vitamin A [26], with South Asia bearing the highest burden of hidden hunger [25].

The primary factors contributing to the rise of hidden hunger in Africa and Asia are geographic disadvantages, including resource allocation, cultural food practices, institutions, and policies [25]. Among these factors, gender equality, in particular female school enrollment, plays a significant role in influencing hidden hunger [25]. Countries with a higher per capita gross domestic product (GDP) tend to experience a reduced burden of both chronic and hidden hunger. Specifically, a 1% increase in GDP is linked with a decrease in the burden of hidden hunger by approximately 0.2–0.3% [27]. A study reported that households with higher wealth and mothers with higher education levels tend to have better under-five survival rates, and in some cases, even overweight children [28].

The burden of hidden hunger is projected to increase by 30 million disability-adjusted life years (DALYs) by 2050 compared to 2010 [29]. While 3.9 million people die due to micronutrient deficiencies, those who survive often suffer from physical and cognitive impairments as they grow [30]. Furthermore, these micronutrient deficiencies put children at risk for various diseases, including visual impairments, recurrent infections, and compromised immune systems [31].

Historically, efforts to enhance food production in response to global population growth have concentrated on maximizing yield and efficiency. In households with limited income, the primary focus often shifts to purchasing economical, energy-dense foods like wheat, rice, and potatoes. This choice reduces dietary diversity and diminishes micronutrient intake [32]. Various strategies have been implemented to bolster micronutrient intake, including supplementation, fortification, biofortification, and diversification of diets. Each of these interventions can yield benefits, yet their effectiveness is constrained by contextual factors and the resource availability to extend their reach and impact. Strategies required to tackle hidden hunger need to be sustainable, cost-effective, and able to deliver benefits in the most remote and marginalized communities.

5 Potential Consequences of Malnutrition During Early Childhood in Later Life Stages

Malnutrition impacts health throughout the life course, with early-life malnutrition being particularly harmful. Various physiological mechanisms propagate the effects of early-life malnutrition across the life course, and malnutrition in adolescence and adulthood can transmit these effects to the next generation. Different forms of malnutrition can interact over a lifetime and across generations. The discovery of metabolic abnormalities in individuals who experienced malnutrition during fetal and early postnatal life carries important public health implications for LMICs, though few studies have examined the relationship between body weight in the first year of life and later metabolic issues.

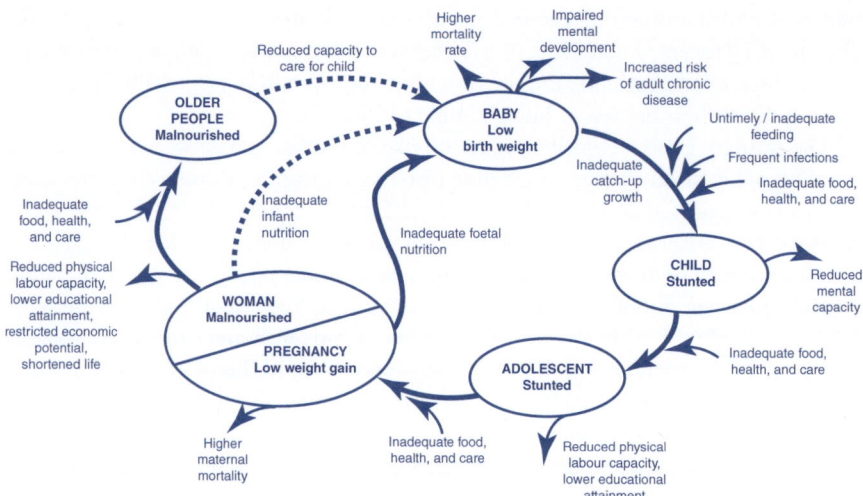

Fig. 3 Consequences of malnutrition. (Adapted from the UN Administrative Committee on Coordination/Sub-Committee on Nutrition (ACC/SCN)-appointed commission on the nutrition challenges of the twenty-first century [35])

Generally, children who suffer from deficiencies in protein, minerals, and vitamins are at increased risk of diseases that can be fatal in severe cases [33]. The impacts of malnutrition (Fig. 3) can be categorized into short-term and long-term effects. Short-term effects include frequent illness, delayed physical and mental development, poor appetite, and low body weight. Long-term effects include stunting, impaired cognitive development, metabolic and cardiovascular diseases [34].

5.1 Increased Mortality

Severe malnutrition has a direct impact on child mortality rates [36]. In many developing economies, hospital case fatality rates for severe malnutrition range from 20% to 30% [37]. Research indicates that the severity of acute malnutrition is positively correlated with an increased risk of death [38]. Children with severe malnutrition are 11.6 times more likely to die than their well-nourished peers [39].

5.2 Increase in Morbidity

Malnutrition results in a higher incidence and greater severity of infections such as pneumonia [40]. It weakens the immune system, making children more vulnerable to severe, frequent, and prolonged infections, which often reduce appetite and nutrient absorption [41]. The relationship between acute malnutrition and infection is often described as a vicious cycle or bidirectional, where infections lead to undernourishment, and vice versa [41]. Malnutrition can cause several immune dysfunction mechanisms. Severe malnutrition has serious physiological consequences, including immunosuppression and concurrent infections [42]. In children with severe malnutrition, the integrity of the skin, respiratory, and gastrointestinal mucosal barriers is often impaired. This impairment is compounded by chronic subclinical enteric dysfunction and alterations to gut microbiota [43].

5.3   Cognitive Development

The detrimental effects of stunting and severe underweight on children's cognitive and neurological development are well-established. According to the 2018 Global Nutrition Report, 189 million children worldwide suffer from both stunting and overweight simultaneously [44]. Severe stunting and underweight significantly hinder children's development, especially in LMICs. These developmental delays manifest as delayed cognitive, behavioral, and motor development, lower IQ, and reduced academic achievement [45, 46]. A scoping review linked length gain to cognitive and neurological development in both normally nourished and stunted children under 24 months. Among stunted children, cognitive and neurodevelopmental deficits may be reversible before the age of eight, particularly with improvements in nutritional status [47].

5.4   Reduced School Performance and Work Capacity

Malnourished children are less likely to reach their full potential in terms of education and economic productivity, earning less income than their well-nourished peers [48]. Adults who were malnourished in early childhood have impaired intellectual performance and reduced capacity for physical work [47]. Briend and Berkley found that poorer school performance among children treated for severe acute malnutrition compared to control groups is a serious concern for the long-term health status of children recovering from severe malnutrition [49].

5.5   Reproductive Performance

The World Health Organization indicated that women's reproductive capacity is affected if they have experienced malnutrition during childhood. There is an increased risk of complicated births and lower birth weight among women who had experienced malnourishment in childhood compared to nourished children [50].

5.6   Noncommunicable Diseases

Severe malnutrition increases the risk of developing chronic diseases in adulthood, such as cardiovascular disease, diabetes, and obesity [51]. Early malnutrition has been significantly linked to chronic diseases later in life. The long-term effects of early-life malnutrition are linked to interconnected biological pathways, including gut microbiome imbalance, inflammation, metabolic dysregulation, and impaired insulin signaling [52]. Exposure to early undernutrition followed by later overweight increases the risk of noncommunicable diseases due to a high metabolic load on an already depleted capacity for homeostasis, and in women, it increases the risk of childbirth complications [52].

A study conducted among children in Brazil found that stunting is associated with reduced lean mass and increased adiposity, especially central abdominal fat, as well as higher insulin sensitivity, elevated cortisol levels, decreased insulin production, and reduced fat oxidation [53]. The adverse effects of overweight on cardio-metabolic markers are more severe in stunted adults. Among overweight adults, stunting is linked to lower levels of triiodothyronine, increased insulin resistance, and higher glycated hemoglobin levels. Proper treatment of childhood undernutrition, leading to recovery in height and weight, may help normalize insulin activity, leptin levels, cortisol stress response, body composition, and bone mineral density [53].

Early postnatal malnutrition, independent of birth weight, adversely affects insulin sensitivity, glucose tolerance, and lipid profile in young men, with these effects worsening as BMI increases, even within the "normal" range [54]. A study evaluating the effects of malnutrition during the first year of life on metabolic parameters in young men reported higher glucose and insulin in individuals with a history of early malnutrition. Higher levels of abdominal adipose tissue were more detrimental to insulin sensitivity in previously malnourished individuals [54].

6 Way Forward

The world is not making sufficient progress to eliminate malnutrition and poverty by 2030. The multi-dimensional crisis, including the pandemics of obesity, undernutrition, and climate change, poses significant threats to child health. Nutrition, health, and the natural environment are interconnected throughout the life course. Frequent climate-change-induced disasters and pandemics weaken global food systems, exacerbating worldwide food insecurity. Current agri-food systems have substantial impacts on the environment, climate, and, consequently, child feeding practices and health.

Persistent inequalities in childhood nutrition highlight the need for a more comprehensive approach to ensure equity and healthy environments, aiming for sustainable and enduring solutions. Early-life nutrition, food environments, and socioeconomic factors should form the foundation for expanding existing initiatives. Therefore, systematic interventions and policies that establish healthy, sustainable, and diverse food systems are imperative. A substantial transformation of the food system is essential to address climate change and safeguard and enhance the lives and futures of children. Current interventions hold the potential for broader expansion to simultaneously tackle issues of undernutrition, overnutrition, and climate change by integrating across education, agriculture, food systems, and social safety nets. Collaborative efforts among various stakeholders are essential to enhance global sustainable nutrition.

References

1. Prentice AM. The triple burden of malnutrition in the era of globalization. 2023. p. 51–61.
2. World Health Organization. Fact sheets- malnutrition. WHO; 2024.
3. Development Initiatives. 2021 global nutrition report: the state of global nutrition, vol. 2021. Global Nutrition Report.
4. Development Initiatives. Global Nutrition report: stronger commitments for greater action. Global Nutrition Report; 2022.
5. The Joint Child Malnutrition Estimates (JME). Levels and trends in child malnutrition: UNICEF/WHO/World Bank Group Joint Child Malnutrition Estimates: Key Findings of the 2023 Edition. UNICEF, World Health Organization and World Bank Group. 2023;24(2).
6. UNICEF. Child Malnutrition [Internet]. 2023 May [cited 2024 Jul 10]. Available from: https://data.unicef.org/topic/nutrition/malnutrition/
7. UNICEF/WHO/WORLD BANK. Levels and trends in child malnutrition UNICEF/WHO/World Bank Group Joint Child Malnutrition Estimates Key findings of the 2021 edition. World Health Organization; 2021.
8. Black RE, Victora CG, Walker SP, Bhutta ZA, Christian P, De Onis M, et al. Maternal and child undernutrition and overweight in low-income and middle-income countries. Lancet. 2013;382:427.
9. Vuong TN, Van DC, Jagals P, Toze S, Gallegos D, Gatton M. Household food insecurity negatively impacts diet diversity in the Vietnamese Mekong Delta: a cross-sectional study. Asia Pac J Public Health. 2023;35(4):276.
10. World Health Organization. Management of HIV-infected children under 5 years of age with severe acute malnutrition [Internet]. 2023 [cited 2024 Jul 11]. Available from: https://www.who.int/tools/elena/interventions/hiv-sam#:~:text=HIV%2Dinfection%20increases%20susceptibility%20to,for%20severe%20acute%20malnutrition)%2C%20compared.
11. Sofeu CL, Tejiokem MC, Penda CI, Protopopescu C, Ndongo FA, Ndiang ST, et al. Early treated HIV-infected children remain at risk of growth retardation during the first five years of life: results from the ANRS-PEDIACAM cohort in Cameroon. PLoS One. 2019;14(7):e0219960.
12. Okechukwu A. Burden of HIV infection in children with severe acute malnutrition at the University of Abuja Teaching Hospital Gwagwalada. J HIV Clin Sci Res: Nigeria; 2015. p. 055.
13. UNICEF. Global breastfeeding scorecard 2022 – protecting breastfeeding through further investments and policy actions. 2022.
14. Berti C, Socha P. Infant and young Child feeding practices and health. Nutrients. 2023;15(5):1184.
15. White JM, Bégin F, Kumapley R, Murray C, Krasevec J. Complementary feeding practices: current global and regional estimates. Matern Child Nutr. 2017;13:e12505.
16. Prüss-Ustün A, Wolf J, Bartram J, Clasen T, Cumming O, Freeman MC, et al. Burden of disease from inadequate water, sanitation and hygiene for selected adverse health outcomes: an updated analysis with a focus on low- and middle-income countries. Int J Hyg Environ Health. 2019;222(5):765.
17. Cumming O, Cairncross S. Can water, sanitation and hygiene help eliminate stunting? Current evidence and policy implications. Matern Child Nutr. 2016;12:91.
18. Caleyachetty R, Lufumpa N, Kumar N, Mohammed NI, Bekele H, Kurmi O, et al. Exposure to household air pollution from solid cookfuels and childhood stunting: a population-based, cross-sectional study of half a million children in low- and middle-income countries. Int Health. 2022;14(6)

19. Singh G, Jha A. Role of women's empowerment in improving the nutritional status of children under five years of age: an insight from the National Family Health Survey-5. Cureus. 2024
20. Ruel MT, Alderman H. Nutrition-sensitive interventions and programmes: how can they help to accelerate progress in improving maternal and child nutrition? Lancet. 2013;382:536.
21. Bhutta ZA, Das JK, Rizvi A, Gaffey MF, Walker N, Horton S, et al. Evidence-based interventions for improvement of maternal and child nutrition: what can be done and at what cost? Lancet. 2013;382:452.
22. UNICEF. UNICEF Conceptual Framework on Maternal and Child Nutrition. Nutrition and Child development section, programme group 3 United Nations Plaza. New York; 2021.
23. World Health Organization and FAO. 2006. WHO, FAO UN: World Health Organization. Guidelines on food fortification with micronutrients; 2006.
24. Research Institute (IFPRI) IFP. 2014 global hunger index the challenge of hidden hunger. 2014.
25. Lenaerts B, Demont M. The global burden of chronic and hidden hunger revisited: new panel data evidence spanning 1990–2017. Glob Food Sec. 2021;28:100480. Available from: https://www.sciencedirect.com/science/article/pii/S2211912420301334.
26. Stevens GA, Beal T, Mbuya MNN, Luo H, Neufeld LM, Addo OY, et al. Micronutrient deficiencies among preschool-aged children and women of reproductive age worldwide: a pooled analysis of individual-level data from population-representative surveys. Lancet Glob Health. 2022;10(11):e1590–9. Available from: https://www.sciencedirect.com/science/article/pii/S2214109X22003679.
27. Lowe NM. The global challenge of hidden hunger: perspectives from the field. In: Proceedings of the nutrition society; 2021.
28. Ekholuenetale M, Tudeme G, Onikan A, Ekholuenetale CE. Socioeconomic inequalities in hidden hunger, undernutrition, and overweight among under-five children in 35 sub-Saharan Africa countries. J Egypt Public Health Assoc. 2020;95:1–15.
29. Sulser TB, Beach RH, Wiebe KD, Dunston S, Fukagawa NK. Disability-adjusted life years due to chronic and hidden hunger under food system evolution with climate change and adaptation to 2050. Am J Clin Nutr. 2021;114(2):550–63.
30. Biesalski K. Hidden hunger consequences for brain development. In: Bread and brain, education and poverty; 2014.
31. Mehboob R. Hidden hunger, its causes and impact on human life. Pak J Health Sci. 2022; https://doi.org/10.54393/pjhs.v3i04.297.
32. Popkin BM, Corvalan C, Grummer-Strawn LM. Dynamics of the double burden of malnutrition and the changing nutrition reality. Lancet. 2020;395:65.
33. Bhan MK, Sommerfelt H, Strand T. Micronutrient deficiency in children. Br J Nutr. 2001;85(S2):S199–203.
34. Das JK, Lassi ZS, Hoodbhoy Z, Salam RA. Nutrition for the next generation: older children and adolescents. Ann Nutr Metab. 2018;72(Suppl. 3):56–64.
35. United Nation Sub–Committee on Nutrition (ACC/SCN). 4th Report – the world nutrition situation: nutrition throughout the life cycle. 2000.
36. Collins S. Treating severe acute malnutrition seriously. Arch Dis Child. 2007;92(5):453–61.
37. Schofield C, Ashworth A. Why have mortality rates for severe malnutrition remained so high? Bull World Health Organ. 1996;74(2):223.
38. Pelletier DL. The relationship between child anthropometry and mortality in developing countries: implications for policy, programs and future research. J Nutr. 1994;124:2047S–81S.
39. Olofin I, McDonald CM, Ezzati M, Flaxman S, Black RE, Fawzi WW, et al. Associations of suboptimal growth with all-cause and cause-specific mortality in children under five years: a pooled analysis of ten prospective studies. PLoS One. 2013;8(5):e64636.
40. Kirolos A, Blacow RM, Parajuli A, Welton NJ, Khanna A, Allen SJ, et al. The impact of childhood malnutrition on mortality from pneumonia: a systematic review and network meta-analysis, vol. 6. BMJ Global Health. BMJ Publishing Group; 2021.
41. Lenters L, Wazny K, Bhutta ZA. Management of severe and moderate acute malnutrition in children. In: Reproductive, maternal, newborn, and child health: disease control priorities. 3rd ed. Washington, DC: World Bank; 2016. p. 205–23.

42. Collins S, Dent N, Binns P, Bahwere P, Sadler K, Hallam A. Management of severe acute malnutrition in children. Lancet. 2006;368(9551):1992–2000.
43. Bhutta ZA, Berkley JA, Bandsma RHJ, Kerac M, Trehan I, Briend A. Severe childhood malnutrition. Nat Rev Dis Primers. 2017;3(1):1–18.
44. Global Nutrition Report. Global Nutrition Report 2018: Shining a light to spur action on nutrition. 88149; 2018.
45. Miller AC, Murray MB, Thomson DR, Arbour MC. How consistent are associations between stunting and child development? Evidence from a meta-analysis of associations between stunting and multidimensional child development in fifteen low-and middle-income countries. Public Health Nutr. 2016;19(8):1339–47.
46. Prado EL, Larson LM, Cox K, Bettencourt K, Kubes JN, Shankar AH. Do effects of early life interventions on linear growth correspond to effects on neurobehavioural development? A systematic review and meta-analysis. Lancet Glob Health. 2019;7(10):e1398–413.
47. Suryawan A, Jalaludin MY, Poh BK, Sanusi R, Tan VMH, Geurts JM, et al. Malnutrition in early life and its neurodevelopmental and cognitive consequences: a scoping review. Nutr Res Rev. 2022;35(1):136–49.
48. Cashin K, Oot L. Guide to anthropometry: a practical tool for program planners, managers, and implementers. Food Nutr Tech Assist III Proj (FANTA)/FHI. 2018;360:1–231.
49. Briend A, Berkley JA. Long term health status of children recovering from severe acute malnutrition. Lancet Glob Health. 2016;4(9):e590–1.
50. Alflah YM, Alrashidi MA. Severe acute malnutrition and its consequences among malnourished children. J Clin Pediatr Res. 2023;2(1):1–5.
51. Alflah YM. Outpatient therapeutic Programme for malnourished children. Asian J Pediatr Res. 2022;10(2):1–6.
52. Okin D, Medzhitov R. Evolution of inflammatory diseases. Curr Biol. 2012;22:R733.
53. Martins VJB, De Albuquerque MP, Sawaya AL. Endocrine changes in undernutrition, metabolic programming, and nutritional recovery. In: Handbook of famine, starvation, and nutrient deprivation: from biology to policy; 2019.
54. González-Barranco J, Ríos-Torres JM. Early malnutrition and metabolic abnormalities later in life. Nutr Rev. 2004;62:134.

Social Determinants of Health and Nutrition Among School-Age Children and Adolescents

Gizachew A. Tessema, Tesfaye S. Mengistu, Adyya Gupta, Amanuel T. Gebremedhin, Eleanor Dunlop, Molla M. Wassie, and Gavin Pereira

1   Introduction

The WHO defines school-age children and adolescents (SACAs) as those individuals aged between 5 and 19 years. Despite this, the age range varies by country according to their educational system. Approximately 90% of SACAs live in low- and middle-income countries (LMICs), particularly in Africa, Asia and Latin

---

G. A. Tessema (✉)
Curtin School of Population Health, Curtin University, Bentley, WA, Australia

enAble Institute, Curtin University, Bentley, WA, Australia

School of Public Health, University of Adelaide, Adelaide, SA, Australia
e-mail: Gizachew.tessema@curtin.edu.au

T. S. Mengistu
Curtin School of Population Health, Curtin University, Bentley, WA, Australia

School of Public Health, University of Adelaide, Adelaide, SA, Australia
e-mail: t.mengistu@uqconnect.edu.au

A. Gupta
Global Centre for Preventive Health and Nutrition (GLOBE), Institute for Health Transformation, Deakin University, Geelong, VIC, Australia
e-mail: adyya.gupta@deakin.edu.au

A. T. Gebremedhin
Curtin School of Population Health, Curtin University, Bentley, WA, Australia

School of Nursing and Midwifery, Edith Cowan University, Joondalup, WA, Australia

Nutrition and Health Innovation Research Institute, School of Medical and Health Sciences, Edith Cowan University, Joondalup, WA, Australia
e-mail: a.gebremedhin@curtin.edu.au

© The Author(s), under exclusive license to Springer Nature Switzerland AG 2025
Z. S. Lassi, R. A. Salam (eds.), *Nutrition Across Reproductive, Maternal, Neonatal, Child, and Adolescent Health Care*,
https://doi.org/10.1007/978-3-031-95721-5_5

America, constituting up to 50% of the population. The SACA period represents an important timeline in the life-course, characterised by numerous fundamental milestones in growth and development, presenting a vital opportunity for shaping future health.

2 Burden of Diseases and Risk Factors

The burden of non-communicable diseases (NCDs) is a growing global concern [1], persisting as the leading cause of death and disability. It is responsible for an estimated 41 million deaths annually—equivalent to 74% of the total global deaths, of which 77% of these deaths occur in LMICs [2]. NCDs accounted for 86.4% (95% uncertainty interval 83.5–88.8) of all years lived with a disability (YLDs), with 38.8% (37.4%–39.8%) of total deaths in adolescents aged 10–24 years [3]. Other studies have also reported that 24.8% of disability-adjusted life years (DALYs) and 14.6% of deaths in adolescents are attributed to NCDs [2, 4]. The four major NCDs, including cardiovascular diseases, cancers, chronic respiratory diseases, diabetes and kidney disease, account for over 80% of all premature NCD deaths in adolescents [2].

In LMICs, NCD prevalence is rapidly overtaking the burden of infectious diseases, with a substantial economic impact [5] as out-of-pocket spending is the major source of funding to cover medical expenses, which will severely affect people at the lowest socio-economic status (SES), as it will cause catastrophic health expenditure (i.e. medical expenditure surpasses expenditure for essential consumption such as food) and medical impoverishment in most LMICs [6–8]. For example, in Nigeria, 20% of NCD-affected households were pushed below the poverty line due to the out-of-pocket expenses [6].

E. Dunlop
Curtin School of Population Health, Curtin University, Bentley, WA, Australia

Deakin University, Institute for Physical Activity and Nutrition (IPAN),
School of Exercise and Nutrition Sciences, Geelong, VIC, Australia
e-mail: e.dunlop@deakin.edu.au

M. M. Wassie
Global Centre for Preventive Health and Nutrition (GLOBE), Institute for Health Transformation, Deakin University, Geelong, VIC, Australia

Cancer Research, Flinders Health and Medical Research Institute, Flinders University, Bedford Park, SA, Australia
e-mail: molla.wassie@flinders.edu.au

G. Pereira
Curtin School of Population Health, Curtin University, Bentley, WA, Australia

enAble Institute, Curtin University, Bentley, WA, Australia
e-mail: gavin.f.pereira@curtin.edu.au

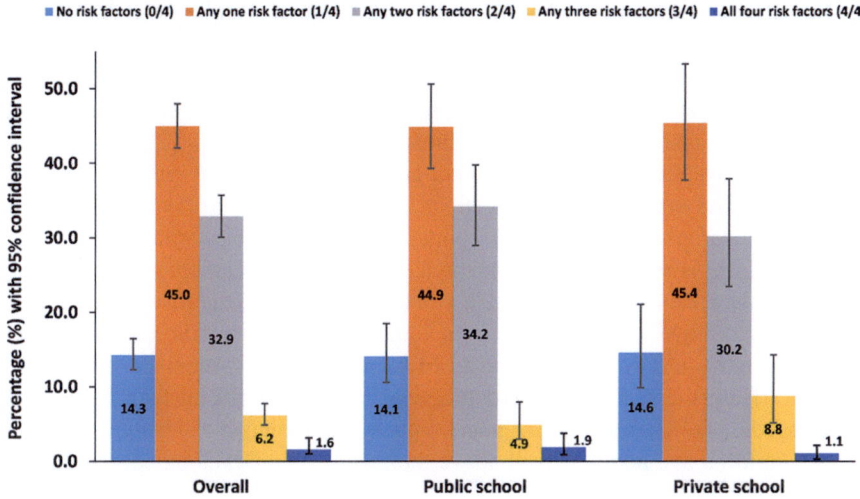

Fig. 1 Prevalence of NCD risk factors among school-going adolescents. (From: Tandon et al. [15]. Published in Open Access open under the terms of the CC BY 4.0 License)

Unhealthy diet and physical inactivity are the main risk factors contributing to NCDs [9, 10]. The rising concern lies in early exposure to these dietary and behavioural risk factors [9]. The simultaneous and rapid change towards unhealthy food choices, declining physical activity patterns and increasing obesity in LMICs has substantially contributed to the increasing NCD burden [11]. The burden of NCDs is growing dramatically, accounting for up to 70% of deaths in LMICs [7, 10]. In China, for instance, obesity prevalence ranges from 7.1% to 16.4%, and overweight/obesity from 29.9% to 50.7%, paralleled by a rise in NCD-related deaths from 80.0% to 88.5% between 2002 and 2019 [12].

The increase in unhealthy dietary patterns and subsequent obesity in SACA is associated with a heightened risk of NCDs, which implies that obesity in SACA is also associated with an increased risk of NCDs [13]. Furthermore, a large population-based study on 140 countries has revealed that the prevalence of multiple NCD risk factors (> = 2 NCD risk factors) has surged up to threefold in adolescents [14]. For example, a study in Kathmandu highlighted that >45% of school adolescents from public and private schools had at least one NCD risk factor, and 30%–34% of school adolescents had at least two risk factors (Fig. 1) [15].

3 Burden of Malnutrition

Malnutrition exists in various forms, including underweight, stunting, wasting, overweight, obesity, anaemia, and other micronutrient deficiencies. Malnutrition among SACAs remains a significant global public health concern influenced by several social, environmental and community-level risk factors [16–18].

Globally, an estimated 149 million under-5 children were stunted (being too short for their age), 45 million were wasted (being too thin for their height) and 38.9 million were overweight or obese, with substantial contribution to higher diseases and disability burden in SACAs (typically aged 5–19 years) [19]. The burden of malnutrition among SACA is predominantly higher in LMICs [20–22], and are largely associated with impaired physical growth and weakened immune systems, making SACAs susceptible to infections and delays in cognitive development [23–25]. This implies that the SACA population is vulnerable to nutritional problems, yet there is an unwavering research gap in this population group that has, consequently, received less attention in global policies [26]. Underweight, stunting, wasting, overweight, obesity, anaemia and other micronutrient deficiencies [27, 28] are major nutritional problems in most LMICs with significant regional and subregional variations [29]. Despite some progress in reducing malnutrition in the past four decades, the prevalence of underweight (or stunting) due to undernutrition among children and adults is well above the Sustainable Development Goal 2030 (SDG-2030) targets.

A substantial increasing trend in the burden of overweight and obesity among SACAs has been observed in LMICs [30]. While there is a slightly modified definition for obesity/overweight in LMICs of the Western Pacific [31] and Asia-Pacific regions [32], the epidemics of overweight and obesity have shown rapid growth among school-age children against the 2025 targets. Previous studies have also predicted that by 2025, nearly 268 million children and adolescents across 200 countries will be overweight, and approximately 124 million of them will be obese [33]. The prevalence of overweight and obesity has increased markedly in many LMICs. For example, the mean prevalence of overweight and obesity in China increased from 5.3% (5.2%–5.4%) to 20.5% (20.4%–20.7%) [34]. More recently, a systematic analysis of data from 11 SEA countries projected that there will be a substantial increase in the prevalence of overweight and obesity among SACAs by 2030, irrespective of the socio-economic positions (SEP) they belong to [30].

Micronutrient deficiencies, also known as *hidden hunger*, are prevalent among SACAs. The most common micronutrient deficiencies among SACAs in LMICs are vitamin A, iron, iodine, and zinc. The prevalence of iron deficiency anaemia (IDA) in LMICs for children aged 6–12 years was 14.2% (95% CI: 10.7%–18.5%). In Indonesia, the prevalence rates of micronutrient deficiencies among children aged 5–17 years were 13.4% for ferritin, 19.7% for zinc, 3% for vitamin A and 12.7% for vitamin D [35]. Furthermore, the prevalence of serum 25(OH)D < 50 nmol/L ranged from 18.9% (95% CI: 8.4%–32.3%) in the African Region to 71.8% (95% CI: 65.4%–77.8%) in the Eastern Mediterranean Region [36]. In South Asian countries, vitamin A deficiency and IDA are predicted to decrease by 84% (95% CI: 50.2%–8%) and 53% (95% CI: 24.1%–11.4%) respectively by 2030; however, the prevalence of vitamin D deficiency is projected to approximately double over the same period [30]. A study from Ethiopia showed that while 9%–33% of children were anaemic, 40%–52% of adolescents were iodine deficient. This study also revealed that vitamin D (42%), zinc (38%), folate (15%), and vitamin A (6.3%) were the most common micronutrient deficiencies in Ethiopian SACAs [37].

Table 1 Prevalence of double burden of malnutrition among adolescents aged 12–15 years by World Health Organization (WHO) region [29]

Region	Pooled prevalence, % (95% CI)	Country-level heterogeneity, I^2 (95% CI)
Africa	1.2 (0.5–2.3)	94.3 (90.6–96.6)
Americas	1.9 (1.2–2.7)	95.9 (94.3–98.9)
Eastern Mediterranean	3.4 (2.1–5.1)	97.5 (96.6–98.1)
European	1.6 (0.9–2.4)	90.9 (83.0–95.2)
South-East Asia	1.8 (1.1–2.8)	96.0 (93.5–97.6)
Western Pacific	1.7 (1.0–2.6)	93.3 (89.9–95.5)
Overall pooled estimate	2.0 (1.7–2.5)	96.0 (95.3–96.5)

The epidemiologic transition to a double burden of malnutrition in this specific group is a critical global public health concern, as it represents considerable potential for future morbidity burden in this generation of SACAs [26, 30, 37, 38]. This includes the increasing risks of developing chronic diseases such as diabetes, cardiovascular diseases and certain cancers and other serious health consequences, including heart attacks, stroke and kidney disease in early adult life [39, 40]. Most LMICs face a double burden of malnutrition, whereby overnutrition and undernutrition coexist within the same individual, household or population [41–43]. Pooled analysis of individual-participant data from 57 LMICs showed that concurrent stunting and overweight/obesity were common among adolescents [29, 38]. Using the Global School-Based Health Behaviour Survey data, the overall prevalence of concurrent stunting and overweight or obesity in adolescents is estimated to be 2.0% (95% CI: 1.7%–2.5%; I^2: 96.0%), with significant difference by region—lowest for Africa (1.2%) and highest for the Eastern Mediterranean region (3.4%) (Table 1) [29]. For the past two decades, there has been a rapidly increasing trend in the double burden of malnutrition in LMICs, as low-cost and energy-dense processed foods have become more widely available [30, 43].

4 Determinants of Health

According to the WHO's Commission on the Social Determinants of Health (CSDH), the social determinants of health (SDH) is defined as the complex social environment in which individuals are born, live, learn, grow, work and play, which affects a wide range of health, functioning and quality-of-life outcomes and risks [44, 45]. Understanding the dynamics of social determinants and their influence on SACAs is vital in designing appropriate prevention initiatives to support better health outcomes during the life-course in LMICs. The CSDH summarised the complex nature of SDH as depicted in Fig. 2 [45]. In this figure, we can see that the health and well-being of SACAs are influenced by arrays of factors, including structural determinants such as socio-economic, political, macro-economic, social/public policies and cultural/societal values. These overarching structural determinants play a crucial role in modifying individual and family-level socio-economic

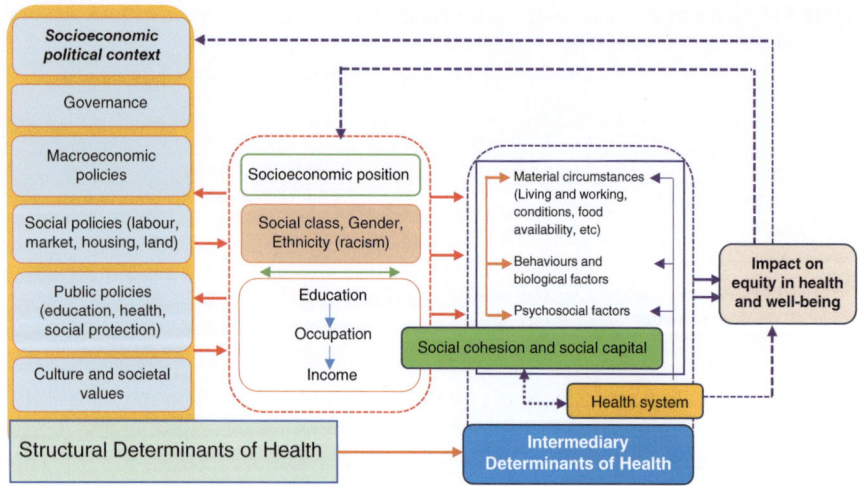

Fig. 2 Social Determinants of Health (SDH) conceptual framework. (Source: Solar and Irwin [45], with permission from WHO)

positions (SEP) and intermediary determinants such as social cohesion, social capital and health system factors impacting the health of SACAs [45].

While the nature and impact of SDH are context-specific, individual or group-level social determinants include gender, race/ethnicity, SES, social class, education, income, occupation, employment status and access to healthy and nutritious foods [21, 45–47]. At the individual level, it is hypothesised that SDHs are responsible for 80% of the factors affecting health outcomes [48]. These social circumstances also contribute to societal stratification, creating perpetual health disparities [39, 45, 48, 49] and intergenerational poverty [50] with a substantial impact on the health and well-being of children and adolescents.

Social determinants influence the health of SACAs through complex interactions and feedback loops [45, 51]. The link between SDH and health outcomes shows a social gradient in both high-income countries (HICs) and LMICs. For example, it is well-established that population groups from lower SEP are more likely to have worse health outcomes than those from a higher SEP. Inequalities in major social determinants such as education, race or ethnic background, income and living standards are the major underlying determinants for poor health outcomes in SACAs.

In LMICs, factors linked with parents' SES, education, occupation, income and access to resources play a substantial role in the overall health and nutritional status of SACAs [52–54]. A longitudinal study showed that body mass index (BMI) trajectories of SACAs aged 7–18 years are significantly associated with SES disparities, including urbanisation, household income, education and occupation [55]. Dong et al. [56] demonstrated an inverse relationship between SES and mean stunting and thinness prevalence, with a positive association between SES and the burden of overweight and obesity [56].

Two studies [57, 58] conducted in LMICs in 2023 have reported that parental SES significantly influences the household food environment. These studies indicated an inverse association between maternal SES and the facilitation of healthy dietary behaviours [58]. Moreover, in addition to accessibility to affordable healthy food, it was shown that providing a better quality diet for children and adolescents remains a considerable challenge [57].

In LMICs, maternal education and other SES characteristics demonstrated consistent associations with the nutritional status of SACAs in many ways [34, 53, 54]. For example, Chen TJ et al., [59] highlighted that higher SES is positively associated with overweight/obesity. Karimi et al., also reported that children from the third tertile of parental SES (i.e. lowest income households) demonstrated lower consumption of fruits, vegetables, nuts, seeds, legumes, whole grains, red and processed meats compared to the wealthiest parents. Furthermore, maternal education is linked with an intergenerational effect on children's and adolescents' health [53, 54]. In a large study by Le et al. [53] using samples from 68 LMICs, child nutritional status, measured by three nutritional status indices (height-for-age, weight-for-height and weight-for-age), was significantly influenced by maternal education [53]. Moreover, a study conducted in India showed that a higher level of maternal education was linked with increased rates of child immunisation, increased access to medical care, lower rates of underweight and lower rates of short-term morbidities [54]. Most recently, an analysis of the Pakistan Demographic and Health Survey (PDHS) showed that higher maternal education, and factors which are most likely to be moderated by maternal education (e.g. maternal employment, family's wealth status (richest), mass media exposure and adequate birth spacing) are strongly linked with positive child health outcomes and decreased risk of child mortality [60].

5 Determinants of Malnutrition

Nutritional status of SACAs is influenced by various factors, including demographic, socio-economic, and household/family attributes [38]. Yet, understanding the potential variations in risk factors for different types of malnutrition is crucial. Jebeile et al. [61] suggested that a socioecological model developed by the Centre for Communicable Diseases Control (CDC) is helpful in understanding the determinants of children's and adolescents' nutrition and the dynamic interrelationships between these factors (Fig. 3) [61]. Subsequent sections summarise the broad determinants of nutritional status in SACAs.

Socio-Demographic and Economic Factors
Evidence from LMICs [16, 30, 38, 62] has demonstrated that socio-demographic (e.g. age and gender) and economic factors play an important role in shaping the nutritional status and well-being of SACAs [30, 55, 62]. Over the past four decades, the global obesity prevalence has tremendously increased in the SACA population with a significant gender difference [16]. Early adolescent girls (aged 10–14 years) were estimated to be twice as likely to be overweight/obese compared to the late

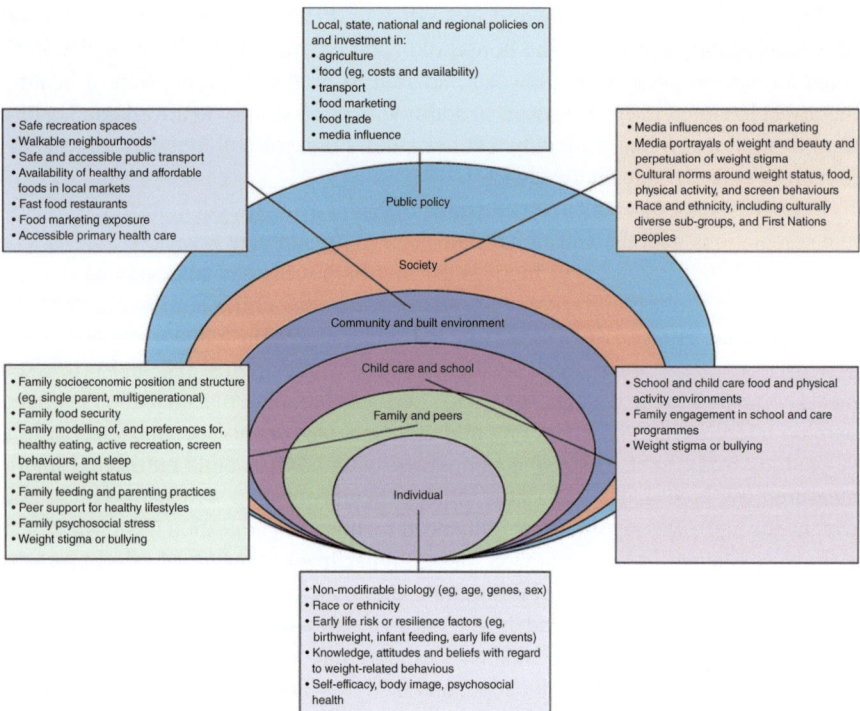

Fig. 3 Socioecological model for understanding of determinants and the dynamic interrelationships between factors influencing child and adolescent obesity. Reprinted from: The Lancet Diabetes & Endocrinology, 10/5, Hiba Jebeile et al. [61], with permission from Elsevier

adolescent group [28]. Studies from Nigeria [38] and Iran [57] showed that parental SES [57], ethnicity [38] and rural residence [38] were important factors associated with SACAs' nutritional status [38] and children's diet quality [57]. Recently, studies show that parental education and wealth status [30, 38] are inversely associated with malnutrition and directly related to overweight and/or obesity, and the double burden of malnutrition in SACAs [28, 30, 38, 56]. For example, inadequate dietary diversity—which is a significant contributor to malnutrition—showed an inverse association with adolescent overweight/obesity, where a low dietary diversity score was correlated with a twofold risk of adolescent overweight/obesity [28]. A national study from Bangladesh also demonstrated that lower parental educational attainment, being a female-headed household and poor household wealth status were associated with increased likelihood of SACAs having inadequate dietary diversity [63].

Family Dynamics and Food Environment

Family dynamics, including family size, household food security, family food choice, diet patterns and food environment, play a substantial role in shaping dietary habits [21, 29, 30] and nutritional status among SACAs. In LMICs, while food insecurity is an important factor associated with a twofold greater risk of undernutrition among SACAs [21], family food diet behaviour also influences the eating behaviours [64, 65].

Food environment parameters such as food availability, accessibility and affordability influence the dietary behaviours and preferences of SACAs towards nutrient-poor foods [26, 66, 67]. Unhealthy food environment leads to a preference for nutrient-poor foods and consumption [66, 67].

There has been a rapid change in food environment across many LMICs, marked by increased access and availability to sugar-sweetened beverages, fast/junk food, sweets/chocolates and refined grains [42, 62]. This rapid change has resulted in an unhealthy food landscape that contributes to the increasing rates of overweight and obesity [26, 29, 63] and micronutrient deficiencies [26, 29, 63]. Studies have demonstrated that food environment parameters such as food availability, accessibility, and affordability influence the dietary behaviours and preferences of SACAs towards nutrient-poor foods [26, 66, 67]. Evidence exploring the impact of food environment on nutritional status among SACAs suggests that increasing autonomy over food choice [68] and high-calorie and obesogenic food environments have accelerated a shift from undernutrition to the increased consumption of sugar-sweetened beverages, junk/fast-food, energy-dense snacks and refined grains were associated with increased odds of overweight/obesity [42] resulting increased double burden of malnutrition in SACAs [49, 58].

School Environment and Media
In LMICs, studies regarding the influence of school environment on nutrition among SACAs are relatively scarce. However, there is increasing evidence that the school environment is a promising avenue [69] for addressing all forms of malnutrition in SACAs by improving food and diet literacy, shaping nutritional choices and promoting healthy eating habits [70–72] through interventions such as school feeding [73] to promote dietary diversity, healthier and more sustainable diet behaviour [72, 74], physical activity [74] and lower body mass index-for-age z-score (BAZ) among SACAs [75]. A recent non-masked, cluster-randomised controlled trial by Kim et al., [69] demonstrated that school-based nutrition education interventions in Ethiopia are feasible to increase dietary diversity, but may have limited feasibility in averting preferences towards junk food consumption [69].

The school environment and media can work in synergy by providing comprehensive nutrition education and balanced, evidence-based nutritional information, resulting in SACAs being more likely to make informed and healthy dietary choices [68]. However, when the media is the predominant source of information, particularly those promoting energy-dense and nutrient-poor foods, it influences children's food preferences and consumption patterns [76]. If unregulated, SACAs are easily targeted with unhealthy food advertisement and marketing via multiple channels, including television, social media and influential celebrities promoting fast foods [77, 78], leading to increased consumption of unhealthy foods. Children who have unhealthy dietary habits and spend more time engaging in screen-based activities (watching television, playing games or using a computer) are more likely to be overweight and obese [30]. This is mainly due to the impact of screen time on physical activity, which reduces or displaces physical activity with increasing energy intake from eating unhealthy snacks while viewing and/or the effects of advertising [79, 80].

Macro-level Factors and Interactions with the Food System

Macro-level factors, including internal conflict, lack of democracy, low gross domestic product (GDP) and urbanization, significantly influence food security and dietary patterns across the life stage. These factors have a greater impact on the health and nutrition of SACAs compared to the adults [29, 81]. Caleyachetty et al., found that 38.4–58.7% of adolescent malnutrition was attributed to macro-level factors [29]. In this study, approximately 43.4% of stunting, 38.4% of thinness and 58.7% of the overweight or obesity were attributed to macro-level factors [29]. In Ethiopia, a country with repeated internal conflict, household food insecurity has been associated with a twofold risk of undernutrition among SACA [21].

The food system encompasses various stages, including safe food production, transportation, consumption and its impact on health and development outcomes. This system plays a critical role in determining the availability of safe and nutritious food, essential for the survival, growth and full developmental potential of SACAs [82, 83]. In LMICs, the intricate interplay between macro-level factors, such as political instability/conflicts, fragility situation and lack of democracy, exerts considerable

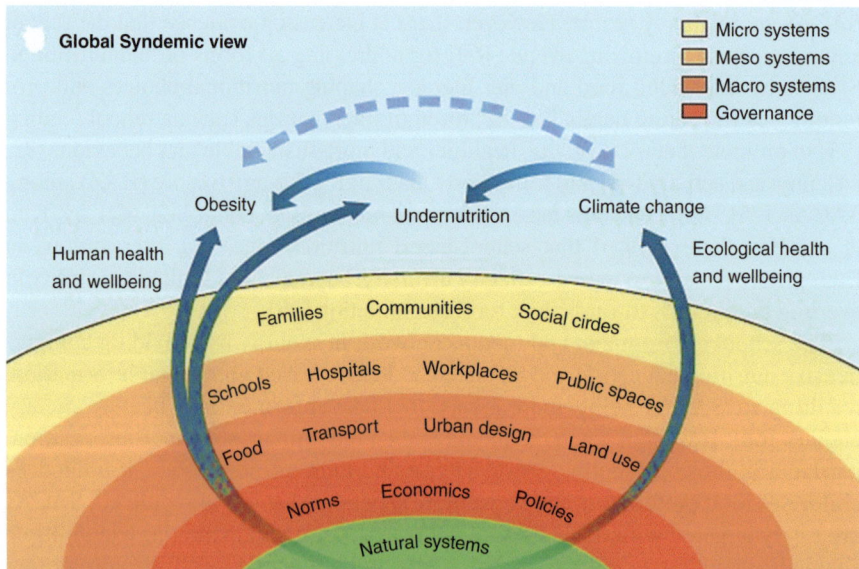

Fig. 4 The global syndemic view of the interaction and common drivers of obesity, undernutrition and climate change. (Reprinted from: The Lancet Diabetes & Endocrinology, 393/10173, Boyd A Swinburn et al. [85], Copyright (2019), with permission from Elsevier)

influence on various components of the food system that have a profound impact on the availability, accessibility and affordability of safe and nutritious food for SACAs [84].

The Global/Planetary Syndemic: Emerging Impact of Climate Change on SACA Nutrition

The Lancet Commission on Obesity summarised the global syndemic of obesity, undernutrition and climate change as drivers at the micro-, meso-, macro-systems and governance level [85]. Public health burden of undernutrition, overweight and obesity and the impact of climate change, together, represents a synergy of epidemics—the global syndemic [85]. Climate change disproportionately affects LMICs [86] and has the potential to cause over 7% reduction in global GDP by 2100 [87]. Overall, the global syndemic exerts its influence on the health of individuals across all countries and regions worldwide [85, 88].

The sweeping impact of climate change is considerably compounded by malnutrition and the natural systems that reinforce human health, often referred to as planetary health [89]. The syndemic of obesity, undernutrition and climate change operates across micro-, meso-, macro-systems and governance levels (Fig. 4) [85]. While further research is required, the existing level of knowledge suggests that double- or triple-duty actions targeting improving school food systems, environmentally sustainable school meals and multilevel community engagement could address the global syndemic [88].

6 Conclusion

In this chapter, we presented the complex influence of multifaceted SDH and nutrition of SACAs in LMICs. Social determinants of health, which encompass a wide array of factors related to an individual's social environment, play a pivotal role in shaping the health outcomes of SACAs. The health and nutrition of SACAs are profoundly influenced by various social factors, including socio-economic factors, family dynamics, food environments, school environments, media influence and macro-level factors such as climate change. The burden of nutritional challenges (undernutrition (stunting and wasting), overweight and obesity, anaemia and other micronutrient deficiencies) among SACAs in LMICs is a public health concern. While malnutrition persists, the prevalence of overweight and obesity is also on the rise, contributing to the double burden of malnutrition in many LMICs.

In summary, addressing the SDH and nutrition among SACAs in LMICs is crucial for improving their overall well-being and prospects. Efforts to reduce health disparities and malnutrition in this vulnerable population must take the multifaceted nature of these determinants and multisectoral approaches into account. With the emerging impact of climate change on nutrition—the global syndemic—it is important to investigate the role of climate change further and mitigate its subsequent impact on nutritional status among SACAs.

References

1. Melkamu K, Jeanne G. The global burden and perspectives on non-communicable diseases (NCDs) and the prevention, data availability and systems approach of NCDs in low-resource countries. In: Edlyne Eze A, Niyi A, editors. Public health in developing countries. Rijeka: IntechOpen; 2019. p. Ch. 2.
2. Noncommunicable Diseases (NCD). 2023. Available from: https://www.who.int/news-room/fact-sheets/detail/noncommunicable-diseases. Accessed 13 Oct 2023.
3. Armocida B, Monasta L, Sawyer S, Bustreo F, Segafredo G, Castelpietra G, et al. Burden of non-communicable diseases among adolescents aged 10-24 years in the EU, 1990-2019: a systematic analysis of the Global Burden of Diseases Study 2019. Lancet Child Adolesc Health. 2022;6(6):367–83.
4. Jain RP, Als D, Vaivada T, Bhutta ZA. Prevention and management of high-burden noncommunicable diseases in school-age children: a systematic review. Pediatrics. 2022;149(Supplement 6):e2021053852F.
5. Kazibwe J, Tran PB, Annerstedt KS. The household financial burden of non-communicable diseases in low-and middle-income countries: a systematic review. Health Res Policy Syst. 2021;19(1):96.
6. Odunyemi A, Rahman T, Alam K. Economic burden of non-communicable diseases on households in Nigeria: evidence from the Nigeria living standard survey 2018-19. BMC Public Health. 2023;23(1):1563.
7. Murphy A, Palafox B, Walli-Attaei M, Powell-Jackson T, Rangarajan S, Alhabib KF, et al. The household economic burden of non-communicable diseases in 18 countries. BMJ Glob Health. 2020;5(2):e002040.
8. Fazal F, Saleem T, Rehman MEU, Haider T, Khalid AR, Tanveer U, et al. The rising cost of healthcare and its contribution to the worsening disease burden in developing countries. Ann Med Surg. 2022;82:104683.
9. Noor AMN, Yap S-F, Liew K-H, Rajah E. Consumer attitudes toward dietary supplements consumption: implications for pharmaceutical marketing. Int J Pharm Healthc Mark. 2014;8(1):6–26.
10. Habib SH, Saha S. Burden of non-communicable disease: global overview. Diabetes Metab Syndr Clin Res Rev. 2010;4(1):41–7.
11. Popkin BM. Nutrition transition and the global diabetes epidemic. Curr Diab Rep. 2015;15:1–8.
12. Peng W, Chen S, Chen X, Ma Y, Wang T, Sun X, et al. Trends in major non-communicable diseases and related risk factors in China 2002–2019: an analysis of nationally representative survey data. Lancet Reg Health–West Pacific. 2023;43:100809.
13. Wang Y, Lim H. The global childhood obesity epidemic and the association between socioeconomic status and childhood obesity. Int Rev Psychiatry. 2012;24(3):176–88.
14. Biswas T, Townsend N, Huda MM, Maravilla J, Begum T, Pervin S, et al. Prevalence of multiple non-communicable diseases risk factors among adolescents in 140 countries: a population-based study. EClinicalMedicine. 2022;52:101591.
15. Tandon K, Adhikari N, Adhikari B, Pradhan PMS. Co-occurrence of non-communicable disease risk factors and its determinants among school-going adolescents of Kathmandu Metropolitan City. PLoS One. 2022;17(8):e0272266.
16. Abarca-Gómez L, Abdeen ZA, Hamid ZA, Abu-Rmeileh NM, Acosta-Cazares B, Acuin C, et al. Worldwide trends in body-mass index, underweight, overweight, and obesity from 1975 to 2016: a pooled analysis of 2416 population-based measurement studies in 128· 9 million children, adolescents, and adults. Lancet. 2017;390(10113):2627–42.
17. Rodriguez-Martinez A, Zhou B, Sophiea MK, Bentham J, Paciorek CJ, Iurilli MLC, et al. Height and body-mass index trajectories of school-aged children and adolescents from 1985 to 2019 in 200 countries and territories: a pooled analysis of 2181 population-based studies with 65 million participants. Lancet. 2020;396(10261):1511–24.

18. Sawyer SM. Global growth trends in school-aged children and adolescents. Lancet. 2020;396(10261):1465–7.
19. Sheets WF. Malnutrition. In: Fact sheets: malnutrition; 2020. p. 1.
20. Ochola S, Masibo PK. Dietary intake of schoolchildren and adolescents in developing countries. Ann Nutr Metab. 2014;64(Suppl. 2):24–40.
21. Tebeje DB, Agitew G, Mengistu NW, Aychiluhm SB. Under-nutrition and its determinants among school-aged children in Northwest Ethiopia. Heliyon. 2022;8(11):e11235.
22. Wrottesley SV, Mates E, Brennan E, Bijalwan V, Menezes R, Ray S, et al. Nutritional status of school-age children and adolescents in low- and middle-income countries across seven global regions: a synthesis of scoping reviews. Public Health Nutr. 2023;26(1):63–95.
23. Berkley JA. Bacterial infections and nutrition: a primer. In: Nutrition and infectious diseases: shifting the clinical paradigm; 2021. p. 113–31.
24. De P, Chattopadhyay N. Effects of malnutrition on child development: evidence from a backward district of India. Clin Epidemiol Glob Health. 2019;7(3):439–45.
25. Dukhi N. Global prevalence of malnutrition: evidence from literature. Malnutrition. 2020;1:1–16.
26. Norris SA, Frongillo EA, Black MM, Dong Y, Fall C, Lampl M, et al. Nutrition in adolescent growth and development. Lancet. 2022;399(10320):172–84.
27. Azzopardi PS, Hearps SJ, Francis KL, Kennedy EC, Mokdad AH, Kassebaum NJ, et al. Progress in adolescent health and wellbeing: tracking 12 headline indicators for 195 countries and territories, 1990–2016. Lancet. 2019;393(10176):1101–18.
28. Gezaw A, Melese W, Getachew B, Belachew T. Double burden of malnutrition and associated factors among adolescent in Ethiopia: a systematic review and meta-analysis. PLoS One. 2023;18(4):e0282240.
29. Caleyachetty R, Thomas GN, Kengne AP, Echouffo-Tcheugui JB, Schilsky S, Khodabocus J, et al. The double burden of malnutrition among adolescents: analysis of data from the global school-based student health and health behavior in school-aged children surveys in 57 low- and middle-income countries. Am J Clin Nutr. 2018;108(2):414–24.
30. Rahman MM, de Silva A, Sassa M, Islam MR, Aktar S, Akter S. A systematic analysis and future projections of the nutritional status and interpretation of its drivers among school-aged children in South-East Asian countries. Lancet Reg Health Southeast Asia. 2023;16:100244.
31. Shiwaku K, Anuurad E, Enkhmaa B, Kitajima K, Yamane Y. Appropriate BMI for Asian populations. Lancet. 2004;363(9414):1077.
32. Lim JU, Lee JH, Kim JS, Hwang YI, Kim TH, Lim SY, et al. Comparison of World Health Organization and Asia-Pacific body mass index classifications in COPD patients. Int J Chron Obstruct Pulmon Dis. 2017;12:2465–75.
33. Afshin A, Reitsma MB, Murray CJ. Health effects of overweight and obesity in 195 countries. N Engl J Med. 2017;377(15):1496–7.
34. Feng Y, Ding L, Tang X, Wang Y, Zhou C. Association between maternal education and school-age children weight status: a study from the China health nutrition survey, 2011. Int J Environ Res Public Health. 2019;16(14):2543.
35. Ernawati F, Efriwati NN, Aji GK, Hapsari Tjandrarini D, Widodo Y, et al. Micronutrients and nutrition status of school-aged children in Indonesia. J Nutr Metab. 2023;2023:4610038.
36. Cui A, Zhang T, Xiao P, Fan Z, Wang H, Zhuang Y. Global and regional prevalence of vitamin D deficiency in population-based studies from 2000 to 2022: a pooled analysis of 7.9 million participants. Frontiers. Nutrition. 2023;10:1070808.
37. Abera M, Workicho A, Berhane M, Hiko D, Ali R, Zinab B, et al. A systematic review and meta-analysis of adolescent nutrition in Ethiopia: transforming adolescent lives through nutrition (TALENT) initiative. PLoS One. 2023;18(4):e0280784.
38. Adeomi A, Fatusi A, Klipstein-Grobusch K. Double burden of malnutrition among school-aged children and adolescents: evidence from a community-based cross-sectional survey in two Nigerian States. AAS Open Res. 2021;4:38.
39. Mohajan D, Mohajan HK. Obesity and its related diseases: a new escalating alarming in Global Health. J Innov Med Res. 2023;2(3):12–23.

40. Lopez-Jimenez F, Almahmeed W, Bays H, Cuevas A, Di Angelantonio E, le Roux CW, et al. Obesity and cardiovascular disease: mechanistic insights and management strategies. A joint position paper by the World Heart Federation and World Obesity Federation. Eur J Prev Cardiol. 2022;29(17):2218–37.
41. Seferidi P, Hone T, Duran AC, Bernabe-Ortiz A, Millett C. Global inequalities in the double burden of malnutrition and associations with globalisation: a multilevel analysis of Demographic and Health Surveys from 55 low-income and middle-income countries, 1992–2018. Lancet Glob Health. 2022;10(4):e482–e90.
42. Jakobsen DD, Brader L, Bruun JM. Association between food, beverages and overweight/obesity in children and adolescents-a systematic review and meta-analysis of observational studies. Nutrients. 2023;15(3)
43. Popkin BM, Corvalan C, Grummer-Strawn LM. Dynamics of the double burden of malnutrition and the changing nutrition reality. Lancet. 2020;395(10217):65–74.
44. Garcia R. Social determinants of health. In: A population health approach to health disparities for nurses: care of vulnerable populations; 2022.
45. Solar O, Irwin A. A conceptual framework for action on the social determinants of health. WHO Document Production Services; 2010.
46. Catalyst N. Social determinants of health (SDOH). NEJM Catalyst. 2017;3(6)
47. Shinde S, Wang D, Moulton GE, Fawzi WW. School-based health and nutrition interventions addressing double burden of malnutrition and educational outcomes of adolescents in low- and middle-income countries: a systematic review. Matern Child Nutr:e13437. https://doi.org/10.1111/mcn.13437.
48. Carter BJ, Jafry MZ, Siddiqi AD, Rogova A, Liaw W, Reitzel LR. Incorporation of social determinants of health into health care practice: a strategy to address health disparities. In: Comprehensive precision medicine. Elsevier; 2023.
49. Lobstein T, Jackson-Leach R, Moodie ML, Hall KD, Gortmaker SL, Swinburn BA, et al. Child and adolescent obesity: part of a bigger picture. Lancet. 2015;385(9986):2510–20.
50. Piketty T. Chapter 8: Theories of persistent inequality and intergenerational mobility. In: Handbook of income distribution, vol. 1. Elsevier; 2000. p. 429–76.
51. Yusni Y, Meutia F. Anthropometry analysis of nutritional indicators in Indonesian adolescents. J Taibah Univ Med Sci. 2019;14(5):460.
52. Gakidou E, Cowling K, Lozano R, Murray CJ. Increased educational attainment and its effect on child mortality in 175 countries between 1970 and 2009: a systematic analysis. Lancet. 2010;376(9745):959–74.
53. Le K, Nguyen M. Shedding light on maternal education and child health in developing countries. World Dev. 2020;133:105005.
54. Vikram K, Vanneman R. Maternal education and the multidimensionality of child health outcomes in India. J Biosoc Sci. 2020;52(1):57–77.
55. Gao M, Wells JC, Johnson W, Li L. Socio-economic disparities in child-to-adolescent growth trajectories in China: findings from the China Health and Nutrition Survey 1991–2015. Lancet Reg Health West Pac. 2022;21:100399.
56. Dong Y, Jan C, Ma Y, Dong B, Zou Z, Yang Y, et al. Economic development and the nutritional status of Chinese school-aged children and adolescents from 1995 to 2014: an analysis of five successive national surveys. Lancet Diabetes Endocrinol. 2019;7(4):288–99.
57. Karimi E, Haghighatdoost F, Mohammadifard N, Najafi F, Farshidi H, Kazemi T, et al. The influential role of parents' socioeconomic status and diet quality on their children's dietary behavior: results from the LIPOKAP study among the Iranian population. BMC Pediatr. 2023;23(1):188.
58. de Vries MM, Rieger M, Sparrow R, Prafiantini E, Agustina R. Behavioural and environmental risk factors associated with primary schoolchildren's overweight and obesity in urban Indonesia. Public Health Nutr. 2023;26(8):1562–75.
59. Chen TJ, Modin B, Ji CY, Hjern A. Regional, socioeconomic and urban-rural disparities in child and adolescent obesity in China: a multilevel analysis. Acta Paediatr. 2011;100(12):1583–9.

60. Asif MF, Ali S, Ali M, Abid G, Lassi ZS. The moderating role of maternal education and employment on child health in Pakistan. Children. 2022;9(10):1559.
61. Jebeile H, Kelly AS, O'Malley G, Baur LA. Obesity in children and adolescents: epidemiology, causes, assessment, and management. Lancet Diabetes Endocrinol. 2022;10:351.
62. Khan DSA, Das JK, Zareen S, Lassi ZS, Salman A, Raashid M, et al. Nutritional status and dietary intake of school-age children and early adolescents: systematic review in a developing country and lessons for the global perspective. Front Nutr. 2021;8:739447.
63. Akter F, Hossain MM, Shamim AA, Khan MSA, Hasan M, Hanif AAM, et al. Prevalence and socio-economic determinants of inadequate dietary diversity among adolescent girls and boys in Bangladesh: findings from a nationwide cross-sectional survey. J Nutr Sci. 2021;10:e103.
64. Sirasa F, Mitchell LJ, Rigby R, Harris N. Family and community factors shaping the eating behaviour of preschool-aged children in low and middle-income countries: a systematic review of interventions. Prev Med. 2019;129:105827.
65. Liu KS, Chen JY, Ng MY, Yeung MH, Bedford LE, Lam CL. How does the family influence adolescent eating habits in terms of knowledge, attitudes and practices? A global systematic review of qualitative studies. Nutrients. 2021;13(11):3717.
66. Popkin BM, Reardon T. Obesity and the food system transformation in Latin America. Obes Rev. 2018;19(8):1028–64.
67. Carducci B, Oh C, Keats EC, Roth DE, Bhutta ZA. Effect of food environment interventions on anthropometric outcomes in school-aged children and adolescents in low- and middle-income countries: a systematic review and meta-analysis. Curr Dev Nutr. 2020;4(7):nzaa098.
68. Neufeld LM, Andrade EB, Suleiman AB, Barker M, Beal T, Blum LS, et al. Food choice in transition: adolescent autonomy, agency, and the food environment. Lancet. 2022;399(10320):185–97.
69. Kim SS, Sununtnasuk C, Berhane HY, Walissa TT, Oumer AA, Asrat YT, et al. Feasibility and impact of school-based nutrition education interventions on the diets of adolescent girls in Ethiopia: a non-masked, cluster-randomised, controlled trial. Lancet Child Adolesc Health 2023;7:686.
70. Hawkins GT, Chung CS, Hertz MF, Antolin N. The school environment and physical and social-emotional well-being: implications for students and school employees. J Sch Health. 2023;93(9):799–812.
71. Ares G, De Rosso S, Mueller C, Philippe K, Pickard A, Nicklaus S, et al. Development of food literacy in children and adolescents: implications for the design of strategies to promote healthier and more sustainable diets. Nutr Rev. 2023;82:536.
72. World Health Organization. Intermittent iron supplementation in preschool and school-age children. Geneva: WHO; 2011.
73. Mohammed B, Belachew T, Kedir S, Abate KH. Effect of School Feeding Program on School Absenteeism of Primary School Adolescents in Addis Ababa, Ethiopia: a Prospective Cohort Study. Food Nutr Bull. 2023; https://doi.org/10.1177/03795721231179264.
74. Verstraeten R, Roberfroid D, Lachat C, Leroy JL, Holdsworth M, Maes L, et al. Effectiveness of preventive school-based obesity interventions in low- and middle-income countries: a systematic review123. Am J Clin Nutr. 2012;96(2):415–38.
75. Mohammed B, Belachew T, Kedir S, Abate KH. Effect of school feeding program on body mass index of primary school adolescents in Addis Ababa, Ethiopia: A prospective cohort study. Front Nutr. 2023;9:1026436.
76. World Health Organization. Marketing of unhealthy foods and drinks: WHO; Available from: https://www.emro.who.int/nutrition/marketing-of-unhealthy-foods/index.html#:~:text=Children%20and%20adolescents%20are%20exposed,and%20drinks%20appeal%20to%20children.
77. Kucharczuk AJ, Oliver TL, Dowdell EB. Social media's influence on adolescents' food choices: a mixed studies systematic literature review. Appetite. 2022;168:105765.
78. van der Bend DLM, Jakstas T, van Kleef E, Shrewsbury VA, Bucher T. Making sense of adolescent-targeted social media food marketing: a qualitative study of expert views on key definitions, priorities and challenges. Appetite. 2022;168:105691.

79. Buchanan LR, Rooks-Peck CR, Finnie RK, Wethington HR, Jacob V, Fulton JE, et al. Reducing recreational sedentary screen time: a community guide systematic review. Am J Prev Med. 2016;50(3):402–15.
80. Robinson TN, Banda JA, Hale L, Lu AS, Fleming-Milici F, Calvert SL, et al. Screen media exposure and obesity in children and adolescents. Pediatrics. 2017;140(Suppl 2):S97–s101.
81. Trask BS. Migration, urbanization, and the family dimension. United Nations Department of Economic and Social; 2022.
82. Fox EL, Timmer A. Children's and adolescents' characteristics and interactions with the food system. Glob Food Sec. 2020;27:100419.
83. Kupka R, Siekmans K, Beal T. The diets of children: overview of available data for children and adolescents. Glob Food Sec. 2020;27:100442.
84. Arslan A, Cavatassi R, Hossain M. Structural and rural transformation and food systems: a quantitative synthesis for LMICs: SSRN; 2022.
85. Swinburn BA, Kraak VI, Allender S, Atkins VJ, Baker PI, Bogard JR, et al. The global Syndemic of obesity, undernutrition, and climate change: the lancet commission report. Lancet. 2019;393(10173):791–846.
86. Erzse A, Balusik A, Kruger P, Thsehla E, Swinburn B, Hofman KJ. Commentary on South Africa's syndemic of undernutrition, obesity, and climate change. S Afr J Sci. 2023;119(3–4):1–5.
87. Kahn ME, Mohaddes K, Ng RN, Pesaran MH, Raissi M, Yang J-C. Long-term macroeconomic effects of climate change: a cross-country analysis. Energy Econ. 2021;104:105624.
88. Venegas Hargous C, Strugnell C, Allender S, Orellana L, Corvalan C, Bell C. Double-and triple-duty actions in childhood for addressing the global syndemic of obesity, undernutrition, and climate change: a scoping review. Obes Rev. 2023;24(4):e13555.
89. Mendenhall E, Singer M. The global syndemic of obesity, undernutrition, and climate change. Lancet. 2019;393(10173):741.

Nutritional Challenges and Issues Relevant to Adolescents

Emily C. Keats, Maya Kshatriya, Christopher Lee, and Zulfiqar A. Bhutta

1   Introduction

Adolescence is the unique life stage between childhood and adulthood, defined by the World Health Organization (WHO) as 10–19 years of age [1]. Adolescents experience rapid physical growth: on average, 20% of adult height and 50% of adult weight is gained during this period [2], underscoring an immense increase in nutrient needs. There is also major psychosocial development occurring, with attitudes, behaviors, and practices learned during this period often setting the stage for health and well-being later in life and intergenerationally. This includes the establishment of dietary habits, especially given adolescents' increased access to foods found outside of the household and increased autonomy in diet choice.

The adolescent cohort is the largest in history, comprising 1.3 billion individuals and making up 16% of the world's population [3], so the actions and experiences of this group will undoubtedly influence the future, including generations to come. Today, we are experiencing significant global shifts due to climate change, COVID-19, and the potential emergence of other pandemics, conflict, and changing food environments; events that will have consequences on nutrition, and many of which will elicit a disproportionate effect on adolescents. Despite all this, relatively

---

E. C. Keats · M. Kshatriya · C. Lee
Centre for Global Child Health, The Hospital for Sick Children, Toronto, ON, Canada
e-mail: ekeats3@jh.edu; maya.kshatriya@sickkids.ca; christopher.lee@sickkids.ca

Z. A. Bhutta (✉)
Centre for Global Child Health, The Hospital for Sick Children, Toronto, ON, Canada

Centre of Excellence in Women and Child Health, The Aga Khan University, Karachi, Pakistan
e-mail: zulfiqar.bhutta@sickkids.ca

© The Author(s), under exclusive license to Springer Nature Switzerland AG 2025
Z. S. Lassi, R. A. Salam (eds.), *Nutrition Across Reproductive, Maternal, Neonatal, Child, and Adolescent Health Care*,
https://doi.org/10.1007/978-3-031-95721-5_6

little attention has been given to adolescent nutrition, which is tightly linked to growth, development, and the attainment of human capital. This is reflected in a lack of understanding of key interventions and delivery platforms to reach adolescents, and subsequently, little practical global guidance on how to meet adolescents' needs.

2 Global Epidemiological Burden of Malnutrition Among Adolescents

Malnutrition, defined by the WHO as deficiencies, excesses, or imbalances in a person's intake of energy or nutrients [4], is one of the most widespread causes of morbidity and mortality among children and adolescents [5, 6]. Although a global issue, malnutrition disproportionately affects those in the Global South, particularly in South and Southeast Asia and Sub-Saharan Africa [7, 8]. In these settings, which have traditionally been rife with undernutrition (i.e., stunting, wasting, underweight, and micronutrient deficiencies), there has been a recent surge of overnutrition (i.e., dietary excess, overweight/obesity, and diet-related noncommunicable diseases), creating a double burden of malnutrition (DBM) [9, 10]. Given that 90% of the world's adolescents live in low- and middle-income countries (LMICs) [11], this is particularly problematic. Malnutrition of any type poses a threat to the rapid nature of physical and psychosocial development during this stage of the life course.

Although relatively less attention has been given to the nutrition of adolescents when compared to mothers and children under-five, recent evidence has emphasized the high burden of malnutrition among adolescents globally, particularly in LMICs, indicating the need for intervention. Regarding undernutrition, findings from the 2013 Global Burden of Disease (GBD) study revealed that protein–energy malnutrition was the ninth leading cause of death among children and adolescents in LMICs in 2013 (~226,000 deaths) [12, 13], equating to approximately 38.5 deaths per 100,000 children and adolescents [12, 13]. Countries that experienced the most child and adolescent deaths from protein–energy malnutrition in 2013 included Nigeria (~43,000), the Democratic Republic of Congo (~33,000), India (~19,500), and Ethiopia (~9600) [13]. A review by Wrottesley et al. [14] focusing on the nutritional status of school-age children and adolescents in LMICs across seven UNICEF-defined global regions (East Asia and Pacific, Europe and Central Asia, South Asia, West and Central Africa, Eastern and Southern Africa, Middle East and North Africa, and Latin America and the Caribbean) notably revealed that prevalence of stunting and thinness remains particularly high among children and adolescents in West and Central Africa, East and Southern Africa, and South Asia. The highest stunting prevalence in these regions ranged from 37% in South Asia to 61% in West and Central Africa, while the highest thinness prevalence ranged from 49% in South Asia to 96% in West and Central Africa [14]. Anemia among children and adolescents was also highly prevalent across all regions, but was most notable in East Asia and the Pacific, West and Central Africa, and Latin America and the Caribbean. The highest anemia prevalence ranged from 81% in Latin America and the Caribbean to 98.5% in East Asia and the Pacific [14]. Most regions also experienced high rates of iodine, vitamin A, vitamin D, and zinc deficiencies among children and adolescents, underscoring the likely coexistence of multiple micronutrient deficiencies [14]. Similar findings, observed by Cusick and Kuch [15], demonstrate that stunting/short stature, underweight/thinness, anemia, and iron deficiency anemia are widespread among adolescents 10–19 years of age in several developing countries including Ecuador, Mexico, Guatemala, Jamaica, Nepal, India, Philippines, Benin, and Cameroon. Anemia was found to be the most significant nutritional problem experienced by adolescents, with a prevalence of 58% in Guatemala, 55% in India, 42% in Nepal, and 32% in Cameroon [15]. In addition, the prevalence of thinness or underweight in adolescents was high in India (53%), Nepal (36%), and Benin (23%) [15–18].

Along with undernutrition, studies have found that there is an increasing burden of overweight and obesity among adolescents in LMICs [14, 15, 19]. Rapid urbanization and other environmental factors have heavily influenced this, including the nutrition transition or shift in consumption of traditional foods to highly processed and energy-dense foods [15, 20]. The burden of overnutrition among adolescents in LMICs was highlighted in the same study by Wrottesley and colleagues [14], who found that overweight and obesity are particularly problematic in the Latin America and Caribbean, East Asia and Pacific, and Middle East and North Africa regions (highest prevalence ranging from 45% in Middle East and North Africa to 59% in East Asia and Pacific), where prevalence rates were consistently high across countries within those regions. Other country-level studies have shown similar findings, including in Brazil, China, Vietnam, Sudan, Botswana, South Africa, and India, where the rise in overweight and obesity among adolescents is mostly attributed to rapid urbanization [15, 21–28]. Additional evidence has demonstrated that the prevalence of overweight and obesity among adolescents was >30–40% in several LMICs in the Pacific Islands, Caribbean Islands, and Arab countries undergoing urbanization between 1990 and 2010 [29, 30]. With LMICs continuing to urbanize and undergo rapid nutrition transitions, it is clear that overnutrition should be prioritized to a similar extent as undernutrition in order to reduce the DBM among adolescents and improve overall health outcomes.

3 Nutritional Challenges and Risk Factors Affecting the Health of Adolescents

Establishing healthy nutritional habits during the formative years of development is a crucial determinant for long-term health and well-being. However, adolescents in LMICs face a range of nutritional challenges that can have a profound impact on their growth and development. For example, nutrition influences immune function, neurodevelopment, and other developmental indices, including pubertal maturation, which, in turn, affects adult stature, the accumulation of muscle and fat mass, and susceptibility to noncommunicable diseases during adulthood. The nutritional challenges experienced by adolescents are interconnected and influenced by a complex interplay of environmental, social, cultural, and economic factors that can vary

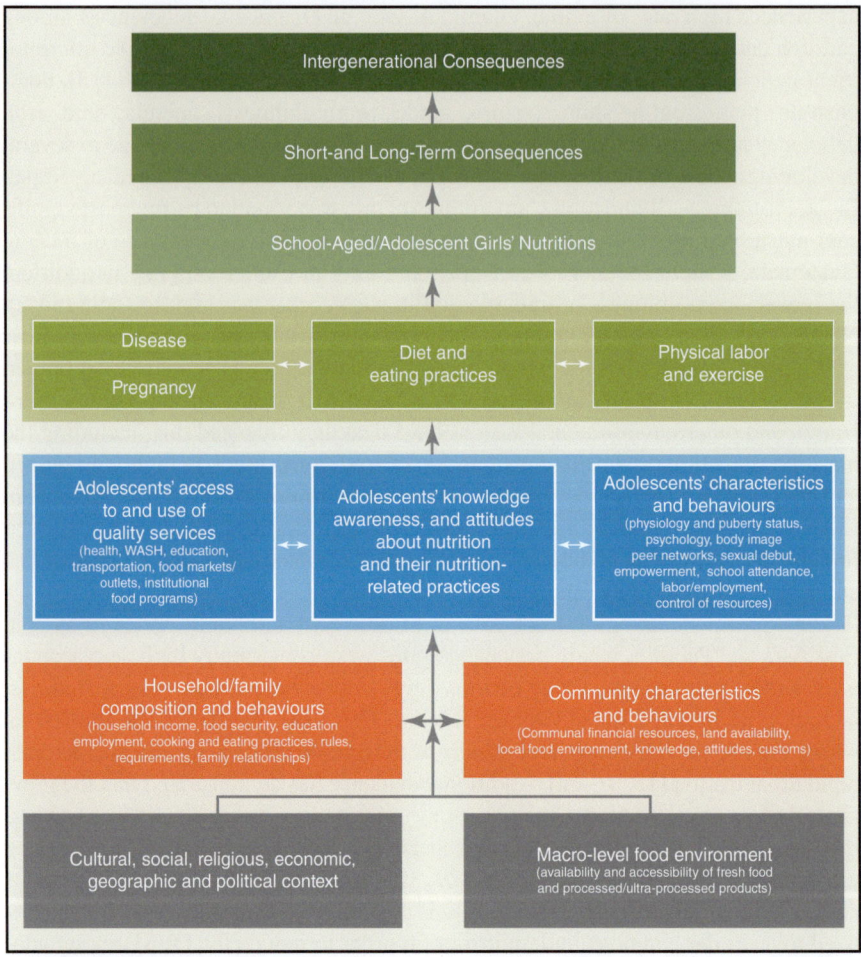

Fig. 1 Conceptual framework illustrating the determinants of adolescent nutrition. ((Reproduced from SPRING, USAID 2016). https://www.advancingnutrition.org/resources/adolescent-resource-bank/conceptual-framework-adolescent-girls-nutrition)

across different settings. Figure 1 highlights the determinants of adolescent girls' dietary intake and related nutritional and health outcomes; this figure can be applied similarly to adolescent boys, though determinants may have varying levels of impact based on gender.

Traditionally, LMICs have been faced with the persistent issue of undernutrition, with a focus on addressing wasting, stunting, underweight/thinness, and micronutrient deficiencies. This has been driven by a number of factors, including poverty, lack of access to nutritious foods, poor health care infrastructure, inadequate sanitation, and in some cases, conflict and humanitarian disasters, all of which lead to a cycle of undernutrition that persists intergenerationally, meaning that infants are born at a disadvantage. In recent years, however, there has been a rise in childhood and adolescent obesity, contributing to the DBM [31]. The 2019 Lancet Series on the DBM reports that while most commonly observed in high-income countries, severe levels of the DBM have now shifted to the poorest LMICs, notably those in South and East Asia and Sub-Saharan Africa [20]. As global food systems undergo significant changes, LMICs are now confronted with new nutritional challenges [31].

Undernutrition poses a significant and persistent public health problem in LMICs, particularly during the adolescent period, where nutritional requirements are increased to support physical maturation, cognitive advancement, and overall health. Micronutrient deficiencies impact individuals across all age-groups, yet their consequences are disproportionately higher among pregnant women, children, and adolescents. The most prevalent deficiencies include iron, zinc, vitamin A, and iodine [32]. The estimated global prevalence of iron deficiency anemia is reportedly highest among adolescent females who live in lower social development index (SDI) countries, at 3.4% as of 2018 [32]. Contrastingly, the prevalence of vitamin A deficiency was found to be higher among adolescent males in middle, low-middle, and low-SDI countries [32].

An additional manifestation of undernutrition is stunting, which originates during prenatal development and persists into infancy, affecting a child's brain and muscle growth [33]. Stunted children who are too short for their age are more likely to become adolescents with short stature, an outcome that is linked to reduced cognitive development and academic achievement, adverse reproductive health outcomes in females, and an overall decrease in economic productivity [34]. Underweight (thinness), classified as having a BMI less than 2 standard deviations (SD) below the median of the WHO growth reference for school-age children and adolescents, is also an indication of undernutrition [35]. Underweight is associated with an increased risk of infectious disease and adverse pregnancy outcomes among girls of reproductive age, including maternal mortality and complications during delivery [36].

On the other hand, the prevalence of obesity and overweight in many LMICs is rapidly rising. This can be attributed to a variety of factors, including the widespread availability and consumption of energy-dense foods, a decline in physical activity, changes in lifestyle, and rapid urbanization [37]. Adolescents who are overweight or obese are more likely to continue carrying excess weight into adulthood, further increasing their risk of obesity-related chronic diseases, such as hypertension, type 2 diabetes, and mortality in later adulthood [34]. Obesity during the adolescent period has also been found to result in negative psychosocial effects and reduced educational achievement [36]. As adolescents are more vulnerable to food marketing and may lack knowledge regarding how to obtain a balanced and nutritious diet, their risk of overweight and obesity is higher [38].

3.1   Early Marriage and Pregnancy

Malnutrition contributes to adverse reproductive health outcomes among adolescent girls [39]. Every day, about 20,000 adolescent girls under 18 years of age in LMICs will give birth [40]. Additionally, half of all adolescent births that take place globally occur in only seven countries, including Bangladesh, Brazil, the Democratic Republic of the Congo, Ethiopia, India, Nigeria, and the United States [40]. Adolescent births also bear a greater burden of disease, despite accounting for only 11% of all births worldwide [40].

Evidence from LMICs indicates that early childbearing can influence a woman's nutritional status in direct and indirect ways [41]. For instance, adolescent girls who are pregnant often do not experience appropriate weight gain during pregnancy, which can lead to poor fetal growth and increase the risk of negative birth outcomes [41]. Pregnancy can also disrupt typical growth patterns observed in adolescent girls, which can have lasting consequences, given that this period is vital for accelerated growth, particularly in populations where malnutrition is prevalent [41]. Pregnant adolescents who are undernourished face an especially high burden of risk that affects their health and that of their infants. Undernourished pregnant adolescents have a heightened risk of experiencing complications during pregnancy and delivery, including preterm birth, stillbirth, anemia, eclampsia, and small for gestational age (SGA) [42]. These adverse outcomes can be attributed to the increased maternal-fetal competition for energy and nutrients during this period [43]. Short stature is one important component of undernutrition that is a risk factor for additional unfavorable and severe pregnancy outcomes among adolescents, including vesicoureteric fistulas and obstructed labor [44].

3.2 Poverty

The consequences of poor nutrition during adolescence are far-reaching, with negative outcomes being exacerbated in LMICs where socioeconomic barriers, limited access to quality health care, and resource constraints are prevalent. A 2022 study examining child and adolescent food insecurity in South Africa found that households that relied on pensions, social grants, remittances, or had no source of income were approximately 1.76–2.15 times more at risk of hunger or experiencing hunger compared to those earning a salary or wage [45]. An additional subanalysis found that households with at least one adolescent aged 15–19 years had nearly 30% higher odds of food insecurity compared to those with only children aged 0–14 years [45]. The constraints of poverty can severely hinder a person's ability to obtain optimal nutrition during critical phases of growth and development, leading to diets that lack diversity and essential nutrients. Resource-limited settings also often lack access to nutrition education, exacerbating the issue. While food supplementation can help improve current nutritional status, it does not address the primary health and nutritional challenges that families living in poverty face [46]. A study by Baxter and colleagues found that among young adolescent girls in Pakistan, a diet lacking in diversity was most significantly predicted by poverty, highlighting restricted purchasing power and/or inadequate access to nutritious foods [47]. Government programs and policy actions should ensure access to healthy school meals, especially in impoverished, food-insecure, or crisis-stricken geographies [48]. Nutrition advocacy should also occur in partnership with youth to ensure it is contextualized for the setting [48].

3.3 Education

Adolescents are vulnerable to external influences that drive their dietary choices and behaviors, including food environments, culture, peers, advertisements, and social media [46]. In particular, adolescents in LMICs have been found to have poorer nutrition-related knowledge, attitudes, and practices due to limited resources, outdated curricula, and lack of trained nutrition educators, leading to susceptibility to illness later in life [49]. Cultural beliefs and practices in some settings can also overshadow scientifically backed nutritional guidelines, particularly where nutrition education is unavailable [50]. Integrating nutrition education into schools can be an effective tool to reach adolescents and teach them about the importance of proper nutrition, healthy eating, and physical activity. Such interventions should start at an early age as a way to raise awareness, not just among children but among their teachers and caregivers as well [51].

In addition to adolescent education, maternal and paternal education levels also serve as predictors of adolescent nutrition. For example, a scoping review on the nutritional status of school-age children and adolescents in LMICs found that lower levels of maternal education predicted stunting and thinness [14]. Additionally, while sedentary behaviors and extended screen time can heighten obesity risks, higher maternal and paternal education was found to mitigate these effects. Current evidence suggests that multicomponent programs that integrate nutrition education alongside diet and physical activity interventions were most effective at improving the nutritional status and dietary behaviors of adolescents [14, 52].

3.4 Empowerment

As children transition into adolescence, the intersection of gender, class, social standing, culture, and context begins to set the stage for their future life trajectory [53]. During adolescence, gender roles and expectations become more deeply rooted, shaping the way they perceive and engage with their surroundings. In many LMICs, gender biases rooted in prevailing patriarchal systems become more pronounced during this period, limiting the choices, opportunities, aspirations, and social connections of young girls compared to their male counterparts [53]. Where vast gender disparities exist, women and girls are more likely to experience nutritional deficiencies, early marriage, and higher fertility rates [54, 55]. However, several studies to date have reported that adolescent girl-specific nutrition education and empowerment programs were not found to be strongly associated with improved nutritional outcomes [56–58]. Hewett and colleagues [56] suggest that addressing additional factors influencing girls' approach to nutrition, including food accessibility and control, relatable information, economic empowerment, and management of household resources, is essential when crafting programs aiming to improve adolescent nutrition outcomes [58]. A recent study aimed to implement a girl-powered nutrition program in four LMICs, which involved codesigning the intervention with adolescent girls [59]. The results were promising, reinforcing and expanding on several established and accepted best practices for engaging with adolescents to enhance their knowledge and attitudes on nutrition.

3.5 Conflict and Displacement

As of May 2022, the United Nations High Commissioner for Refugees (UNHCR) reported that 103 million people in the world have been forcibly displaced due to conflict and persecution [60]. This includes 32.5 million refugees, with more than half being below the age of 18. While data is limited, UNHCR estimates indicate that there are a minimum of 3.4 million refugees and 9.8 million globally displaced adolescents between 12 and 17 years old [61]. Due to adolescence being a period of rapid development, this group is particularly vulnerable to conflict-induced adverse health outcomes, including severe malnutrition and psychiatric disorders such as post-traumatic stress disorder, anxiety, and depression [62]. A study conducted by Acharya and colleagues [63] looking at the impact of conflict-related violence on the nutritional status of children in Iraq found that a child exposed to the maximum number of attack incidents experienced a 0.51 SD reduction in height-for-age z-score (HAZ; a measure of chronic malnutrition) compared to children who were not exposed to any incidents. The strongest association between violence and HAZ was found in regions with higher conflict levels.

Furthermore, in refugee settings, the prevalence of macro and micronutrient deficiencies is common due to displacement, rationing of food, limited access to nutritious food, and lack of income [62, 64, 65]. A study conducted in refugee camps located in Kenya and Nepal found that anemia, iron deficiency, and vitamin A deficiency were common among adolescent refugees [66]. The prevalence of anemia was notably high, reported at 46% and 24% in Kenyan and Nepalese adolescent refugees, respectively [66]. While there is a need to increase the uptake of nutrients among this subgroup, the lack of routine access to food presents a significant challenge to program implementation in these settings.

Interventions to address nutritional challenges in conflict settings are provided by governments and relief agencies and typically include supplementary feeding programs for at-risk groups, general food and micronutrient supplementation distribution, agricultural support, and infant and young child feeding groups [62]. Interventions aimed at addressing malnutrition and micronutrient deficiencies were found to be most effective during the stable and developmental periods of emergencies [62, 67].

Unfortunately, there is an overall lack of scientific investigation into the social determinants of nutrition among adolescents in LMICs. Solutions to explore and address adolescent nutrition must be multifaceted and context-specific to establish a foundation of good health and well-being that will persist into adulthood.

4 Eating and Lifestyle Behaviors, Along with Psychosocial Factors Affecting the Dietary Habits of Adolescents

The choices that adolescents make around eating and lifestyle behaviors will set a foundation for healthy—or unhealthy—habits later in life. Despite this knowledge, there are critical data gaps when trying to determine what adolescents are consuming and how patterns may differ by subgroup (e.g., sex, socioeconomic status, urban/rural, and region) and over time, which makes policy and programmatic recommendations challenging. Data from India's Comprehensive National Nutrition Survey (2016–2018) found that a higher proportion of girls and boys from wealthy and urban subgroups consumed more nutrient-rich foods, like fruits, vegetables, dairy, meat and, eggs, than poor and rural subgroups of adolescents, but that they tended to consume more nutrient-poor and energy-dense foods too [68]. Further analysis of this data demonstrated substantial differences across India's states, highlighting the complexity of drawing conclusions based on aggregate data. A 2018 systematic review of dietary intake and habits among adolescent girls in LMICs [69] found low self-reported consumption of nutritious foods such as dairy, meats (including poultry and fish), fruits, and vegetables. In contrast, adolescent girls reported frequently consuming (4–6 times per week) energy-dense and nutrient-poor foods such as sweet and salty snacks, sugar-sweetened beverages, and fast foods. Authors also noted regional variation in consumption habits, with 40% of girls in Latin America and the Caribbean and 25% in South Asia reporting daily consumption of fast foods, for example. The review supports the nutrition transition hypothesis, whereby more "Westernized" diets are gradually replacing traditional foods in LMICs; a finding that has been mirrored in other work on adolescent diets [69–71]. The Global School-based Student Health Survey (GSHS), the only source of adolescent dietary intake data that is comparable across LMICs, also demonstrates poor dietary habits that are widespread, like daily consumption of carbonated beverages and weekly fast foods, despite variability within and across regions [68]. Overall, these findings underscore the importance of interventions to improve the food environments of adolescents to combat the increasing double burden of malnutrition and noncommunicable diseases associated with unhealthy diets.

Neufeld and colleagues explored the various influences on adolescent diets, acknowledging the intersecting factors found at the individual, social, community, and macro levels that play a role, such as biological and psychosocial changes, peer and family influence, the physical food environment, and social/cultural norms and social media [72]. It's also important to note that gendered roles, whether becoming a wife or mother or taking on additional caregiving responsibilities, often play a role in food choice, purchasing, preparation, and access for adolescents in many contexts [73]. Using qualitative data from 11 countries and a literature review, the authors found differences in the relative importance of desirability vs. affordability vs. availability between traditional, mixed, and modern food environment contexts.[1] Adolescents' increased autonomy and agency, combined with social cues, can

---

[1] Based on the criteria of the High Level Panel of Experts on Food Security and Nutrition [74].

negatively impact dietary choices through desirability in modern and some mixed environments, whereas adolescents experiencing food insecurity and poverty[2] view food as a basic need (not a choice), and one that concerns the community above the individual [68]. Among these latter groups, there is a greater influence of availability and affordability, with affordability reflecting an ability—or not—to pay for food that often leads to adolescents seeking income opportunities for food purchase [68]. The convenience of foods was also examined, but was found only to apply to modern and mixed food environments. Convenience was reported to be relatively less important when compared to desirability in a modern food environment and of lesser importance when compared to availability, desirability, and affordability in a mixed food environment. Importantly, despite vastly different food environment contexts, the social aspect of eating with friends and family was consistently highlighted as being important to adolescents [68].

5   Data and Nutrition Monitoring

Given this unique and sensitive life course stage, it's clear that multiple strategies across multiple sectors, including education, health, technology, social protection, and the food system, will be required to improve adolescent nutrition. Unfortunately, standardized data to monitor the nutritional status of adolescents is fragmented, which hinders our ability to inform priority national and local actions and develop global targets. Hargreaves and colleagues summarized available global databases related to adolescent health (Fig. 2), of which nutrition-focused data are a very small component [48]. While some of these data represent the determinants of good nutrition, or proxies thereof, the only LMIC-relevant nutrition-specific indicators pictured include iron supplementation, dietary diversity scores, anemia prevalence, and anthropometry from Demographic and Health Surveys (DHS), which omit adolescents aged 14 years and below. Physical activity-focused data is lacking across the board, underscoring our inability to draw conclusions on how improved (or unimproved) physical activity is impacting adolescent overweight and obesity. Of note, this figure has omitted the Global Burden of Disease (GBD) and the Institute for Health Metrics and Evaluation (IHME) data that encompass adolescent-specific risk factors and outcomes.

In addition to this paucity of data, there can be a lack of agreement on what constitutes the adolescent period (though the most widely used definition is 10–19 years), and no consensus on anthropometric definitions of malnutrition in adolescents, including those for use in emergency settings [75]. Without clear definitions, this adds to the complexity of setting targets, tracking trends, and establishing thresholds for programmatic activities. However, reliable data is required to set targets, and without targets, there is less incentive to collect data, creating a chicken-and-egg scenario. There is a clear push from the nutrition community to revisit and

---

[2]All included studies from traditional food environments were in the context of extreme poverty.

Domains	Population Council Adolescent Data Hub	Demographic and Health Survey (DHS) data	Health Behavior in School Age Children (HBSC)	United States Adolescent Health	WHO Maternal, Newborn, Child and Adolescent Health data portal	UNICEF adolescent health data (Multiple Indicator Cluster Survey)
Databases	• 127 LMICs • 473 datasets (453 observational, 20 experimental, 358 national representative data) • Age 10–14, 15–19, and 20–24 years	• All DHS surveys conducted from 2000 to 2017 with availability of data for girls or boys age 15–19 years	• WHO collaborative cross-sectional national survey • Data was collected every 4 years on 11–15-year-olds in 49 countries and regions across Europe and North America	• US national and state level • Age 9–20 years	• Global health data, including regional and country data • Age 10–19 years	• More than 100 countries around the world • Age 15–19 years
Natural systems and planetary health	No data	No data	No data	No data	No data	No data
Social, cultural, and gender norms	• Gender attitudes and beliefs • Community engagement • Crime • Social networks • Subjective expectations	No data	• Social environments	• Healthy relationships	• National policies	No data
Economic development, urbanisation, and food and agriculture systems	• Economics • Health-care access and utilisation • Migration and mobility	• Iron supplementation	No data	No data	No data	No data
Household, school, and peer dietary and activity patterns	• Demographic characteristics • Education • Family and household structure • Time use	No data	No data	• Demographics	No data	• Education • Marriage • Early demographics • Participation
Individuals — Physical activity	No data	No data	No data	No data	No data	No data
Individuals — Cognitive and emotional growth	• Mental health	No data	No data	• Mental health	No data	• Mental health
Individuals — Food choice and dietary intake	No data	• Women's diet diversity score	No data	No data	No data	No data
Other relevant outcomes	• Physical health • Reproductive health	• Anaemia • Anthropometry • Adolescent childbearing	• Health and wellbeing • Health behaviours	• Reproductive health • Physical health and nutrition • Substance abuse	• Adolescent sexual and reproductive health • Morbidity • Mortality and cause of death	• Childbearing • Violence

Fig. 2 Databases that include adolescent health-related data [48]. (Reprinted from: The Lancet, 399/10320, Dougal Hargreaves et al., Strategies and interventions for healthy adolescent growth, nutrition, and development, 198/210, Copyright (2022), with permission from Elsevier")

reestablish valid indicators, references, and cutoffs for anthropometry in adolescents to improve measurement and, ultimately, status [76].

Of course, context specificity will be required to effectively learn from collected data and adapt multisectoral actions in a way that is appropriate for a given food environment. A country-level situational analysis should be conducted that takes into account all the factors that play a role in adolescent nutrition, including assessments of: nutritional status (anthropometry, micronutrient status), dietary intake and habits; food environments (at school, home, and in the community), physical activity and health service access, and availability and uptake of nutrition-related national policies and guidelines [48]. The disaggregation of available country or regional-level data by key subgroup, including adolescent boys vs girls, younger vs. older adolescents, those who live in urban vs. rural settings, those who are attending vs. not attending school, among others, will be key to reach those who likely need intervention most.

6   Current and Emerging Initiatives and Strategies

Recently, there has been recognition of the importance of better understanding the adolescent period through data. The creation of some global initiatives has followed, including the 2016 Lancet Commission on Adolescent Health and Wellbeing, which provides evidence-informed recommendations that underscore the importance of investing in adolescent health to derive benefits today, into adulthood, and within future generations [77]. This series also highlights that, beyond accounting for the social and economic rights of adolescents and the need to consider sustainable development, there are substantial country-level economic returns that can be realized through improving the health and nutrition of the adolescent cohort [78], a finding that is particularly salient in low-income settings and is a crucial metric for policymakers.

Adolescent nutrition has been incorporated directly within Sustainable Development Goal (SDG) 2, that is, to end all forms of malnutrition by 2030, including addressing the nutritional needs of adolescent girls. In addition, it's widely recognized that in order to achieve many or most of the SDGs' (17 goals, 169 targets, and 231 indicators) targets, improving adolescent health and nutrition will be crucial. Effects on health, particularly negative insults, can compound over the life course from birth up until old age. Therefore, poor health and nutrition during the adolescent period could lead to lower education levels, chronic disease, poor productivity, reduced earnings, and less attainment of human capital. With this in mind, improving adolescent health will be especially necessary to achieve SDGs targeting poverty, health security, education, and the reduction of inequalities [79]. Despite the acknowledgement of the importance of this life stage, the Gender and Adolescence: Global Evidence (GAGE) research program identified that out of 232 SDG indicators (in 2019), less than 8% are gender-, adolescent-, or youth-specific [80]. These 8% (18 indicators) cover just six goals relating to poverty, health and well-being, education, gender equality, work and economic growth, and sustainable cities and communities. GAGE also reports that country data for these 18 indicators is limited, and that data quality is unknown for many [80].

As a step forward, the Global Strategy for Women's, Children's and Adolescents' Health (2016–2030) was created in order to translate the SDG agenda into concrete guidance. The goal of this global strategy was to mobilize international and national action by governments, multilateral organizations, civil society, and the private sector to improve the health and well-being and end preventable deaths of women, children, and adolescents. The strategy promotes a monitoring framework with 16 key indicators (60 total), including those for mortality, birth rates, education, violence, and the sexual and reproductive health of adolescents [81]. Since its inception, several reports on progress have been published, and a data portal has been created for visualization and comparison of trends across countries. Country profiles were also generated for each WHO member state in order to easily assess progress across all targets in one dashboard. Progress should be made with these efforts closely monitored, such that the global community, country stakeholders, and local communities are all more accountable.

Noticeably, these initiatives focus on adolescent health broadly, with nutrition often occupying a small subcomponent of health. As a response to this, the Emergency Nutrition Network convened the Global Adolescent Nutrition Network (GANN) that is composed of 100+ members from across academia, nongovernmental organization, donors, UN agencies, and government agencies, all with the core mission of advancing the nutrition of adolescents through advocacy, research and collaboration, and sharing of learnings. In addition, a 2021 Lancet Series on Adolescent Nutrition, with contributions by many GANN members [82], was published outlining the consequences of poor nutrition and effective interventions to prevent and manage nutritional disorders during adolescence. The series highlights the need for better data, multisectoral coordination, and gender- and environment-responsive action, and above all, increased attention to adolescent nutrition within global nutrition policy frameworks.

7 Discussion/Conclusion

7.1 Implications for Global and Regional (Specifically LMICs) Policies and Practices

Indeed, while adolescent health and, to a lesser extent, nutrition, have gained some global traction over the last decade, more can be done. There have been global initiatives that call for the improvement of adolescent health and well-being, and, at the country level, adolescents are beginning to show up in some stand-alone policies and strategies. However, more common is the inclusion of adolescents within target groups—either lumped in with women of reproductive age or school-age children—despite the continued realization that adolescents are a unique group that requires unique targeting strategies. In addition, it's clear that national and subnational programs and implementation studies specifically targeting adolescent nutrition are lagging behind any political commitments (which are also lagging, in many cases). A 2015 review of policies and programs specific to adolescent nutrition in Scaling Up Nutrition (SUN) countries found that only seven (out of 22 countries with national nutrition plans available) included the improvement of adolescent nutrition as a strategic objective. Of these, only two reported an assessment of adolescent nutrition, and none included adolescents within their monitoring and evaluation plans. While an updated review would likely show some progress, the recent Lancet Series confirms the requirement of countries to strengthen their focus on adolescent nutrition, beyond micronutrient supplementation strategies, to ensure that both undernutrition and overweight/obesity, and the structural systems that allow them to prevail, are assessed. This series also calls for more adolescent-specific data, better research on delivery platforms, and the inclusion of adolescent themselves in the planning and review of such strategies.

7.2 Implications for the SDGs

SDG-2 specifies the need to "address the nutritional needs of adolescent girls," but it will be impossible to do this without a number of criteria being met. Firstly, adolescents—both boys and girls—need to be incorporated into country-level nutrition plans and strategies that cut across sectors for maximal impact. Secondly, in order to understand the nutritional needs of adolescents, appropriate age and gender disaggregated data are required, along with a better understanding of the complex drivers of both undernutrition and overnutrition in this age-group. Finally, additional research on the impact of adolescent nutrition-specific policies and programs will be crucial to course correct and ensure that interventions are effective, in terms of both impact and cost, and appropriately delivered.

7.3 Conclusions and Priorities Moving Forward

As demonstrated throughout this chapter, adolescent nutrition will require strong commitment at the global and national levels in order to see progress (Table 1). With the continued high burden of undernutrition and the growing burden of overweight/obesity and related noncommunicable diseases among adolescents in LMICs, a multipronged approach is urgently needed. To effectively improve nutrition in this age-group, both direct and indirect nutrition interventions will be required, meaning that sectors including health (and particularly mental and reproductive health), education, agriculture, social protection, and water, sanitation, and hygiene should be involved, at a minimum. There is a need for a more pointed focus on adolescent nutrition in country-led policies and programs, along with creating policies and programs that improve adolescents' food environments. Micronutrient supplementation, the promotion of healthy diets, and the promotion of active lifestyles are

Table 1 Way forward to improve adolescent nutrition

1. Create stand-alone adolescent nutrition policies globally and at the country level with embedded targets.
2. Ensure that rigorous adolescent nutrition-specific research is conducted, including on delivery platforms and drivers of undernutrition and overweight/obesity, and that data is sex- and age-disaggregated.
3. Develop multi-sectoral programming for improving adolescent nutrition that encompasses scalable monitoring and evaluation schemes.
4. Use human-centered design approaches to ensure that adolescents are included in the design and implementation planning of nutrition research and strategies.

three evidence-based interventions that would make a good start. However, more research is needed to determine context-specific adolescent needs and how to effectively achieve progress. Additionally, standardized data for monitoring and evaluation is lacking, hindering national and global target-setting and accountability. Data need to be both age- (10–14 and 15–19, at minimum) and gender-disaggregated in order to make proper assessments. Finally, it is critical that adolescents themselves need to be included in program design for effective and efficient intervention targeting, delivery, uptake, and program sustainability.

References

1. WHO: Adolescent health. https://www.who.int/health-topics/adolescent-health#tab=tab_1. 2023. Accessed.
2. Norris SA, Frongillo EA, Black MM, Dong Y, Fall C, Lampl M, et al. Nutrition in adolescent growth and development. Lancet. 2022;399(10320):172–84. https://doi.org/10.1016/s0140-6736(21)01590-7.
3. UNICEF: Adolescents. https://data.unicef.org/topic/adolescents/overview/ (2022). Accessed.
4. WHO: Malnutrition - Key Facts. https://www.who.int/news-room/fact-sheets/detail/malnutrition (2021). Accessed.
5. Pal A, Pari AK, Sinha A, Dhara PC. Prevalence of undernutrition and associated factors: a cross-sectional study among rural adolescents in West Bengal, India. Int J Pediatr Adolesc Med. 2017;4(1):9–18. https://doi.org/10.1016/j.ijpam.2016.08.009.
6. UNICEF. The State of the World's Children 2005- Childhood under threat. 2005.
7. Müller O, Krawinkel M. Malnutrition and health in developing countries. CMAJ. 2005;173(3):279–86. https://doi.org/10.1503/cmaj.050342.
8. WHO. The world health report 2002: reducing risks, promoting healthy life. World Health Organization; 2002.
9. Seferidi P, Hone T, Duran AC, Bernabe-Ortiz A, Millett C. Global inequalities in the double burden of malnutrition and associations with globalisation: a multilevel analysis of Demographic and Health Surveys from 55 low-income and middle-income countries, 1992-2018. Lancet Glob Health. 2022;10(4):e482–e90. https://doi.org/10.1016/S2214-109X(21)00594-5.
10. WHO. The double burden of malnutrition: policy brief. World Health Organization; 2017.
11. Cappa C, Wardlaw T, Langevin-Falcon C, Diers J. Progress for children: a report card on adolescents. Lancet. 2012;379(9834):2323–5. https://doi.org/10.1016/S0140-6736(12)60531-5.
12. Das JK, Salam RA, Thornburg KL, Prentice AM, Campisi S, Lassi ZS, et al. Nutrition in adolescents: physiology, metabolism, and nutritional needs. Ann N Y Acad Sci. 2017;1393(1):21–33. https://doi.org/10.1111/nyas.13330.
13. Global Burden of Disease Pediatrics Collaboration. Global and national burden of diseases and injuries among children and adolescents between 1990 and 2013: findings from the global burden of disease 2013 study. JAMA Pediatr. 2016;170(3):267–87. https://doi.org/10.1001/jamapediatrics.2015.4276.
14. Wrottesley SV, Mates E, Brennan E, Bijalwan V, Menezes R, Ray S, et al. Nutritional status of school-age children and adolescents in low- and middle-income countries across seven global regions: a synthesis of scoping reviews. Public Health Nutr. 2023;26(1):63–95. https://doi.org/10.1017/S1368980022000350.
15. Cusick SE, Kuch AE. Determinants of undernutrition and overnutrition among adolescents in developing countries. Adolesc Med State Art Rev. 2012;23(3):440–56.
16. Kurz KM. Adolescent nutritional status in developing countries. Proc Nutr Soc. 1996;55(1b):321–31.

17. Nguyen PH, Scott S, Neupane S, Tran LM, Menon P. Social, biological, and programmatic factors linking adolescent pregnancy and early childhood undernutrition: a path analysis of India's 2016 National Family and Health Survey. Lancet Child Adolesc Health. 2019;3(7):463–73. https://doi.org/10.1016/S2352-4642(19)30110-5.
18. Patton GC, Neufeld LM, Dogra S, Frongillo EA, Hargreaves D, He S, et al. Nourishing our future: the Lancet Series on adolescent nutrition. Lancet. 2022;399(10320):123–5. https://doi.org/10.1016/s0140-6736(21)02140-1.
19. Bhattarai S, Bhusal CK. Prevalence and associated factors of malnutrition among school going adolescents of Dang district. Nepal AIMS Public Health. 2019;6(3):291–306. https://doi.org/10.3934/publichealth.2019.3.291.
20. Popkin BM, Corvalan C, Grummer-Strawn LM. Dynamics of the double burden of malnutrition and the changing nutrition reality. Lancet. 2020;395(10217):65–74. https://doi.org/10.1016/S0140-6736(19)32497-3.
21. Cui Z, Dibley MJ. Trends in dietary energy, fat, carbohydrate and protein intake in Chinese children and adolescents from 1991 to 2009. Br J Nutr. 2012;108(7):1292–9. https://doi.org/10.1017/s0007114511006891.
22. Gupta DK, Shah P, Misra A, Bharadwaj S, Gulati S, Gupta N, et al. Secular trends in prevalence of overweight and obesity from 2006 to 2009 in urban Asian Indian adolescents aged 14-17 years. PLoS One. 2011;6(2):e17221. https://doi.org/10.1371/journal.pone.0017221.
23. Kac G, Velasquez-Melendez G, Schlussel MM, Segall-Correa AM, Silva AA, Perez-Escamilla R. Severe food insecurity is associated with obesity among Brazilian adolescent females. Public Health Nutr. 2012;15(10):1854–60. https://doi.org/10.1017/S1368980011003582.
24. Kimani-Murage EW, Kahn K, Pettifor JM, Tollman SM, Dunger DB, Gomez-Olive XF, et al. The prevalence of stunting, overweight and obesity, and metabolic disease risk in rural south African children. BMC Public Health. 2010;10:158. https://doi.org/10.1186/1471-2458-10-158.
25. Maruapula SD, Jackson JC, Holsten J, Shaibu S, Malete L, Wrotniak B, et al. Socio-economic status and urbanization are linked to snacks and obesity in adolescents in Botswana. Public Health Nutr. 2011;14(12):2260–7. https://doi.org/10.1017/s1368980011001339.
26. Nagwa MA, Elhussein AM, Azza M, Abdulhadi NH. Alarming high prevalence of overweight/obesity among Sudanese children. Eur J Clin Nutr. 2011;65(3):409–11. https://doi.org/10.1038/ejcn.2010.253.
27. Tang HK, Dibley MJ, Sibbritt D, Tran HM. Gender and socio-economic differences in BMI of secondary high school students in Ho Chi Minh city. Asia Pac J Clin Nutr. 2007;16(1):74–83.
28. Wrotniak BH, Malete L, Maruapula SD, Jackson J, Shaibu S, Ratcliffe S, et al. Association between socioeconomic status indicators and obesity in adolescent students in Botswana, an African country in rapid nutrition transition. Pediatr Obes. 2012;7(2):e9–e13. https://doi.org/10.1111/j.2047-6310.2011.00023.x.
29. Popkin BM, Adair LS, Ng SW. Global nutrition transition and the pandemic of obesity in developing countries. Nutr Rev. 2012;70(1):3–21. https://doi.org/10.1111/j.1753-4887.2011.00456.x.
30. Yang L, Bovet P, Ma C, Zhao M, Liang Y, Xi B. Prevalence of underweight and overweight among young adolescents aged 12-15 years in 58 low-income and middle-income countries. Pediatr Obes. 2019;14(3):e12468. https://doi.org/10.1111/ijpo.12468.
31. Estecha Querol S, Iqbal R, Kudrna L, Al-Khudairy L, Gill P. The double burden of malnutrition and associated factors among south Asian adolescents: findings from the global school-based student health survey. Nutrients. 2021;13(8) https://doi.org/10.3390/nu13082867.
32. Salam RA, Das JK, Bhutta ZA. Multiple micronutrient supplementation during pregnancy and lactation in low-to-middle-income developing country settings: impact on pregnancy outcomes. Ann Nutr Metab. 2014;65(1):4–12. https://doi.org/10.1159/000365792.
33. WHO: Stunting in a Nutshell. https://www.who.int/news/item/19-11-2015-stunting-in-a-nutshell#:~:text=Children%20are%20defined%20as%20stunted,WHO%20Child%20Growth%20Standards%20median. 2015. Accessed.

34. Caleyachetty R, Thomas GN, Kengne AP, Echouffo-Tcheugui JB, Schilsky S, Khodabocus J, et al. The double burden of malnutrition among adolescents: analysis of data from the global school-based student health and health behavior in school-aged children surveys in 57 low- and middle-income countries. Am J Clin Nutr. 2018;108(2):414–24. https://doi.org/10.1093/ajcn/nqy105.
35. WHO Global Health Observatory. Prevalence of thinness among children and adolescents, BMI < −2 standard deviations below the median. https://www.who.int/data/gho/indicator-metadata-registry/imr-details/4805#:~:text=Definition%3A,school%2Dage%20children%20and%20adolescents.&text=Based%20on%20measured%20height%20and%20weight. Accessed.
36. Abarca-Gómez L, Abdeen ZA, Hamid ZA, Abu-Rmeileh NM, Acosta-Cazares B, Acuin C, et al. Worldwide trends in body-mass index, underweight, overweight, and obesity from 1975 to 2016: a pooled analysis of 2416 population-based measurement studies in 128 9 million children, adolescents, and adults. Lancet. 2017;390(10113):2627–42. https://doi.org/10.1016/S0140-6736(17)32129-3.
37. Keats EC, Rappaport AI, Shah S, Oh C, Jain R, Bhutta ZA. The dietary intake and practices of adolescent girls in low- and middle-income countries: a systematic review. Nutrients. 2018;10(12) https://doi.org/10.3390/nu10121978.
38. Kraak VI, Vandevijvere S, Sacks G, Brinsden H, Hawkes C, Barquera S, et al. Progress achieved in restricting the marketing of high-fat, sugary and salty food and beverage products to children. Bull World Health Organ. 2016;94(7):540–8. https://doi.org/10.2471/BLT.15.158667.
39. Victora CG, Christian P, Vidaletti LP, Gatica-Dominguez G, Menon P, Black RE. Revisiting maternal and child undernutrition in low-income and middle-income countries: variable progress towards an unfinished agenda. Lancet. 2021;397(10282):1388–99. https://doi.org/10.1016/S0140-6736(21)00394-9.
40. Prentice AM. Nutrition challenges and issues of relevance to adolescents an low and middle-income countries. In: Health and nutrition in adolescents and young women: Preparing for the next generation: 80th Nestlé Nutrition Institute Workshop, Bali, November 2013. 80. S.Karger AG. 2014. https://doi.org/10.1159/000360252. Accessed 9/14/2023.
41. Goli S, Rammohan A, Singh D. The effect of early marriages and early childbearing on women's nutritional status in India. Matern Child Health J. 2015;19(8):1864–80. https://doi.org/10.1007/s10995-015-1700-7.
42. Keats EC, Akseer N, Thurairajah P, Cousens S, Bhutta ZA, Global Young Women's Nutrition Investigators G. Multiple-micronutrient supplementation in pregnant adolescents in low- and middle-income countries: a systematic review and a meta-analysis of individual participant data. Nutr Rev. 2022;80(2):141–56. https://doi.org/10.1093/nutrit/nuab004.
43. Wallace JM. Competition for nutrients in pregnant adolescents: consequences for maternal, conceptus and offspring endocrine systems. J Endocrinol. 2019;242(1):T1–T19. https://doi.org/10.1530/JOE-18-0670.
44. Bhutta ZA, Das JK, Rizvi A, Gaffey MF, Walker N, Horton S, et al. Evidence-based interventions for improvement of maternal and child nutrition: what can be done and at what cost? Lancet. 2013;382(9890):452–77. https://doi.org/10.1016/S0140-6736(13)60996-4.
45. Mkhize S, Libhaber E, Sewpaul R, Reddy P, Baldwin-Ragaven L. Child and adolescent food insecurity in South Africa: a household-level analysis of hunger. PLoS One. 2022;17(12):e0278191. https://doi.org/10.1371/journal.pone.0278191.
46. Salam RA, Das JK, Irfan O, Ahmed W, Sheikh SS, Bhutta ZA. Effects of preventive nutrition interventions among adolescents on health and nutritional status in low- and middle-income countries: a systematic review. Campbell Syst Rev. 2020;16(2):e1085. https://doi.org/10.1002/cl2.1085.
47. Baxter JB, Wasan Y, Islam M, Cousens S, Soofi SB, Ahmed I, et al. Dietary diversity and social determinants of nutrition among late adolescent girls in rural Pakistan. Matern Child Nutr. 2022;18(1):e13265. https://doi.org/10.1111/mcn.13265.

48. Hargreaves D, Mates E, Menon P, Alderman H, Devakumar D, Fawzi W, et al. Strategies and interventions for healthy adolescent growth, nutrition, and development. Lancet. 2022;399(10320):198–210. https://doi.org/10.1016/s0140-6736(21)01593-2.
49. Charles Shapu R, Ismail S, Ahmad N, Lim PY, Abubakar Njodi I. Systematic review: effect of health education intervention on improving knowledge, attitudes and practices of adolescents on malnutrition. Nutrients. 2020;12(8) https://doi.org/10.3390/nu12082426.
50. Adeomi AA, Fatusi A, Klipstein-Grobusch K. Children eat all things here': a qualitative study of mothers' perceptions and cultural beliefs about underweight and overweight children and adolescents in selected communities in two Nigerian states. BMJ Open. 2022;12(4):e059020. https://doi.org/10.1136/bmjopen-2021-059020.
51. Bhutta ZA, Lassi ZS, Bergeron G, Koletzko B, Salam R, Diaz A, et al. Delivering an action agenda for nutrition interventions addressing adolescent girls and young women: priorities for implementation and research. Ann N Y Acad Sci. 2017;1393(1):61–71. https://doi.org/10.1111/nyas.13352.
52. Aguayo VM, Paintal K. Nutrition in adolescent girls in South Asia. BMJ. 2017;357:j1309. https://doi.org/10.1136/bmj.j1309.
53. Kabeer N. Gender, livelihood capabilities and women's economic empowerment: reviewing evidence over the life course. 2018.
54. Akseer N, Al-Gashm S, Mehta S, Mokdad A, Bhutta ZA. Global and regional trends in the nutritional status of young people: a critical and neglected age group. Ann N Y Acad Sci. 2017;1393(1):3–20. https://doi.org/10.1111/nyas.13336.
55. Riddle AY, Kroeger CM, Ramage AK, Bhutta ZA, Kristjansson E, Vlassoff C, et al. PROTOCOL: the effects of empowerment-based nutrition interventions on the nutritional status of adolescent girls in low- and middle-income countries. Campbell Syst Rev. 2019;15(3) https://doi.org/10.1002/cl2.1042.
56. Hewett PC, Willig AL, Digitale J, Soler-Hampejsek E, Behrman JR, Austrian K. Assessment of an adolescent-girl-focused nutritional educational intervention within a girls' empowerment programme: a cluster randomised evaluation in Zambia. Public Health Nutr. 2020;24:651. https://doi.org/10.1017/s1368980020001263.
57. Leroy JL, Ruel M, Sununtnasuk C, Ahmed A. Understanding the determinants of adolescent nutrition in Bangladesh. Ann N Y Acad Sci. 2018;1416:18. https://doi.org/10.1111/nyas.13530.
58. Hewett PC, Willig AL, Digitale J, Soler-Hampejsek E, Hachonda NJ, Behrman JR, et al. Adolescent Girls Empowerment Program (AGEP): Nutrition.
59. Dyke E, Penicaud S, Hatchard J, Dawson AM, Munishi O, Jalal C. Girl-powered nutrition program: key themes from a formative evaluation of a nutrition program co-designed and implemented by adolescent girls in low- and middle-income countries. Curr Dev Nutr. 2021;5(7):nzab083. https://doi.org/10.1093/cdn/nzab083.
60. UNHCR. More than 100 million people are forcibly displaced. https://www.unhcr.org/refugee-statistics/insights/explainers/100-million-forcibly-displaced.html. 2022. Accessed.
61. Ataullahjan A, Gaffey MF, Spiegel PB, Bhutta ZA. The health impacts of displacement due to conflict on adolescents. In: Allotey P, Reidpath D, editors. The health of refugees: public health perspectives from crisis to settlement. Oxford University Press; 2019. p. 0.
62. Carroll GJ, Lama SD, Martinez-Brockman JL, Perez-Escamilla R. Evaluation of nutrition interventions in children in conflict zones: a narrative review. Adv Nutr. 2017;8(5):770–9. https://doi.org/10.3945/an.117.016121.
63. Acharya Y, Luke N, Naz S, Sharma D. Exposure to conflict-related violence and nutritional status of children in Iraq. SSM Popul Health. 2020;11:100585. https://doi.org/10.1016/j.ssmph.2020.100585.
64. Bilukha OO, Jayasekaran D, Burton A, Faender G, King'ori J, Amiri M, et al. Nutritional status of women and child refugees from Syria-Jordan, April-may 2014. MMWR Morb Mortal Wkly Rep. 2014;63(29):638–9.
65. Engidaw MT, Gebremariam AD. Prevalence and associated factors of stunting and thinness among adolescent Somalian refugee girls living in eastern Somali refugee camps, Somali regional state, Southeast Ethiopia. Confl Heal. 2019;13(1):17. https://doi.org/10.1186/s13031-019-0203-3.

66. Woodruff BA, Blanck HM, Slutsker L, Cookson ST, Larson MK, Duffield A, et al. Anaemia, iron status and vitamin a deficiency among adolescent refugees in Kenya and Nepal. Public Health Nutr. 2006;9(1):26–34. https://doi.org/10.1079/phn2005825.
67. Blanchet K, Sistenich V, Ramesh A, Frison S, Warren E, Smith J, et al. An evidence review of research on health interventions in humanitarian crises. Enhancing Learning and Research in Humanitarian Assistance. 2015.
68. Neufeld LM, Andrade EB, Ballonoff Suleiman A, Barker M, Beal T, Blum LS, et al. Food choice in transition: adolescent autonomy, agency, and the food environment. Lancet. 2022;399(10320):185–97. https://doi.org/10.1016/S0140-6736(21)01687-1.
69. Ochola S, Masibo PK. Dietary intake of schoolchildren and adolescents in developing countries. Ann Nutr Metab. 2014;64(Suppl 2):24–40. https://doi.org/10.1159/000365125.
70. Aurino E, Fernandes M, Penny ME. The nutrition transition and adolescents' diets in low- and middle-income countries: a cross-cohort comparison. Public Health Nutr. 2017;20(1):72–81. https://doi.org/10.1017/S1368980016001865.
71. Beal T, Morris SS, Tumilowicz A. Global patterns of adolescent fruit, vegetable, carbonated soft drink, and fast-food consumption: a meta-analysis of global school-based student health surveys. Food Nutr Bull. 2019;40(4):444–59. https://doi.org/10.1177/0379572119848287.
72. Story M, Kaphingst KM, Robinson-O'Brien R, Glanz K. Creating healthy food and eating environments: policy and environmental approaches. Annu Rev Public Health. 2008;29:253–72. https://doi.org/10.1146/annurev.publhealth.29.020907.090926.
73. Aurino E. Do boys eat better than girls in India? Longitudinal evidence on dietary diversity and food consumption disparities among children and adolescents. Econ Hum Biol. 2017;25:99–111. https://doi.org/10.1016/j.ehb.2016.10.007.
74. HLPE. Nutrition and food systems. A report by the high-level panel of experts on food security and nutrition of the committee on world food security. Rome: Food and Agrilcture Organization of the United Nations; 2017.
75. Zakari Ali NLSW, Emily M. Adolescent nutrition mapping study: A global stakeholder survey of policies, research, interventions and data gaps. 2020.
76. Lelijveld N, Benedict RK, Wrottesley SV, Bhutta ZA, Borghi E, Cole TJ, et al. Towards standardised and valid anthropometric indicators of nutritional status in middle childhood and adolescence. Lancet Child Adolesc Health. 2022;6(10):738–46. https://doi.org/10.1016/S2352-4642(22)00196-1.
77. Patton GC, Sawyer SM, Santelli JS, Ross DA, Afifi R, Allen NB, et al. Our future: a lancet commission on adolescent health and wellbeing. Lancet. 2016;387(10036):2423–78. https://doi.org/10.1016/s0140-6736(16)00579-1.
78. Sheehan P, Sweeny K, Rasmussen B, Wils A, Friedman HS, Mahon J, et al. Building the foundations for sustainable development: a case for global investment in the capabilities of adolescents. Lancet. 2017;390(10104):1792–806. https://doi.org/10.1016/S0140-6736(17)30872-3.
79. WHO. Child and adolescent health. Denmark: World Health Organization Regional Office for Europe; 2017.
80. Guglielmi S, Jones N. The invisibility of adolescents within the SDGs. Assessing gaps in gender and age disaggregation to leave no adolescent behind. London: Gender and Adolescence: Global Evidence; 2019.
81. WHO. Indicator and monitoring framework for the global strategy for women's, children's and adolescents' health (2016-2030). World Health Organization; 2016.
82. The Lancet: Adolescent Nutrition. https://www.thelancet.com/series/adolescent-nutrition. 2021. Accessed.

Health Sector Interventions

Family Planning

Fatima Haider, Mishaal Zulfiqar, and Zahid Ali Memon

1 Overview

The World Health Organization (WHO) defines family planning as "the ability of individuals and couples to anticipate and attain their desired number of children and the spacing and timing of their births (48). It is achieved through the use of contraceptive methods and the treatment of involuntary infertility"(World Health Organization). According to the WHO, a woman should wait at least 24 months after a live birth before getting pregnant again. Ensuring access to the people for their choice of contraceptive methods promotes several human rights such as freedom of opinion and expression, and the liberty to work and education. Additionally, it substantially improves the health and well-being of mothers and children, along with imparting other socioeconomic advantages (50).

Various initiatives to improve family planning services and decrease unmet needs are being implemented globally, especially in the low- and middle-income countries (LMICs); however, there is still a long way to go as the women's unmet need for family planning remains high in most of the LMICs, particularly in sub-Saharan Africa (26). In 1994, the United Nations organized an International Conference on Population and Development (ICPD) in Cairo, inviting governments,

F. Haider · M. Zulfiqar
Center of Excellence Women and Child Health, Aga Khan University, Karachi, Pakistan
e-mail: fatima.haider@aku.edu; mishaal.ali@aku.edu

Z. Ali Memon (✉)
Institute of Global Health and Development, Aga Khan University, Karachi, Pakistan
e-mail: zahid.memon@aku.edu

© The Author(s), under exclusive license to Springer Nature Switzerland AG 2025
Z. S. Lassi, R. A. Salam (eds.), *Nutrition Across Reproductive, Maternal, Neonatal, Child, and Adolescent Health Care*,
https://doi.org/10.1007/978-3-031-95721-5_7

non-governmental organizations, media representatives, and other relevant stakeholders to discuss solutions to significant issues such as immigration, population, family planning, birth control, education of women, etc. At ICPD, more than 179 countries agreed that: "(a) All couples and individuals have the right to decide freely and responsibly the number, spacing and timing of their children, and to have the information and means to do so; (b) Decisions concerning reproduction should be made free from discrimination, coercion and violence."

I. Building on the goals from the ICPD conference, the Millennium Summit in 2000 (introduction of the Millennium Development Goals), the World Summit in 2005 and 2007, United Nations Population Fund strategic plan 2008–2011, and the Sustainable Development Goals (SDGs) 2030, there has been a continuous process of recognizing family planning issues. The 2030 Agenda for the SDGs emphasizes achieving universal access to reproductive health-care services, including family planning, information and education, and integration of family planning into national programs (43). Moreover, out of the 17 SDGs and 169 targets of the 2030 agenda, many targets are related to women empowerment, gender equality, and health, where family planning plays an important role in achieving most of these targets. Among the SDGs, Goal 3—on guaranteeing good health and well-being for all—and Goal 5—on promoting gender equality and the empowerment of women and girls—specifically point toward family planning. The benefits that family planning offers to individuals, communities, and societies are of immense importance, the critical ones being: (i) avoiding unintended pregnancies; (ii) reducing the spread of sexually transmitted diseases (STDs); and (iii) while addressing the problem of STDs, it helps reduce rates of infertility (25). All these developments on the field and agenda have further emphasized on improving of family planning and sexual and reproductive health. Moreover, these global interactions continue to reflect on the gaps between strategies, identify priorities, outline the approaches and principles related to family planning and sexual and reproductive health's strategic outcomes.

2 Global Trends

Many countries conduct national surveys to collect data on family planning practices, contraceptive use, unmet needs, and related indicators. These surveys, such as the Demographic and Health Surveys (DHS) and Multiple Indicator Cluster Surveys (MICS), provide valuable epidemiological data on family planning at national and regional levels.

Globally, 966 million women of reproductive age (15–49 years) out of the total 1.9 billion women are using some method of contraception (Fig. 1). About 874 million women use a modern contraceptive method and 92 million use traditional

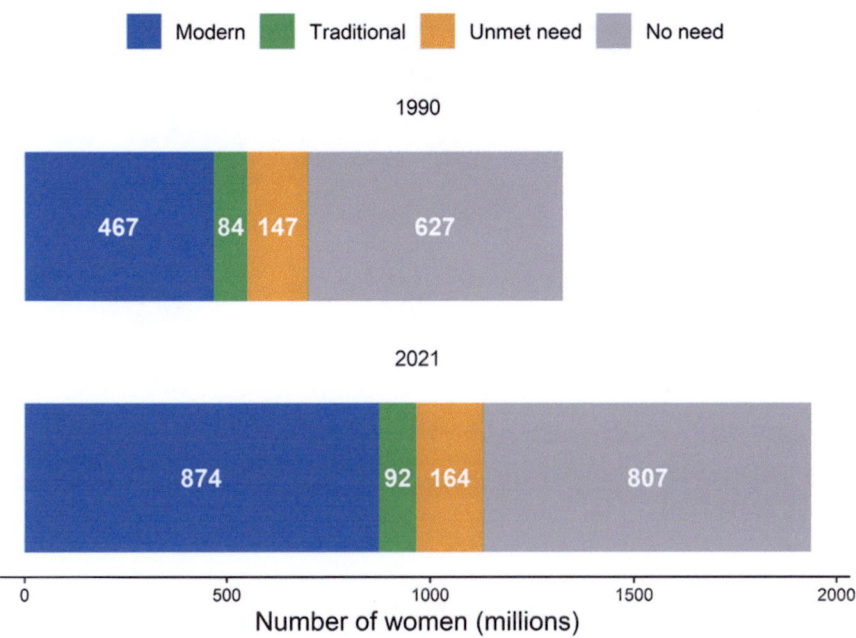

Fig. 1 Global number of women of reproductive age (15–49 years) who use modern and traditional contraceptives (44)

contraceptive methods. There are still 164 million women who wish to avoid pregnancy but are not using any contraceptive methods (unmet need for family planning) (44). An additional 70 million women are projected to be added to this figure by 2030 (50).

The low and lower-middle-income countries have the largest gaps in meeting the needs for family planning. Although, eight out of ten countries that witnessed the largest increase in the use of modern contraceptive methods from 1991 to 2021 are from sub-Saharan Africa, this still accounts for only 56% of the women in this region in need for family planning (Fig. 2). Moreover, many countries with high proportion of unmet needs for family planning are projected to witness a rapid growth in the population of women aged 14–49 years through 2030, which will create additional challenges to keep pace with the growing demand (43).

The global contraceptive utilization trend shows that the highest proportion of women who want to avoid pregnancy and are using any method of contraception falls between 25 and 44 years. However, despite the increase in adolescent (15–19 years) population from 45% in 2000 to 61% in 2020, the proportion of women with satisfied need for family planning remains low among this age group as compared to other ages (44).

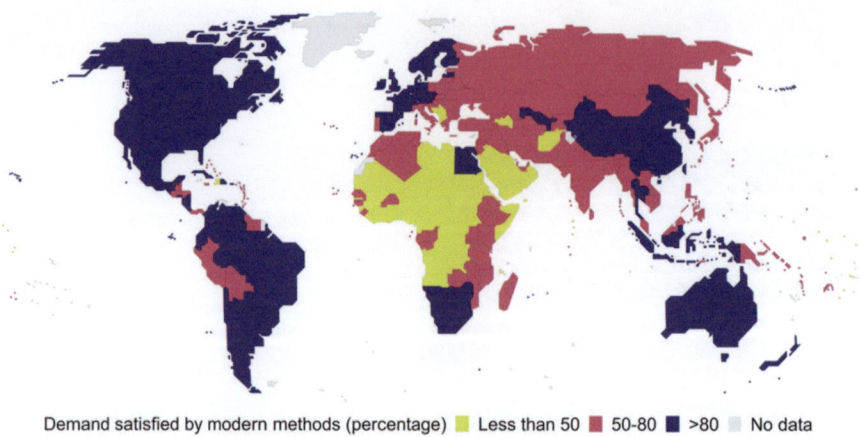

Fig. 2 Proportion of women of reproductive age (15–49 years) who have their need for family planning satisfied (44)

3 Advantages of Family Planning

The effective fulfillment of the demand for family planning through the utilization of modern contraceptive methods can yield significant economic, social, and individual health advantages for developing nations. Meeting the demand for family planning could alleviate strain on natural resources and promote attainment of SDGs related to environmental sustainability and food security (40). A reduced rate of population growth simplifies the provision of sustainable infrastructure, such as clean water and sanitation, promotes responsible land usage, and helps curb pollution stemming from industrial operations (15). Furthermore, the anticipated decline in the proportion of young individuals presents a favorable circumstance for accelerated economic progress, as a larger portion of the population enters economically productive stages. This advantageous situation is commonly referred to as the demographic dividend (15). Moreover, improving women's ability to delay childbearing brings about increased possibilities for mothers to pursue education and early employment opportunities (40).

It also has potential positive impacts on maternal and child health. Adequate birth spacing allows mothers to recover physically and emotionally from the previous pregnancy and childbirth. It lowers the maternal mortality and the risk of maternal complications, such as anemia, high blood pressure, and postpartum depression. Mothers can regain their strength while also promoting improved health outcomes for both themselves and their children (2). Moreover, birth spacing empowers women by giving them greater control over their reproductive choices. It enables women to pursue education, employment, and personal goals, thereby enhancing their social and economic opportunities. Women who can space their pregnancies have more agency and autonomy in making decisions that affect their lives (5, 40). Children born with sufficient spacing between pregnancies have a higher chance of receiving proper nutrition, health care, and attention from their parents. This leads to improved physical and cognitive development, reducing the risk of stunting, malnutrition, and developmental delays (42). Birth spacing helps families maintain a balance between their financial resources, time, and energy. It allows parents to provide adequate attention, care, and support to each child, fostering stronger parent-child relationships. Families can plan and invest in their children's education, health care, and overall upbringing more effectively (34).

4 Methods of Contraception

There are various methods of contraception available, each with its own benefits and considerations. It is important to consult a health-care provider to determine the most suitable method based on individual's health, lifestyle and preferences. Table 1 provides an overview of the various methods of contraception available along with their mechanism of action and failure rates.

Table 1 List of methods of contraception by mechanism, duration of protection, and failure rate (6, 50)

Type of contraceptive	Mechanism	Duration of protection	Failure rate %
Intrauterine contraception			
Levonorgestrel intrauterine system (LNG IUD)	It prevents pregnancy by releasing a small amount of progestin each day.	From 3 to 8 years	0.1–0.4
Copper T intrauterine device (IUD)	Placed inside the uterus to prevent pregnancy.	Up to 10 years	0.8
Hormonal methods			
Implant	Inserted under the skin of a woman's upper arm.	3 years	0.1
Injectables	The shots of the hormone progestin are to be administered in the buttocks or arm of the woman.	1 or 3 months	4
Combined oral contraceptives	Prevents the release of eggs from the ovaries (ovulation).	Daily	7
Progestin only pill	Thickens cervical mucous to block sperm and egg from meeting and prevents ovulation.	Daily	7
Patch	This skin patch is worn on the lower abdomen, buttocks, or upper body (but not on the breasts). It releases hormones progestin and estrogen into the bloodstream.	The patch is worn once a week for 3 weeks. Taken out in the week when periods are expected.	7

(continued)

Table 1 (continued)

Type of contraceptive	Mechanism	Duration of protection	Failure rate %
Hormonal vaginal ring	The ring releases the hormones progestin and estrogen. It is placed inside the vagina.	The ring is worn for 3 weeks, taken out in the week when periods are expected.	7
Emergency contraception			
Copper IUD	The copper T IUD is inserted within 5 days of unprotected sex.	[a]NA	NA
Emergency contraceptive pill	Women can take emergency contraceptive pills up to 5 days after unprotected sex, but the sooner the pills are taken, the better they will work.	NA	NA
Barrier methods			
Diaphragm or cervical cap	It is used before sexual intercourse, along with spermicide, to block or kill sperm.		17
Sponge	The sponge works for up to 24 hours and must be left in the vagina for at least 6 hours after the last act of intercourse.	24 hours	14
Male condom	A male condom keeps sperm from getting into a woman's body.	[a]NA	13
Female condom	The female condom prevents sperm from getting inside the body. It can be inserted up to eight hours before sexual intercourse.	[a]NA	21
Spermicides	These products work by killing sperm and come in several forms—Foam, gel, cream, film, suppository, or tablet. They are placed in the vagina no more than one hour before intercourse. They are left in place for at least six to eight hours after intercourse.	[a]NA	21
Fertility awareness-based methods			
Calendar or rhythm method	The couple prevents pregnancy by avoiding unprotected vaginal sex during the first and last estimated fertile days, by abstaining.	[a]NA	2–23
Withdrawal or coitus interruptus	The sperm are released outside woman's body, preventing fertilization.	[a]NA	
Lactational amenorrhea method	For women who have recently had a baby and are breastfeeding, the Lactational amenorrhea method can be used as birth control when three conditions are met: (1) amenorrhea (not having any menstrual periods after delivering a baby), (2) fully or nearly fully breastfeeding, and (3) less than 6 months after delivering a baby.		
Permanent methods			
Female sterilization or tubal ligation	The fallopian tubes are tied (or closed) so that sperm and eggs cannot meet for fertilization.	[a]NA	0.5
Male sterilization or vasectomy	This operation keeps a man's sperm from going to his penis, so his ejaculate never has any sperm that can fertilize an egg.	[a]NA	0.15

[a]Not applicable

5 FP 2030 and Family Planning Core Indicators

FP2030 which follows FP2020, is a global initiative that started from 2012 in London with the goal of achieving a target of 120 million additional women and girls in 69 of the world's poorest counties to use modern contraception by 2020 (13). For the last 8 years, it has served as a primary hub for family planning, offering a central platform for stakeholders to come together, coordinate efforts, exchange information, facilitate resource allocation, and promote progress in the field. FP2030, builds on and expands FP2020 agenda which involves:

- Global partnerships fostering shared learning and mutual responsibility for commitments and outcomes.
- Family planning approaches prioritizing individuals' rights and promoting equity.
- A dedication to promoting gender equality by empowering women and girls, involving men, boys, and communities in the process.
- Equitable collaborations with adolescents, youths, and marginalized populations, addressing their specific needs based on accurate and disaggregated data collection and use (13).

There are 17 core indicators that serve as the foundation of the measurement agenda and strive to capture multiple important dimensions of family planning including, equity, availability, access, quality, empowerment, and informed choice (12).

6 Family Planning Challenges in Lower-Middle-Income Countries

Despite numerous investments and initiatives to improve utilization of modern contraceptives in LMICs, the countries have struggled to reduce the fertility rates. The challenges faced in achieving global family planning goals and outcomes vary as per each country's context however a few major challenges are listed below:

1. *Limited Access to Contraceptive Services*
    Limited access and the poor quality of family planning services has been largely responsible for low modern contraceptive prevalence rate (mCPR) in LMICs. Many LMICs lack adequate infrastructure, resources, and trained health-care professionals to provide comprehensive family planning services. Over the past decades, international donors have supported in designing and implementing family planning programs to promote access to appropriate methods of contraception, as well as counseling, and awareness on reproductive health for couples and individuals. Yet, an estimated 218 million women of reproductive age (15–49 years) in LMICs have an unmet need for modern contraceptives, resulting in unsafe abortion, unintended pregnancy, and STDs (36). LMICs have limited financial resources with competing priorities in sectors such

as infrastructure development, education, defense, and poverty alleviation. With limited funding allocated to the health-care sector, family planning stands as the last priority (47). Insufficient funding hinders the development of an efficient health-care system, training of health-care professionals and maintenance of contraceptives stock (38). Rural areas often have limited access to health-care facilities and skilled health-care professionals and the geographical disparities further exacerbate the challenges faced in delivering family planning services (16).

2. *Health System Strengthening*

The health systems in LMICs are weak, which negatively affects the quality of family planning services. Many studies show that clients do not utilize family planning services at public health facilities as health providers are rude, available for limited work hours, confidentiality of patients is not maintained, lack of trust in services or clinical competency, poor distribution of outlets, and lack of family planning information in local language (46, 51). LMICs often experience higher unmet need for contraception, which means that individuals who want to prevent or delay pregnancy are unable to access or use modern contraceptive methods due to various reasons. Determinants of unmet need from supply side include inadequate quantity and quality of family planning methods and information materials, occasional stockouts of contraceptives, and lack of client's preferred family planning method. Due to insufficient funding, health-care providers are not trained, and along with the lack of essential commodities and weak supply chain mechanism, the *availability* and effectiveness of family planning programs are undermined.

3. *Sociocultural Barriers*

Cultural norms, gender inequalities and traditional beliefs act as a barrier to family planning in LMICs. The societal settings do not expose young girls and boys to family planning concept and services due to which they have limited knowledge on the possible options and importance of birth spacing (32). Women face cultural and social barriers, such as restrictions on mobility and lack of transportation limiting their access to health care services. Studies show that older women in Rwanda and Eastern Sudan, are more likely to engage in family planning discussions with their partner compared to younger women (4). Despite younger women showing preference for birth spacing, they often have limited knowledge about modern family planning options and are less likely to discuss family planning with health-care providers in comparison to older women. This reluctance to express their family planning needs can be partly attributed to the stigma associated with contraceptive use among young females, including concerns about perceived infidelity, extramarital relationships (17, 27, 37), religious beliefs that discourage interference with God's reproductive plans, and distrust in the confidentiality of health-care workers (49). However, post ICPD conference, many countries have adopted the model of community health worker (CHW) program to create awareness regarding family planning among women of reproductive age in these settings.

Family Planning 109

4. *Women's Agency*: The lack of women's agency has a significant impact on family planning service utilization in LMICs. Women's agency refers to their ability to make decisions and control their own lives, including accessing health-care services and information. The lack of agency can lead to women being unable to make decisions about their own health, informed choice of family planning method and size and time of family. In LMICs, women have limited awareness and knowledge about contraceptive methods, their benefits, and proper usage, which poses a significant challenge. Inadequate sex education and reproductive health information lead to misconceptions, myths, and stigmatization surrounding family planning, discouraging its uptake. Moreover, the husband—and in some cases, the mother-in-law—acts as the gatekeeper for a woman's family planning journey. As such, the agency of women is hindered by the patriarchal societal norms, where men hold the power and decision-making authority to access health-care services and making it difficult for women to make decisions or acquire family planning services without their consent (49). This acts as a barrier for women to access health-care services for themselves.
5. *Legal and Policy Constraints*: In some LMICs, legal and policy frameworks may restrict access to certain contraceptive methods or limit the provision of family planning services. For example, in some countries, oral contraceptive pills are allowed only on prescription, which hinders access to oral contraceptive pills. In some parts of Africa, women receive family planning methods from community based workers, and factors such as age restrictions or spousal consent requirements, can create obstacles for individuals seeking contraception.

Addressing these challenges requires a multifaceted approach involving government commitment, increased investment in health-care systems, comprehensive sex education, community engagement, and efforts to overcome cultural and gender barriers. Additionally, strengthening partnerships with international organizations and increasing access to affordable and diverse contraceptive options can help improve family planning outcomes in LMICs.

7   High Impact Practices

High Impact Practices (HIPs) refer to a group of evidence-based family planning practices that have been carefully evaluated by experts and have proven to be a successful best practice in achieving family planning goals (22, 24) (Fig. 3). Each HIP is quantifiable and exhibits a noticeable impact in achieving diverse family planning outcomes (11) These outcomes include increasing the uptake of modern contraceptives, reducing unintended pregnancies, decreasing overall fertility rates, or addressing at least one of the primary factors influencing fertility (such as delaying marriage or sexual initiation among adolescents, promoting birth spacing, encouraging exclusive breastfeeding, or advocating for postpartum abstinence).

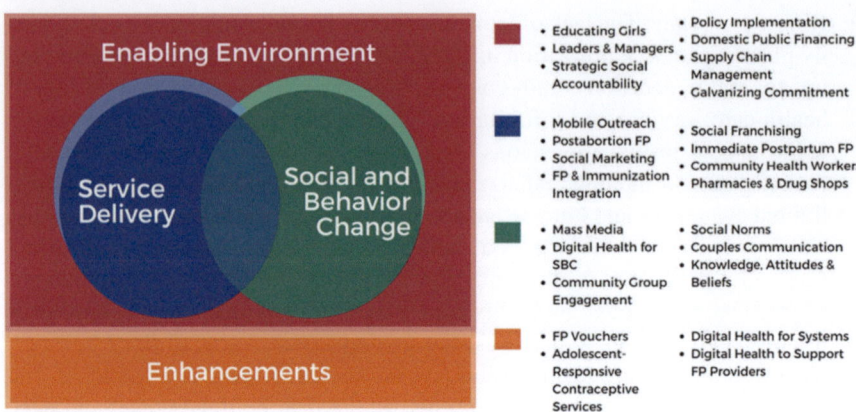

Fig. 3 High impact practices in family planning. (Reproduced from HIPs, August 2022)

7.1 Enabling Environment

To support the family planning outcomes, it is imperative to have an enabling environment. Enabling environment refers to an ideal state, where policies, social norms, budgetary allocations, availability and affordability of necessary products, political commitment, leadership, and coalition building are present across sectors. Political commitment, domestic public financing, and implementation of policies are linked to concrete results yielding improved family planning outcomes (21). The support of decision makers is considered of great importance to implement family planning policies, allocate funds, set out streams of domestic funding, inclusion of family planning in national insurance policies, and leverage other sources of funding and collaborative government support to promote family planning at the national and subnational level (17). An enabling environment focuses on different ways to support family planning goals and ensure equitable access for all. For example, the government of Guatemala repurposed the tax on alcoholic beverages to be used for reproductive health and the purchase of family planning commodities. Similarly, the state of Madagascar approved of family planning law, while reversing the colonial French law prohibiting the youth or married woman without the spousal consent to access contraceptives (8). It is the collaborative role societal agencies such as government, civil society and other stakeholders play to advocate for the legal and financial change to improve access to family planning (Fig. 4 [19]).

7.2 Service Delivery

In LMICs, higher unmet need for family planning is attributable to lower access and geographic and social barriers to utilization of family planning services. CHW models have been successful in LMICs as they reduce inequities by bringing services, information, and supplies to women and men in the communities where they reside

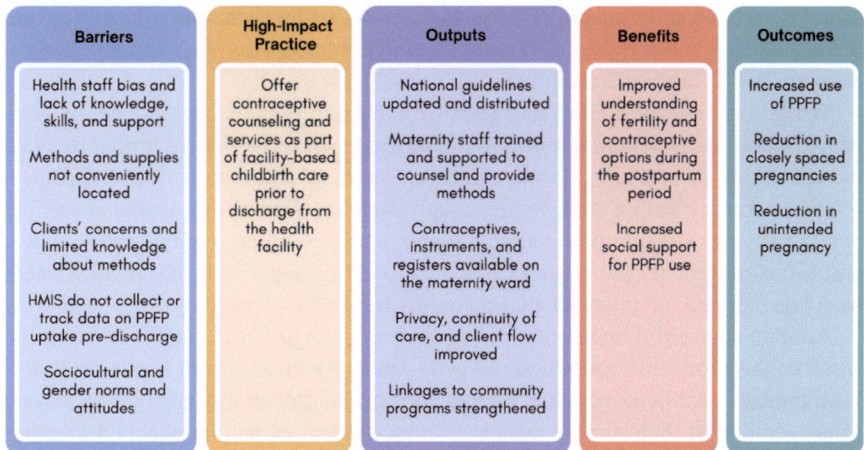

Fig. 4 Offering family planning counseling and services at the same time and location as facility-based childbirth care: Theory of change. (High Impact Practices in Family Planning (HIPs), 2022 May)

instead of requiring them to visit otherwise inaccessible health facilities. The CHWs are trained for sharing information, providing services, and referrals on a need basis. Another important achievement has been the integration of family planning at every stage of encounter within maternal and child health services. Capacity building and training of health-care providers encourage them to counsel clients on adoption of possible family planning methods during antenatal care, postabortion, and postpartum encounters (28). Approximately 61% of postpartum women have an unmet need for contraceptives in LMICs (41), due to sociocultural barriers such as myths related to use of contraceptives while breastfeeding (14, 35), timing of return to menses (1), sexual activity (7), and lack of access to contraceptives. Providing family planning as a part of care during and immediately after childbirth has proven to be a high-impact practice to address gaps and improve postpartum family planning uptake. For example, a hospital in northern Nigeria utilized couples' counseling to increase the immediate postpartum family planning uptake from 29% to 49% (10). In Rwanda, the postpartum family planning counseling session is utilized to design an individualistic plan to coincide the child's immunization appointments with the family planning sessions, that led to an increase in the proportion of women who adopted a method predischarge and the proportion of women who left the facility with a plan (45).

Within service delivery, another successful best practice that has stood out is *social marketing*. Social marketing moves beyond knowledge and instead focuses on behavior change, through market research and consumer insight to inform the delivery of health information, products, and services tailored to clients' needs, values, and preferences. For example, the Dimpa program in India helped introduce injectable contraceptives as an option in private health facilities, leading to the inclusion of injectables in the national family planning program (30). Similarly, social marketing programs in Nigeria work along with private providers to ensure the availability and provision of implants, oral contraceptive pills, and intrauterine devices (IUDs) in private facilities (45).

While inclusion of CHWs and social franchising models have added value in provision of family planning services, mobile outreach services have further reduced the inequities in accessing family planning services and commodities. Outreach models offer a flexible and strategic approach to allocate resources, including health-care providers, family planning commodities, supplies, equipment, vehicles, and infrastructure. These resources are deployed to areas with the greatest need, based on demand, in a manner that optimally meets the demand.

Another successful intervention is *mobile outreach facilities,* as this expands the reach of the product in areas that are geographically distant from health facilities. Furthermore, mobile outreach facilities confirm confidentiality of the clients and offer methods of their choice, which reduces the fear of stigma attached to using family planning facilities. Another successful example is of Malawi, where from 2004 to 2010, the prevalence of modern contraceptive use among married women increased by 14%, rising from 28% to 42% (9). A case study examining Malawi's experience determined that the mobile outreach service delivery program was instrumental in attaining this achievement (18).

7.3 Social Behavior Change

Social and behavior change (SBC) is another successful model, which aims to enhance and sustain changes in individual behaviors, social norms, and the overall enabling environment. As described in Fig. 5, SBC approaches design and implement interventions at the individual, community, and societal levels, promoting the adoption of healthy practices. These programs integrate insights from various disciplines, including communication, social psychology, anthropology, behavioral economics, sociology, human-centered design, and social marketing, leveraging a comprehensive understanding of human behavior. The interdisciplinary SBC approach addresses the influence of acceptance and continuation of family planning methods, facilitating individuals and couples in achieving their reproductive goals. These factors include social and gender roles, societal norms related to family, sexuality, and fertility, communication within couples, perceived costs at personal and social levels, method-specific barriers (e.g., misconceptions, fear of side effects), perceived low pregnancy risks, uncertain or conflicting fertility preferences, and general disapproval of contraception. Research shows that SBC interventions are essential to inform high-quality and sustainable family planning interventions. Along with couples counseling, tailored communication, forms of performing art, digital, social, and mass media have been described as the most influential in shaping social norms and increasing support for family planning practices. Moreover, SBC interventions have been proven to contribute to improving the interaction between clients and providers, enhancing perceptions of quality services, building trust in the health-care system, and fostering linkages with other health areas. By

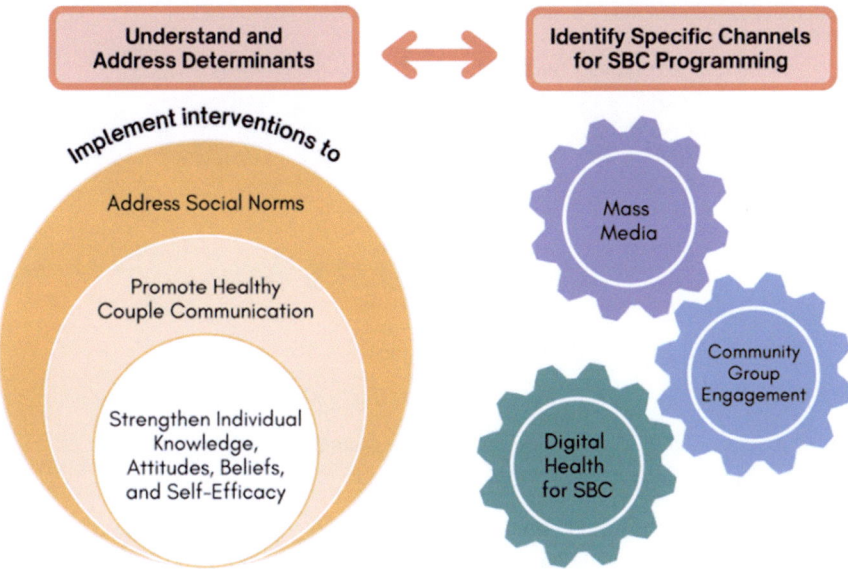

Fig. 5 Integrated framework for effective implementation of the social and behavior change (23)

complementing service delivery and the enabling environment, SBC forms a network of interconnected HIPs to strengthen family planning programs. A successful example is of Urban Reproductive Health Initiative (NURHI) project, which was conducted in six cities in Nigeria. The NURHI project, focused on changing cultural perceptions of modern contraception in Nigeria via SBC communication through diverse demand generation activities using multiple communication and media channels to disseminate the messages on family planning (39). This transmedia intervention led to a pronounced 10% increase in the use of modern contraceptive methods and a similar increase in the desire for contraception products in three million women of reproductive age, through a network of 244 primary health care facilities in Nigeria (31).

7.4 Enhancements

Enhancements refers to the continuous new and relevant innovations and effective practices which have been successful in promoting family planning practices such as inclusion of adolescents, utilization of digital health services support system and providers and family planning vouchers.

According to the WHO, the age between 10 and 19 is an important phase in an adolescent's life, which encompasses social, physical, and cognitive changes and often the age for sexual debut (49). As adolescents transition to adulthood, it is important to provide them with correct knowledge about family planning and

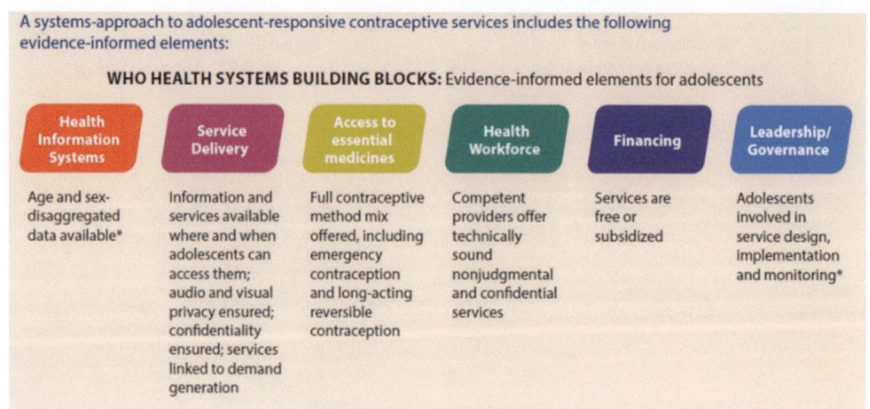

Fig. 6 A systems-approach to adolescent-responsive contraceptives (20)

services to ensure informed choices. Many countries are not supportive of expanding this spectrum of knowledge to adolescents for sociocultural and political beliefs, however, the consequences of such policies have led to unsafe abortions, STDs, teenage pregnancies, etc. HIPs propose a systems-approach that works toward making existing contraceptive services accessible. The systems-approach below (Fig. 6) implies that policies, procedures, and programs across the health system should respond to the needs and preferences of adolescents.

Universally family planning vouchers or coupons have also been deemed successful in reducing the barriers to family planning services. These vouchers are referrals which clients can present to the health-care providers to obtain any service and payment is made after the service is utilized. By focusing on specific population groups, voucher programs can enhance client awareness of contraceptive options and provide information on where and when services can be accessed. Moreover, vouchers can assist health-care providers in improving service quality through accreditation processes and expanding the availability of contraceptive methods. For example, in Nicaragua, adolescents who were provided with vouchers had 3.1 times greater chances of utilizing participating health centers compared to those who did not receive vouchers. Furthermore, sexually active adolescents who received vouchers had twice the likelihood of using modern contraception and 2.5 times higher odds of reporting condom use during their last sexual encounter, in comparison to adolescents who did not have access to vouchers (33).

7.5   Digital Technologies in Family Planning

Lastly, digital technologies have helped enhance HIPs in family planning as digital applications, through cellphones, tablets, and computers, improve access and efficiency. With the rise in mobile phone users in LMICs, mHealth interventions have seen widespread acceptance worldwide as a platform for sexual and reproductive health and family planning education. Moreover, it removes logistical hurdles for individuals, enabling them to conveniently access information related to family planning while maintaining confidentiality. A systematic review conducted to assess the effectiveness of mHealth interventions in improving family planning uptake and adherence in LMICs showed promising results in improving family planning outcomes (3). Another study looked at the effect of technology-based contraceptive decision aids and also concluded that digital applications can manage logistic issues and reduce contraceptive stockouts (29). In Malawi, CHWs utilize cellphones to update the stock status, whereby the system automatically calculates the need for supply as per the stock consumed and sends the request for supply to the health center, enabling health center staff to prepare orders for CHWs (29). Similarly, countries have invested in better health management information systems for the timely analysis and reporting of stocks and family planning indicators. Additionally, technology is also being used for counseling, workshops, refresher trainings, convenient client-provider interactions, purchasing contraceptives of their choice, extending information and services to far-flung areas, and improving efficiency, accountability, and transparency of financial services and stocks.

8 Conclusion

In conclusion, family planning is an indispensable component of global health and development efforts. By empowering individuals to take control of their reproductive health, family planning programs can contribute to numerous benefits, including improved maternal and child health, reduced poverty, increased educational and economic opportunities for women, and environmental sustainability. Additionally, by reducing unintended pregnancies, family planning plays a crucial role in achieving broader global goals, such as gender equality, human rights, and social justice.

However, barriers to access, cultural and religious opposition, and inadequate funding continues to challenge family planning services. Addressing these challenges require a multifaceted approach that includes political commitment, increased investment in health-care infrastructure, comprehensive sexuality education, and efforts to combat stigma and misinformation. In moving forward, governments, civil society organizations, health-care providers, and international partners need to collaborate effectively to ensure that HIPs in family planning are adopted and incorporated in the policies, particularly in LMICs. By prioritizing family planning as a fundamental human right and an integral component of sustainable development, the outcomes for family planning can be improved significantly.

References

1. Abdulkadir Z, Grema BA, Michael GC, Omeiza SY. Effect of antenatal couple counselling on postpartum uptake of contraception among antenatal clients and their spouses attending antenatal Clinic of a Northern Nigeria Tertiary Hospital: a randomized controlled trial. West Afr J Med. 2020;37(6):695–702. Available from: http://europepmc.org/abstract/MED/33185269.

2. Ahmed S, Li Q, Liu L, Tsui AO. Maternal deaths averted by contraceptive use: an analysis of 172 countries. Lancet. 2012;380(9837):111–25.
3. Aung B, Mitchell JW, Braun KL. Effectiveness of mHealth interventions for improving contraceptive use in low-and middle-income countries: a systematic review. Global Health: Science and Practice. 2020;8(4):813–26.
4. Bawah AA, et al. Women's fears and men's anxieties: the impact of family planning on gender relations in Northern Ghana. Stud Fam Plan. 1999;30(1):54–66. https://doi.org/10.1111/j.1728-4465.1999.00054.x.
5. Canning D, Schultz TP. The economic consequences of reproductive health and family planning. Lancet. 2012;380(9837):165–71. https://doi.org/10.1016/s0140-6736(12)60827-7.
6. Center for Disease Control and Prevention. Contraception. 2023. Available from: https://www.cdc.gov/reproductivehealth/contraception/index.htm
7. Chandani Y, Andersson S, Heaton A, Noel M, Shieshia M, Mwirotsi A, et al. Making products available among community health workers: Evidence for improving community health supply chains from Ethiopia, Malawi, and Rwanda. J Glob Health. 2014;4:2047–978 (Print). https://doi.org/10.7189/jogh.04.020405.
8. Chebet JJ, McMahon SA, Greenspan JA, Mosha IH, Callaghan-Koru JA, Killewo J, et al. "Every method seems to have its problems" - Perspectives on side effects of hormonal contraceptives in Morogoro region, Tanzania. BMC Womens Health. 2015;15(1):97. https://doi.org/10.1186/s12905-015-0255-5.
9. Chintsanya J. Trends and correlates of contraceptive use among married women in Malawi: evidence from 2000–2010 Malawi demographic and health surveys. Calverton: DHS Program; 2013. Available from: https://dhsprogram.com/pubs/pdf/WP87/WP87.pdf.
10. Dalious M, Ganesan R. Expanding family planning options in India: lessons from the Dimpa program. Bethesda: Strengthening Health Outcomes through the Private Sector.
11. EngenderHealth. The SEED assessment guide for family planning programming. New York; 2011. Available from: https://www.engenderhealth.org/wp-content/uploads/2021/10/SEED-Assessment-Guide-for-Family-Planning-Programming.pdf
12. FP2020. Measurement-Estimate Tables. Available from: http://2015-2016progress.familyplanning2020.org/page/measurement/estimate-tables
13. FP2030. About FP2030. Available from: https://fp2030.org/about
14. Gahungu J, Vahdaninia M, Regmi PR. The unmet needs for modern family planning methods among postpartum women in sub-Saharan Africa: a systematic review of the literature. Reprod Health. 2021;18(1):35. https://doi.org/10.1186/s12978-021-01089-9.
15. Goodkind D, Lollock L, Choi Y, McDevitt T, West L. The demographic impact and development benefits of meeting demand for family planning with modern contraceptive methods. Glob Health Action. 2018;11(1):1423861. https://doi.org/10.1080/16549716.2018.1423861.
16. Habib SS, Jamal WA, Zaidi SMA, Siddiqui JA, Khan HM, Creswell J, et al. Barriers to access of healthcare services for rural women—applying gender lens on TB in a rural district of Sindh, Pakistan. Int J Environ Res Public Health. 2021;18(19):10102. https://doi.org/10.3390/ijerph181910102.
17. Hardee K, Wright K, Spicehandler J. Family planning policy, program, and practice decision-making: the role of research evidence and other factors. Washington, DC; 2015. Available from: https://knowledgecommons.popcouncil.org/departments_sbsr-rh/724/.
18. Higgs ES, Goldberg AB, Labrique AB, Cook SH, Schmid C, Cole CF, et al. Understanding the role of mHealth and other media interventions for behavior change to enhance child survival and development in low- and middle-income countries: an evidence review. J Health Commun. 2014;19:164–89. https://doi.org/10.1080/10810730.2014.929763.
19. High Impact Practices in Family Planning (HIPs). High impact practice briefs; 2017. Available from: https://www.fphighimpactpractices.org/briefs/
20. High Impact Practices in Family Planning (HIPs). Adolescent-Responsive Contraceptive Services: Institutionalizing adolescent-responsive elements to expand access and choice. 2021. Available from: http://www.fphighimpactpractices.org/briefs/adolescent-responsive-contraceptive-services

21. High Impact Practices in Family Planning (HIPs). Family Planning Enabling Environment Overview Brief. 2022. Available from: https://www.fphighimpactpractices.org/briefs/enabling-environment-overview/
22. High Impact Practices in Family Planning (HIPs). Family Planning High Impact Practices List. 2022. Available from: https://www.fphighimpactpractices.org/briefs/family-planning-high-impact-practices-list/
23. High Impact Practices in Family Planning (HIPs). SBC Overview: Integrated Framework for Effective Implementation of the Social and Behavior Change High Impact Practices in Family Planning. 2022. Available from: https://www.fphighimpactpractices.org/briefs/sbc-overview/
24. High Impact Practices in Family Planning (HIPs). Immediate Postpartum Family Planning: A key component of childbirth care. 2022. Available from: https://www.fphighimpactpractices.org/briefs/immediate-postpartumfamily-planning/
25. Institute of Medicine (US). In: Butler WC, Stith AB, editors. Committee on a Comprehensive Review of the HHS Office of Family Planning Title X Program. A Review of the HHS Family Planning Program: Mission, Management, and Measurement of Results. Washington, DC: National Academies Press (US); 2009.
26. Izugbara CO. Family planning in East Africa: trends and dynamics. Nairobi: African Population and Health Research Center; 2018.
27. Kaida A, et al. Male participation in family planning: results from a qualitative study in Mpigi District, Uganda. J Biosoc Sci. 2005;37(3):269–86. https://doi.org/10.1017/s0021932004007035.
28. Kouyate LAM. The transition barrier analysis: Sylhet. Bangladesh: Jhpiego; 2010.
29. Levine R, Corbacio A, Konopka S, et al. mHealth compendium, volume 5. Arlington, VA: African Strategies for Health, Management Sciences for Health; 2016.
30. Macro NSO. Malawi demographic and health survey 2010. Zomba, Malawi, and Calverton: DHS Program; 2010. Available from: https://dhsprogram.com/pubs/pdf/FR247/FR247.pdf.
31. Evaluation of the Nigerian urban reproductive health initiative (NURHI) program. Stud Fam Plan. 2017;48(3):253–68. https://doi.org/10.1111/sifp.12027.
32. Mekonnen W, Worku A. Determinants of low family planning use and high unmet need in Butajira District, south Central Ethiopia. Reprod Health. 2011;8:37. Available from:https://link.gale.com/apps/doc/A275938124/AONE?u=anon~99e7484a&sid=googleScholar&xid=511ffbd1.
33. Meuwissen LE, Gorter AC, Knottnerus AJA. Impact of accessible sexual and reproductive health care on poor and underserved adolescents in Managua, Nicaragua: a quasi-experimental intervention study. J Adolesc Health. 2006;38(1):56.e1. https://doi.org/10.1016/j.jadohealth.2005.01.009.
34. Miller G, Babiarz KS. Family planning: program effects. In: Wright JD, editor. International encyclopedia of the social & behavioral sciences. 2nd ed. Oxford: Elsevier; 2015. p. 786–93.
35. Borda MR, McKaig C. Return to sexual activity and modern family planning use in the extended postpartum period: an analysis of findings from seventeen countries. Afr J Reprod Health. 2010;14(4)
36. Pillai VA, Nagoshi JL. Unmet family planning need and intimate partner violence in The Democratic Republic of the Congo: results from a Nationwide Survey. Afr J Reprod Health. 2018;22(1):90–9. Available from: https://www.ajrh.info/index.php/ajrh/article/view/161.
37. Plummer ML, et al. Farming with your hoe in a sack: condom attitudes, access, and use in rural Tanzania. Stud Fam Plan. 2006;37(1):29–40. https://doi.org/10.1111/j.1728-4465.2006.00081.x.
38. Prata N. Making family planning accessible in resource-poor settings. Philos Trans R Soc B. 2009;364(1532):3093–9. https://doi.org/10.1098/rstb.2009.0172.
39. SBC, The Compass for Social and Behavior Change. NURHI 2 Social Mobilization Tools. Available from: https://thecompassforsbc.org/project-examples/nurhi-2-social-mobilization-tools
40. Starbird E, Norton M, Marcus R. Investing in family planning: key to achieving the sustainable development goals. Glob Health Sci Pract. 2016;4(2):191–210.

41. Tran NT, Yameogo WME, Gaffield ME, Langwana F, Kiarie J, Kulimba DM, Kouanda S. Postpartum family-planning barriers and catalysts in Burkina Faso and the Democratic Republic of Congo: a multiperspective study. Open Access J Contracept. 2018;9:63–74. https://doi.org/10.2147/OAJC.S170150.
42. UNICEF. Key Practice: Spacing between pregnancies. Available from: https://www.unicef.org/uganda/key-practice-spacing-between-pregnancies
43. United Nations. Family Planning and the 2030 Forward Agenda for Sustainable Development Data Booklet 2019.
44. United Nations Department of Economic and Social Affairs, Population Division. World family planning 2022: meeting the changing needs for family planning: contraceptive use by age and method. New York; 2022. Available from: file:///C:/Users/fatima.haider/Documents/SMK/REFERENCE%20PAPERS/undesa_pd_2022_world-family-planning%20(1).pdf.
45. USAID. Three successful sub-Saharan Africa family planning programs: lessons for meeting the MDGs. Washington; 2012. Available from: https://pdf.usaid.gov/pdf_docs/PA00HQSV.pdf
46. Ward VM, Bertrand JT, Puac F. Exploring sociocultural barriers to family planning among Mayans in Guatemala. Int Fam Plan Perspect. 1992;18(2):59–65. https://doi.org/10.2307/2133395.
47. Woog V, Singh S, Browne A, Philbin J. Adolescent women's need for and use of sexual and reproductive health services in developing countries. Available from: www.guttmacher.org/pubs/AdolescentSRHS-Need-Developing-Countries.pdf
48. World Health Organization. Contraception. Available from: https://www.who.int/health-topics/contraception#tab=tab_1
49. World Health Organization. Consolidated guideline on sexual and reproductive health and rights of women living with HIV. Geneva; 2017.
50. World Health Organization. Family Planning/Contraception Methods. 2020. Available from: https://www.who.int/news-room/fact-sheets/detail/family-planning-contraception
51. Wulifan JK, Brenner S, Jahn A, De Allegri M. A scoping review on determinants of unmet need for family planning among women of reproductive age in low and middle income countries. BMC Womens Health. 2016;16(1):2. https://doi.org/10.1186/s12905-015-0281-3.

Nutrition Intervention During Pregnancy and Lactation

Komal Abdul Rahim, Zahra Ali Padhani, and Zohra S. Lassi

1 Introduction

Malnutrition in women is a global health issue that includes both undernutrition and overnutrition [1]. The burden of malnutrition among women is increasing globally, particularly in low- and middle-income countries (LMICs) due to rising poverty and inequalities [2]. Since the year 2000, there has been no change in the prevalence of underweight among adolescent girls (i.e., 8%) and a very small reduction from 12% in 2000 to 10% in 2022 among women (20–49 years) [2]. Overweight and obesity, on the other end of the continuum, are also a matter of growing concern. Globally, obesity prevalence among women was 18.5% in the year 2022, which is almost a 10% increase since 1990 [3], with prevalence exceeding 60% in eight countries. In Uganda, the prevalence of overweight/obesity among women of reproductive age was 57.4%, in Nigeria, the rate was 66.7%, in Tanzania, it was 74.1%, the Maldives

K. Abdul Rahim (✉)
Centre of Excellence in Trauma and Emergencies (CETE), Aga Khan University Hospital, Karachi, Pakistan

Dean's Office, Medical College, Aga Khan University Hospital, Karachi, Pakistan
e-mail: komal.rahim@aku.edu

Z. A. Padhani
School of Public Health, Faculty of Health and Medical Sciences, The University of Adelaide, Adelaide, SA, Australia
e-mail: zahraali.padhani@adelaide.edu.au

Z. S. Lassi
School of Public Health, University of Adelaide, Adelaide, SA, Australia

Robinson Research Institute, Adelaide Medical School, The University of Adelaide, Adelaide, SA, Australia
e-mail: zohra.lassi@adelaide.edu.au

© The Author(s), under exclusive license to Springer Nature Switzerland AG 2025
Z. S. Lassi, R. A. Salam (eds.), *Nutrition Across Reproductive, Maternal, Neonatal, Child, and Adolescent Health Care*,
https://doi.org/10.1007/978-3-031-95721-5_8

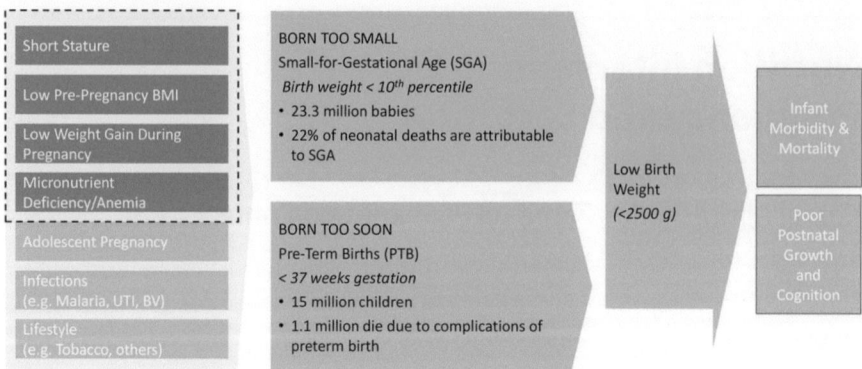

Fig. 1 Maternal nutrition and other factors influencing adverse birth outcomes. BMI body mass index; UTI urinary tract infection; BV bacterial vaginosis

had a prevalence of 63%, while South Africa reported a prevalence of 87% [4–7]. Acute malnutrition during pregnancy and breastfeeding also remains a concern that requires treatment once yearly; the estimates have suggested a 25% increase in acute malnutrition during pregnancy and breastfeeding from 2020 to 2022 (5.5 million versus 6.9 million, respectively) globally [2]. In LMICs, 240 million mothers are underweight as defined by a body mass index (BMI) of less than 18.5 [8], 450 million have short stature [9], and 468 million are anemic. Among all the countries, the highest burden of maternal malnutrition is seen in India, with 100 million adult women being underweight [8].

Figure 1 depicts the pathway for how maternal malnutrition leads to adverse birth and child health outcomes. The growing burden of maternal malnutrition has long been neglected due to gender-based inequities and resource allocation. The first 1000 days are given significance; the first 280 days from conception till birth are given preference and considered a critical window for future growth [10]. Despite this biological necessity, most resources dedicated to maternal and child health have been focused on the child [11], with minimal consideration for a woman's nutritional status before pregnancy.

Given the factors and consequences associated with poor nutrition in women, several targets set by the Sustainable Development Goals (SDGs) are directed to improve women's nutrition, health, and well-being. SDG Goal 2, "Zero Hunger," aims to provide access to safe and nutritious food for all, while SDG Goal 3, "Good Health and Well-Being," aims for a one-third reduction in premature deaths from noncommunicable diseases by 2030. The same goal addresses the need to reduce global maternal mortality by improving women's health, closely linked to proper nutrition during pregnancy and lactation. SDG Goal 5 focuses on gender equality, ensuring universal access to sexual and reproductive health, including access to nutrition education and services for women during preconception, pregnancy, and lactation [12].

The guidelines by the World Health Organization (WHO) on maternal nutrition emphasize proper nutrition during preconception, pregnancy, and lactation [13]. The global movement of Scaling Up Nutrition (SUN) united governments, civilians, businesses, and donors to address malnutrition in all its forms [14]. The United Nations Children's Fund (UNICEF) Nutrition Strategy (2020–2030) aims to improve maternal and child nutrition, including nutrition during pregnancy and lactation [15]. The United Nations Decade of Action on Nutrition (2016–2025) is also committed to intensifying efforts to alleviate hunger and prevent all forms of malnutrition globally, including that of women and children [16]. All the global policies mirror the international community's commitment to addressing women's nutritional needs. This chapter sheds light on interventions targeted toward maternal nutrition to improve maternal and child outcomes.

2 Five Programming Priorities

To improve nutrition in women, UNICEF has provided a strategic framework with five priorities. These priorities include programming for (1) women's nutrition before pregnancy, (2) women's nutrition during pregnancy (3), and women's nutrition during the breastfeeding period. In all contexts, particular emphasis will be given to the (4) nutrition of adolescent mothers and other nutritionally at-risk women, and (5) innovations for maternal nutrition [17].

The first priority is to prepare mothers for a healthy pregnancy by addressing nutritional status and ensuring access to a well-balanced diet, preserving maternal and fetal health, and promoting a balanced diet. The second priority is to help mothers through prenatal supplementation, education, and access to diverse, nutritious food options for the fetus's health and the mother's well-being. The third priority of nutrition during breastfeeding focuses on breastmilk being a vital source of nutrients for infants. Ensuring adequate nutrition during this period helps provide the child with a good quantity of quality milk. The fourth priority of nutrition for adolescent mothers and at-risk women acknowledges the specific vulnerabilities of certain groups and establishes tailored interventions to address their requirements. These groups are vulnerable to undernutrition due to preexisting health conditions or limited resource access, necessitating tailored interventions to address their needs. The last priority includes innovations for maternal nutrition, in which implementing new strategies, technologies, and interventions can enhance access to nutritional support for women [17]. Together, these priorities constitute a holistic strategy for enhancing women's nutritional well-being, spanning from prepregnancy to the breastfeeding phase.

3 Nutritional Interventions and Their Impact (Table 1)

3.1 Nutritional Education/Counseling

Maintaining a healthy diet, accessing essential services, and adopting optimal practices during pregnancy improve pregnancy outcomes. Nutritional counseling is integral to ensure that well-nourished mothers meet their nutrient needs during breastfeeding and replenish body stores [18]. Maternal nutrition counseling is an

Table 1 Summary of evidence-based interventions and their impact on the outcomes

Interventions	Outcomes (MD/RR; 95% CI)			
	Food intake	Child outcome	Maternal outcomes	Mortality outcome
Nutrition education	Protein intake: MD: 10.44 g, 95% CI, 1.83–19.05		Weight gain: RR: 2.84; 95% CI, 1.10–3.09	
Nutritional supplementation				
Balanced energy protein supplementation		*Stillbirth*: RR: 0.39; 95% CI, 0.19–0.80 *LBW*: RR: 0.60; 95% CI, 0.41–0.86 *SGA*: RR: 0.71; 95% CI, 0.54–0.94		*Perinatal mortality*: RR: 0.50; 95% CI, 0.30–0.84
Lipid-based nutrient supplements		*BW*: MD: 53.28 g, 95% CI, 28.22–78.33 *BL*: MD: 0.24 cm, 95% CI, 0.11–0.36		
Micronutrient supplementation				
Vitamin A			*Maternal anemia*: RR: 0.64; 95% CI, 0.43–0.93	*Maternal mortality*: RR: 0.88; 95% CI, 0.65–1.20 *Perinatal mortality*: RR: 1.01; 95% CI, 0.95–1.07
Zinc		*Preterm birth*: RR: 0.87; 95% CI, 0.74–1.03 *Stillbirth*: RR: 1.22; 95% CI, 0.80–1.88 *LBW*: RR: 1.08; 95% CI, 0.94–1.25		*Perinatal deaths*: RR: 1.10; 95% CI, 0.81–1.51
Iron and folic acid		*LBW*: RR: 0.88; 95% CI, 0.78–0.99	*Maternal anemia*: RR: 0.52; 95% CI, 0.41–0.66	

(continued)

Table 1 (continued)

Interventions	Outcomes (MD/RR; 95% CI)			
	Food intake	Child outcome	Maternal outcomes	Mortality outcome
Multiple micronutrient supplementation		*Preterm birth*: RR: 0.95; 95% CI, 0.90–1.01 *SGA*: RR: 0.92; 95% CI, 0.88–0.97		
Food fortification		*NTD*: RR: 0.57; 95% CI, 0.45–0.73		

Abbreviations: *MD* Mean difference; *RR* Relative risk; *LBW* Low birth weight; *BW* Birth weight; *BL* Birth length; *SGA* Small for gestational age; *NTD* Neural tube defects

interactive process between a service provider and a woman and her family, facilitating information exchange and support for decision-making and nutrition improvement [19].

A recent systematic review showed that nutritional counseling among pregnant women is effective in improving dietary intake [20]. The pooled estimates suggested that nutritional education may improve dietary caloric intake (mean difference [MD]: 81.65; 95% confidence interval (CI), 15.37–147.93; $n = 3$), protein intake (MD: 10.44 g, 95% CI, 1.83–19.05; $n = 2$), and gestational weight gain (relative risk [RR]: 1.84; 95% CI, 1.10–3.09; $n = 3$). In addition, nutritional counseling probably led to the immediate initiation of breastfeeding after birth, but did not affect anemia and the risk of stillbirths [20].

The WHO emphasizes counseling in preconception care, and nutrition education and counseling are also an integral part of the UNICEF's nutritional strategies for 2020–2030 [21]. However, many women in LMICs lack access to quality counseling services due to poor policies, financial resources, and a lack of knowledge. In many LMIC settings, counseling methods and resources do not align with local conditions, and programs lack targets, progress monitoring, and accountability from community healthcare workers [19].

3.2 Nutritional Supplementation

A combination of adequate dietary intake and nutritional supplements has the potential to address the specific nutritional demands during these crucial periods.

3.2.1 Balanced Energy Protein

Balanced energy protein (BEP) supplements are ready-to-use supplements that offer a balanced composition of multiple micronutrients (MMNs), provide energy and protein, ensuring that protein constitutes less than 25% of the total caloric content [22].

The pooled estimates from a systematic review showed that BEP supplementation may reduce stillbirth (RR: 0.39; 95% CI, 0.19–0.80; $n = 3$), perinatal mortality (RR: 0.50; 95% CI, 0.30–0.84; $n = 1$), low birth weight (LBW) infants (RR: 0.60; 95% CI, 0.41–0.86; $n = 3$), and small for gestational age (SGA) (RR: 0.71; 95% CI, 0.54–0.94; $n = 5$). BEP supplementation also led to increased birth weight by 107.28 g but did not affect preterm birth, miscarriage, neonatal and infant mortality, birth length, and head circumference [23].

The WHO has recommended the use of BEP supplementation for pregnant and lactating mothers in countries where malnourishment is prevalent. However, even in countries with adequate maternal nutritional indicators, women with specific risk factors can benefit from BEP supplementation. This includes women with a history of recurrent LBW babies, multiple pregnancies, short intervals between pregnancies, preexisting maternal malnutrition, substance abuse, and limited access to adequate food sources. BEP supplementation is generally advised for women during their second trimester, and its use may be continued up to 6 months postpartum [24].

3.2.2 Fortified Blended Food

Fortified blended foods (FBFs), also referred to as multiple micronutrients fortified blended foods, are formulated food blends designed to supply pregnant and lactating women with a comprehensive array of vital nutrients to promote their health and the optimal development of their infants [25]. FBFs are fortified blends of grains, legumes, nuts, seeds, and oils, recommended by the WHO, to supplement the diets of pregnant and lactating women, both malnourished and adequately nourished [26].

FBFs come in various forms: ready-to-use blends are prepackaged blends that require no cooking or preparation, and these can be consumed directly. Home-based blends are prepared using local ingredients and fortified with micronutrients. Extruded blends are made from a mixture of legumes, grains, and micronutrients available in ready-to-eat form [26]. FBF supplementation is generally advised for women during their second and third trimesters, and its use may be continued up to 6 months postpartum [24].

3.2.3 Lipid-Based Nutrient Supplements

The term "lipid-based nutrient supplements" (LNS) is a generic term encompassing various fortified, lipid-based products that provide the majority of energy from lipids (>50%, including essential fatty acids) but also include protein, carbohydrates, and micronutrients.

Traditionally, LNS is available in three formulations: Large-quantity LNS or ready-to-use therapeutic foods (RUTF), which provide 180–280 g/d of supplementary food and are used for severe acute malnutrition [27]; ready-to-use supplementary foods (RUSF) or medium-quantity LNS, which provides 45–90 g/d of supplementary food and is used to treat (or sometimes prevent) moderate acute malnutrition; and home fortification of local foods or small-quantity LNS, which provides 20 g of food per day and is meant to complement food in the diet [28]. According to UNICEF, the recommended period of LNS supplementation is from

Week 12 of gestation for the remaining duration of pregnancy. It shall be continued for 1 month postpartum during lactation [29].

Evidence from a systematic review highlighted no difference between LNS and iron and folic acid (IFA) groups for maternal gestation weight gain and maternal mortality [30]. However, positive birth outcomes were noted with slightly higher birth weight (MD: 53.28 g, 95% CI, 28.22–78.33; $n = 3$) and birth length (MD: 0.24 cm, 95% CI, 0.11–0.36; $n = 3$) in the LNS group. A reduction in the proportion of SGA infants and stunting was also seen in the LNS group [30].

3.3 Micronutrient Supplementation

Micronutrient deficiencies, particularly in animal-source foods, are primarily caused by substandard diets, particularly in developing countries. Diseases like malaria and intestinal parasite infections can also impair micronutrient metabolism [31]. Micronutrient deficiencies, such as folate, iron, and iodine, can lead to abnormal prenatal development and pregnancy outcomes [31]. However, B vitamins, vitamin D, and iodine deficiencies are less recognized. Research is needed to understand the adverse effects of poor maternal vitamin A and zinc status during pregnancy [32]. In addition, maternal antioxidant status may prevent abnormal pregnancy outcomes [33]. In lactation, the maternal status of these same micronutrients (excluding zinc) influences their concentrations in breast milk. Limited attention has been directed toward the adverse consequences of micronutrient depletion on maternal health and function during this period [31].

3.3.1 Calcium Supplementation

Calcium is crucial for bone development and maintenance throughout life. Maternal bones can be compromised during pregnancy and breastfeeding due to increased calcium absorption from the intestine. The placenta actively transports calcium to the fetus. Insufficient calcium intake can lead to reduced maternal bone mineral density (BMD), increased risk of delayed bone maturation in the newborn, and potential reduction in BMD or tooth solidity for offspring later in life [34]. Calcium-related maternal metabolic stress negatively impacts fetal growth and can lead to complications like preeclampsia and eclampsia in mothers and bone diseases like rickets in infants.

Calcium intake is recommended by the WHO since 2011 as it reduces the risk of preeclampsia in populations who consume a low dietary intake [35]. Multiple systematic reviews and meta-analyses have highlighted that calcium supplementation significantly reduces hypertensive diseases such as preeclampsia and eclampsia [36–38]. Pregnant women should consume 1000 mg of calcium daily, while lactating women should consume 1200 mg [39].

3.3.2 Vitamin A Supplementation

Vitamin A is essential for normal vision, gene expression, growth, immune function, and reproduction. Vitamin A deficiency during pregnancy has been associated with night blindness, growth retardation, and fetal/neonatal and maternal death [40]. Moreover, increased risk of adverse perinatal outcomes, including anemia, pregnancy-induced hypertension, preterm delivery, LBW, fetal deformities, and intrauterine growth restriction (IUGR), has been observed in women without vitamin A supplementation during pregnancy [41]. A systematic review assessed the effectiveness of vitamin A supplementation on pregnancy outcomes and suggested that when the supplementation was provided during pregnancy and puerperium, it improved the immune system and decreased night blindness; however, there was no impact on the birth outcomes and child mortality. In addition, supplementation before, during, and after pregnancy showed additional improvement in the lung function of preschool children [42]. Another meta-analysis highlighted that vitamin A supplementation does not affect the risk of maternal mortality (RR: 0.88; 95% CI, 0.65–1.20; $n = 4$; GRADE = high), perinatal mortality (RR: 1.01; 95% CI, 0.95–1.07; $n = 1$), neonatal mortality, stillbirth, neonatal anemia, and preterm birth. In addition, evidence showed that vitamin A supplementation may reduce maternal clinical infection and maternal anemia (RR: 0.64; 95% CI, 0.43–0.93; $n = 3$; GRADE = moderate) [43].

The recommended daily intake of Vitamin A is 770 mcg of retinol equivalent (mcg RE) in pregnant women and 1300 mcg RE in lactating women [44].

3.3.3 Zinc Supplementation

Zinc is crucial for cell division, differentiation, and tissue growth. Zinc deficiency during pregnancy can lead to irreversible effects on newborns, including growth impairment, congenital malformations, spontaneous abortion, LBW, IUGR, preeclampsia, premature labor, postpartum bleeding, and delayed immune system development [45]. Although rare globally, mild to moderate zinc deficiency is widespread among pregnant and lactating women [46]. Pooled estimates highlighted that zinc supplementation may have little to no difference on preterm birth (RR: 0.87; 95% CI, 0.74–1.03; $n = 21$; GRADE = low), stillbirth (RR: 1.22; 95% CI, 0.80–1.88; $n = 7$; GRADE = low), and perinatal deaths (RR: 1.10; 95% CI, 0.81–1.51; $n = 2$ GRADE = low). For the birth outcome, zinc supplementation may have little to no impact on mean birth weight, LBW, and SGA [47]. Another systematic review showed no impact of zinc supplementation on the risk of LBW baby (RR: 1.08; 95% CI, 0.94–1.25; $n = 10$; GRADE = moderate) [48].

In low-income countries, zinc supplementation during pregnancy can decrease the likelihood of preterm birth [49].

3.3.4 Iron and Folic Acid Supplementation

Iron deficiency anemia is regarded as the most common micronutrient deficiency worldwide among pregnant women. Southeast Asia has the highest prevalence of anemia among pregnant women (48.2%), followed by Africa with the second highest prevalence (46.16%) in the year 2016. Several observational studies have shown that folate deficiency-related anemia, that is, megaloblastic anemia, was noted in pregnant mothers who were not supplemented with folic acid during their prenatal period [50, 51]. A deficiency of folate during pregnancy is a cause of neural tube defects in the fetus, such as spina bifida [52].

A meta-analysis revealed that IFA supplementation reduced the prevalence of anemia by 69% and LBW by 20% [53]. In addition, it decreased neonatal deaths by 34% in Pakistan [54] and 45% in Nepal [55]. Evidence comparing the effectiveness of IFA supplementation versus folic acid supplementation showed a 48% reduction in the risk of maternal anemia during the third trimester of pregnancy (RR: 0.52; 95% CI, 0.41–0.66; $n = 5$; GRADE = moderate), and a 12% reduction in LBW (RR: 0.88; 95% CI, 0.78–0.99). However, it did not reduce the risk of perinatal mortality [48]. Literature has shown that IFA supplementation is effective in reducing preterm birth [56, 57], prenatal mortality [58], neonatal mortality [59, 60], and infant mortality [61].

Since iron and folic acid are two essential nutrients in pregnancy and lactation, there are recommended dosages to prevent their deficiency. IFA supplementation must be started before conception and continued throughout the pregnancy and 3 months after the delivery if the mother is breastfeeding. The recommended daily dose of iron is 30–60 mg, while the recommended daily dose of folic acid is 400–800 mcg [62]. The Lancet nutrition series from 2021 also advocates for antenatal IFA supplementation, along with multiple micronutrients, as critical nutritional interventions during the "first 1000 days of life" [63].

3.4 Multiple Micronutrient Supplementation

Micronutrient deficiencies rarely exist in isolation [64] and to ascertain a preclinical or clinical condition of a single nutrient deficiency is challenging. Thus, multiple micronutrient (MMN) supplementation is potentially the most cost-effective way to respond to micronutrient deficiencies at the population level [65].

Evidence from systematic review suggested that MMN supplementation with IFA can result in a slight reduction in preterm births (RR: 0.95; 95% CI, 0.90–1.01; $n = 18$), SGA infants (RR: 0.92; 95% CI, 0.88–0.97; $n = 17$), and LBW infants (RR: 0.88; 95% CI, 0.85–0.91; $n = 18$) [66]. There were no significant differences between groups for perinatal mortality, stillbirths, or neonatal mortality. There was little difference in maternal anemia, maternal mortality, miscarriage, caesarean section delivery, and congenital anomalies [66].

While MMN supplementation is crucial, it should not be mistaken for a substitute for a balanced diet; instead, MMN should complement a healthy and balanced diet, rich in fruits, vegetables, whole grains, and lean proteins. UNICEF, United Nations University, and the WHO collaborated to develop a comprehensive MMN tablet named United Nations International Multiple Micronutrient Antenatal Preparation (UNIMMAP) [67]. However, the WHO does not universally recommend its use over the current practice of IFA supplementation; its use is limited to the context of rigorous research.

3.5 Agricultural Interventions/Kitchen Garden

Agricultural interventions, such as kitchen gardens, enhance nutrition, food security, and livelihoods in community or household settings by promoting sustainable practices, empowering individuals to grow food, promoting self-sufficiency, dietary diversity, and economic stability. Kitchen gardens, also known as home gardens, are small plots of land where individuals grow fruits, vegetables, herbs, and livestock to provide households with fresh, locally grown produce, improving nutrition by increasing access to diverse, nutrient-dense foods. [68]. Agricultural interventions are programs and practices that improve farming communities' productivity, sustainability, and well-being by enhancing crop yields, market access, and mitigating climate change's impact on agricultural systems [69].

Agricultural interventions and kitchen gardens during pregnancy and lactation can positively impact both mother and fetus by providing nutrient-dense food, improving diet quality, and allowing essential vitamins and minerals to be included in the mother's diet [70]. This Intervention improves dietary diversity for pregnant women, ensuring they have access to diverse food items to meet increased nutritional demands during pregnancy and lactation, contributing to breast milk's nutritional content. [71].

3.6 Food Fortification

Food fortification enhances food content by adding essential micronutrients to staple foods and potentially addressing population-level micronutrient deficiencies [25] [72]. However, the success of fortification programs depends on factors like food selection, nutrient bioavailability, and population acceptance [25]. Folic acid is the most commonly used vitamin in food fortification. As indicated by the Food and Drug Administration, commonly fortified foods include breads, cereals, and pasta.

A systematic review assessed the impact of micronutrient fortification and showed that iron fortification significantly increased serum ferritin and hemoglobin levels in women of reproductive age and pregnant women, while folate fortification reduced the incidence of congenital anomalies like neural tube defects (RR: 0.57; 95% CI, 0.45–0.73) [73]. Another systematic review from 2015 found no difference in maternal anemia and hemoglobin in food fortification versus MMN supplementation groups [74].

To reduce the risk of neural tube defects in pregnant women, it is recommended that women take folate from fortified foods [75].

3.7 Antenatal and Postnatal Care

Antenatal and postnatal care during pregnancy and lactation are crucial for the mother's and baby's health and well-being. It helps in the early detection and management of pregnancy complications like gestational diabetes, preeclampsia, and anemia, leading to improved maternal and birth outcomes. Prenatal screening and tests during antenatal care help identify potential problems early, allowing for informed decisions and timely interventions [76]. During antenatal care visits, mothers are advised on their nutritional intake to ensure their health and the baby's development. This includes advice on a balanced diet and supplementation needs. Regular checkups, ultrasounds, and fetal monitoring are also required to detect issues promptly [75]. Home visits during pregnancy and lactation are crucial for maternal and child healthcare strategies, providing personalized care and support. These visits, conducted by healthcare professionals or community workers, promote maternal and child well-being through multifaceted interventions. They contribute to comprehensive antenatal care, monitoring expectant mothers' health, assessing fetal development, and addressing concerns or complications. Education and counseling sessions cover nutrition, prenatal care, and birth planning, reducing complications during pregnancy and childbirth [77]. A Nepalese systematic review highlighted that birth preparedness classes increased the uptake of antenatal and postnatal care, compliance with MMN supplementation, and increased awareness of danger signs of pregnancy [78].

Postnatal care is crucial for a mother's physical and emotional recovery post-childbirth, reducing the risk of postnatal complications like depression and infections. It also helps identify and address potential risks like cardiovascular diseases, osteoporosis, and mental health conditions, leading to improved maternal long-term outcomes [79]. Postnatal care involves breastfeeding counseling, where healthcare professionals guide mothers on latching, milk supply, common challenges, and successful breastfeeding. It also covers family planning and contraceptive options, enabling couples to make informed decisions about subsequent pregnancies. [80]. An African systematic review highlighted that family planning counseling interventions improved postpartum modern contraceptive uptake [81]. Home visits during the postpartum period can enhance breastfeeding by guiding mothers on proper latching techniques and troubleshooting common challenges. Monitoring maternal recovery and conducting regular assessments of newborn's health is integral to home visits that can also be extended to immunization administration and nutritional guidance, ensuring both mother's and infant's well-being and optimal development [82]. Home visits improve healthcare accessibility for women in remote areas, overcoming geographical and logistical barriers. The individualized care provided during these visits fosters trust and engagement within the community, contributing to the effectiveness of maternal and child health initiatives [83].

3.8 Social Protection Programs

The main aim of social protection programs is to reduce the income constraints on low-income groups, which is the primary social determinant for them to have poor nutritional access. This provides them with cash, food, vouchers, and assets to fulfill their basic needs, increase their resilience, and support their livelihoods.

Cash assistance is a humanitarian aid program that provides cash directly to the recipients in exchange for goods and services. Cash assistance during pregnancy and lactation facilitates regular prenatal checkups, early detection of complications, and access to necessary maternity-related supplies. It also covers childbirth expenses, reducing barriers to healthcare facilities. Cash assistance has the potential to improve maternal nutrition, foster optimal fetal development, and support breastfeeding initiatives. It also allows mothers to take time off work without financial strain, promoting better mental health and early bonding with the newborn [84]. Doocy et al.'s (2020) study from Somalia food crisis showed that cash vouchers significantly increase mid-upper arm circumference (0.9 cm; 95% CI, 0.6–1.3) among pregnant and lactating women [84].

Food assistance is also a humanitarian aid designed to provide food aid to vulnerable populations, especially those facing food insecurity or poverty. Food assistance during pregnancy and lactation provides nutritional support to pregnant women and their developing fetus. It aims to address unique dietary needs during this critical period, providing essential minerals and vitamins. Nutrient-rich food is provided, overcoming economic barriers to access nutritious food. This includes fruits, vegetables, whole grains, and lean proteins, ensuring mothers can consume healthy foods [85]. Mshanga et al.'s (2019) study findings showed an improvement in serum retinol of 20 umol L^{-1} in Maasai-pregnant women who were given a food basket intervention compared to control (p-value <0.001) [85], suggesting that the food basket helps improve micronutrient deficiency.

Food assistance can help prevent deficiencies and reduce maternal outcomes like anemia by supplementing micronutrients like IFA or fortified foods. It is crucial for promoting breastfeeding, as adequate nutrition is essential for optimal infant growth and development. Addressing nutritional needs through food assistance can alleviate poverty by reducing the economic burden associated with access to nutrient-dense foods during pregnancy and lactation [86]. The beneficial effects of food assistance are seen when combined with nutritional education, as the provision of a food basket does not mean that there is food security for the individual; individuals with a higher need may not be able to eat enough due to the way food gets distributed. Thus, it is crucial to provide nutritional education along with a food basket to pregnant women [87].

4 Future Implications

Nutritional interventions during pregnancy and lactation are pivotal determinants that have far-reaching implications on the mother's and child's overall health and well-being. The importance of these interventions ranges across varied domains, influencing maternal and child health, disease prevention, and breastfeeding practices, and carrying implications for future generations. Beyond immediate health benefits, it sets the stage for the child's development. Adequate intake of essential nutrients supports fetal growth during pregnancy and nourishes infant development during lactation. This has a lasting impact on the child's physical and cognitive development.

Access to diverse and nutritious food promotes breastfeeding practices, establishing the basis for a child's health and reducing the risk of infections and chronic diseases. Beyond individual benefits, breastfeeding practices have economic and public health implications that contribute to a healthier and more productive population. Also, the intergenerational impact of maternal nutrition is notable. The nutritional status of a pregnant woman not only influences the immediate offspring but can shape the health and health trajectory of subsequent generations. This underscores the importance of viewing nutrition interventions as an investment in communities' long-term health and prosperity. Furthermore, nutritional interventions align with the global SDG maternal and child health targets. By achieving positive outcomes, nations can excel in their health and well-being, contributing to a healthier, sustainable, and resilient future.

References

1. Hossain MI, Rahman A, Uddin MSG, Zinia FA. Double burden of malnutrition among women of reproductive age in Bangladesh: a comparative study of classical and Bayesian logistic regression approach. Food Sci Nutr. 2023;11(4):1785–96.
2. United Nations Children's Fund. Undernourished and overlooked: a global nutrition crisis in adolescent girls and women. UNICEF: New York; 2022.
3. NCD Risk Factor Collaboration (NCD-RisC). Worldwide trends in underweight and obesity from 1990 to 2022: a pooled analysis of 3663 population-representative studies with 222 million children, adolescents, and adults. Lancet. 2024;403(10431):1027–50.
4. Ajayi IO, Adebamowo C, Adami HO, Dalal S, Diamond MB, Bajunirwe F, et al. Urban-rural and geographic differences in overweight and obesity in four sub-Saharan African adult populations: a multi-country cross-sectional study. BMC Public Health. 2016;16(1):1126.
5. Hashan MR, Rabbi MF, Haider SS, Das GR. Prevalence and associated factors of underweight, overweight and obesity among women of reproductive age group in the Maldives: evidence from a nationally representative study. PLoS One. 2020;15(10):e0241621.
6. Khanam M, Osuagwu UL, Sanin KI, Haque MA, Rita RS, Agho KE, et al. Underweight, overweight and obesity among reproductive Bangladeshi women: a Nationwide survey. Nutrients. 2021;13(12)
7. Mengesha Kassie A, Beletew Abate B, Wudu Kassaw M, Gebremeskel AT. Prevalence of underweight and its associated factors among reproductive age group women in Ethiopia: analysis of the 2016 Ethiopian demographic and health survey data. J Environ Public Health. 2020;2020:9718714.
8. Collaboration NRF. Trends in adult body-mass index in 200 countries from 1975 to 2014: a pooled analysis of 1698 population-based measurement studies with 19·2 million participants. Lancet. 2016;387(10026):1377–96.
9. Kozuki N, Katz J, Lee ACC, Vogel JP, Silveira MF, Sania A, et al. Short maternal stature increases risk of small-for-gestational-age and preterm births in low-and middle-income countries: individual participant data meta-analysis and population attributable fraction. J Nutr. 2015;145(11):2542–50.
10. Alem AZ, Yeshaw Y, Liyew AM, Tessema ZT, Worku MG, Tesema GA, et al. Double burden of malnutrition and its associated factors among women in low and middle income countries: findings from 52 nationally representative data. BMC Public Health. 2023;23(1):1479.
11. Grollman C, Arregoces L, Martínez-Álvarez M, Pitt C, Mills A, Borghi J. 11 years of tracking aid to reproductive, maternal, newborn, and child health: estimates and analysis for 2003-13 from the Countdown to 2015. Lancet Glob Health. 2017;5(1):e104–e14.

12. United Nations. Sustainable development goals. 2015.
13. WHO. Nutrition: Nutrition of women in the preconception period, during pregnancy and the breastfeeding period 2011.
14. United Nations. Scaling up nutrition (SUN) movement. 2020.
15. UNICEF. UNICEF Nutrition Strategy 2020.
16. United Nations. United Nations Decade of Action on Nutrition (2016–2025)
17. UNICEF. UNICEF Programming Guidance. Prevention of malnutrition in women before and during pregnancy and while breastfeeding. New York; 2021.
18. Marshall NE, Abrams B, Barbour LA, Catalano P, Christian P, Friedman JE, et al. The importance of nutrition in pregnancy and lactation: lifelong consequences. Am J Obstet Gynecol. 2022;226(5):607–32.
19. UNICEF. COUNSELLING TO IMPROVE MATERNAL NUTRITION: Considerations for programming with quality, equity and scale. A TECHNICAL BRIEF 2022.
20. Dewidar O, John J, Baqar A, Madani MT, Saad A, Riddle A, et al. Effectiveness of nutrition counseling for pregnant women in low- and middle-income countries to improve maternal and infant behavioral, nutritional, and health outcomes: a systematic review. Campbell Syst Rev. 2023;19(4):e1361.
21. UNICEF. Nutrition, for every child. UNICEF. Nutrition Strategy 2020–2030 New York: UNICEF; 2020. Available from: https://www.unicef.org/reports/nutrition-strategy-2020-2030.
22. de Kok B, Argaw A, Hanley-Cook G, Toe LC, Ouédraogo M, Dailey-Chwalibóg T, et al. Fortified balanced energy-protein supplements increase nutrient adequacy without displacing food intake in pregnant women in rural Burkina Faso. J Nutr. 2021;151(12):3831–40.
23. Lassi ZS, Padhani ZA, Rabbani A, Rind F, Salam RA, Bhutta ZA. Effects of nutritional interventions during pregnancy on birth, child health and development outcomes: a systematic review of evidence from low- and middle-income countries. Campbell Syst Rev. 2021;17(2):e1150.
24. WHO. e-Library of Evidence for Nutrition Actions (eLENA) 2023 [Available from: https://www.who.int/tools/elena/interventions/energy-protein-pregnancy#:~:text=WHO%20Recommendations,small%20for%20gestational%20age%20neonates.
25. Yang Z, Huffman SL. Review of fortified food and beverage products for pregnant and lactating women and their impact on nutritional status. Matern Child Nutr. 2011;7 Suppl 3(Suppl 3):19–43.
26. WHO. Specialized Nutritious Foods [Available from: https://www.wfp.org/specialized-nutritious-food#:~:text=Fortified%20Blended%20Foods%20(FBFs),-What%20are%20they&text=FBFs%20are%20blends%20of%20partially,vegetable%20oil%20or%20milk%20powder.
27. Diop el HI, Dossou NI, Ndour MM, Briend A, Wade S. Comparison of the efficacy of a solid ready-to-use food and a liquid, milk-based diet for the rehabilitation of severely malnourished children: a randomized trial. Am J Clin Nutr. 2003;78(2):302–7.
28. Arimond M, Zeilani M, Jungjohann S, Brown KH, Ashorn P, Allen LH, et al. Considerations in developing lipid-based nutrient supplements for prevention of undernutrition: experience from the International Lipid-Based Nutrient Supplements (iLiNS) Project Matern Child Nutr. 2015;11 Suppl 4(Suppl 4):31–61.
29. UNICEF. Product Specification Sheet. 2022.
30. Das JK, Hoodbhoy Z, Salam RA, Bhutta AZ, Valenzuela-Rubio NG, Weise Prinzo Z, et al. Lipid-based nutrient supplements for maternal, birth, and infant developmental outcomes. Cochrane Database Syst Rev. 2018;8(8):Cd012610.
31. Allen LH. Multiple micronutrients in pregnancy and lactation: an overview2. Am J Clin Nutr. 2005;81(5):1206S–12S.
32. Gernand AD, Schulze KJ, Stewart CP, West KP Jr, Christian P. Micronutrient deficiencies in pregnancy worldwide: health effects and prevention. Nat Rev Endocrinol. 2016;12(5):274–89.
33. Sebastiani G, Navarro-Tapia E, Almeida-Toledano L, Serra-Delgado M, Paltrinieri AL, García-Algar Ó, et al. Effects of antioxidant intake on fetal development and maternal/neonatal health during pregnancy. Antioxidants (Basel). 2022;11(4)

34. Tihtonen K, Korhonen P, Isojärvi J, Ojala R, Ashorn U, Ashorn P, et al. Calcium supplementation during pregnancy and maternal and offspring bone health: a systematic review and meta-analysis. Ann N Y Acad Sci. 2022;1509(1):23–36.
35. World Health Organization. WHO recommendations for prevention and treatment of pre-eclampsia and eclampsia. 2011. Available from: https://apps.who.int/iris/bitstream/handle/10665/44703/9789241548335_eng.pdf.
36. Imdad A, Bhutta ZA. Effects of calcium supplementation during pregnancy on maternal, fetal and birth outcomes. Paediatr Perinat Epidemiol. 2012;26(Suppl 1):138–52.
37. Hofmeyr GJ, Lawrie TA, Atallah Á N, Torloni MR. Calcium supplementation during pregnancy for preventing hypertensive disorders and related problems. Cochrane Database Syst Rev. 2018;10(10):Cd001059.
38. Hofmeyr GJ, Manyame S, Medley N, Williams MJ. Calcium supplementation commencing before or early in pregnancy, for preventing hypertensive disorders of pregnancy. Cochrane Database Syst Rev. 2019;9(9):Cd011192.
39. Willemse J, Meertens LJE, Scheepers HCJ, Achten NMJ, Eussen SJ, van Dongen MC, et al. Calcium intake from diet and supplement use during early pregnancy: the expect study I. Eur J Nutr. 2020;59(1):167–74.
40. van den Broek N, Dou L, Othman M, Neilson JP, Gates S, Gülmezoglu AM. Vitamin A supplementation during pregnancy for maternal and newborn outcomes. Cochrane Database Syst Rev. 2010;11:Cd008666.
41. Huang Y, Zheng S. The effect of vitamin a deficiency during pregnancy on anorectal malformations. J Pediatr Surg. 2011;46(7):1400–5.
42. Cruz S, da Cruz SP, Ramalho A. Impact of vitamin A supplementation on pregnant women and on women who have just given birth: a systematic review. J Am Coll Nutr. 2018;37(3):243–50.
43. McCauley ME, van den Broek N, Dou L, Othman M. Vitamin A supplementation during pregnancy for maternal and newborn outcomes. Cochrane Database Syst Rev. 2015;10
44. Gluckman SP, Hanson M, Seng CY, Bardsley A. 47 Vitamin A in pregnancy and breastfeeding. 2014 [cited 12/14/2023]. In: Nutrition and lifestyle for pregnancy and breastfeeding [Internet]. Oxford University Press, [cited 12/14/2023]; [0]. Available from: https://doi.org/10.1093/med/9780198722700.003.0006.
45. Agedew E, Tsegaye B, Bante A, Zerihun E, Aklilu A, Girma M, et al. Zinc deficiency and associated factors among pregnant women's attending antenatal clinics in public health facilities of Konso Zone, Southern Ethiopia. PLoS One. 2022;17(7):e0270971.
46. Brown KH, Rivera JA, Bhutta Z, Gibson RS, King JC, Lönnerdal B, et al. International Zinc Nutrition Consultative Group (IZiNCG) technical document #1. Assessment of the risk of zinc deficiency in populations and options for its control. Food Nutr Bull. 2004;25(1 Suppl 2):S99–203.
47. Carducci B, Keats EC, Bhutta ZA. Zinc supplementation for improving pregnancy and infant outcome. Cochrane Database Syst Rev. 2021;3(3):Cd000230.
48. Oh C, Keats EC, Bhutta ZA. Vitamin and mineral supplementation during pregnancy on maternal, birth, child health and development outcomes in low- and middle-income countries: a systematic review and meta-analysis. Nutrients. 2020;12(2)
49. Krebs NF. Update on zinc deficiency and excess in clinical pediatric practice. Ann Nutr Metab. 2013;62(Suppl 1):19–29.
50. Willoughby ML, Jewell FG. Folate status throughout pregnancy and in postpartum period. Br Med J. 1968;4(5627):356–60.
51. Metz J. Folate deficiency conditioned by lactation. Am J Clin Nutr. 1970;23(6):843–7.
52. Wald NJ. Folic acid and neural tube defects: discovery, debate and the need for policy change. J Med Screen. 2022;29(3):138–46.
53. Imdad A, Bhutta ZA. Routine iron/folate supplementation during pregnancy: effect on maternal anaemia and birth outcomes. Paediatr Perinat Epidemiol. 2012;26(Suppl 1):168–77.
54. Nisar YB, Dibley MJ. Earlier initiation and use of a greater number of iron-folic acid supplements during pregnancy prevents early neonatal deaths in Nepal and Pakistan. PLoS One. 2014;9(11):e112446.

55. Nisar YB, Dibley MJ, Mebrahtu S, Paudyal N, Devkota M. Antenatal iron-folic acid supplementation reduces neonatal and Under-5 mortality in Nepal. J Nutr. 2015;145(8):1873–83.
56. Haider BA, Olofin I, Wang M, Spiegelman D, Ezzati M, Fawzi WW. Anaemia, prenatal iron use, and risk of adverse pregnancy outcomes: systematic review and meta-analysis. BMJ : British Medical Journal. 2013;346:f3443.
57. Iqbal S, Ekmekcioglu C. Maternal and neonatal outcomes related to iron supplementation or iron status: a summary of meta-analyses. J Matern Fetal Neonatal Med. 2019;32(9):1528–40.
58. Yeboah A, Ainuson-Quampah J, Nkumsah-Riverson P, Asah-Opoku K. Maternal dietary iron and folate intake in the third trimester and birth outcomes: a prospective cohort study at a teaching Hospital in Accra. Ghana Am J Trop Med Hyg. 2022;106(4):1072–7.
59. Rai RK, De Neve JW, Geldsetzer P, Vollmer S. Maternal iron-and-folic-acid supplementation and its association with low-birth weight and neonatal mortality in India. Public Health Nutr. 2022;25(3):623–33.
60. Nisar YB, Dibley MJ. Iron/folic acid supplementation during pregnancy prevents neonatal and under-five mortality in Pakistan: propensity score matched sample from two Pakistan demographic and health surveys. Glob Health Action. 2016;9:29621.
61. Dibley MJ, Titaley CR, d'Este C, Agho K. Iron and folic acid supplements in pregnancy improve child survival in Indonesia. Am J Clin Nutr. 2012;95(1):220–30.
62. WHO. WHO recommendations on antenatal care for a positive pregnancy experience. Geneva: World Health Organization; 2016.
63. Bhutta ZA, Das JK, Rizvi A, Gaffey MF, Walker N, Horton S, et al. Evidence-based interventions for improvement of maternal and child nutrition: what can be done and at what cost? Lancet. 2013;382(9890):452–77.
64. Darnton-Hill I. Public health aspects in the prevention and control of vitamin deficiencies. Curr Dev Nutr. 2019;3(9):nzz075.
65. McArdle HJ, Ashworth CJ. Micronutrients in fetal growth and development. Br Med Bull. 1999;55(3):499–510.
66. Keats EC, Haider BA, Tam E, Bhutta ZA. Multiple-micronutrient supplementation for women during pregnancy. Cochrane Database Syst Rev. 2019;3(3):Cd004905.
67. WHO. Composition of a multi-micronutrient supplement to be used in pilot programmes among pregnant women in developing countries. New York: World Health Organization; 1999.
68. Galhena DH, Freed R, Maredia KM. Home gardens: a promising approach to enhance household food security and wellbeing. Agric Food Secur. 2013;2(1):8.
69. Edoardo M, Lawrence H, Alexander C, Jairo I-C. Effectiveness of agricultural interventions that aim to improve nutritional status of children: systematic review. BMJ. 2012;344:d8222.
70. Habtu M, Agena AG, Umugwaneza M, Mochama M, Munyanshongore C. Effect and challenges of an integrated nutrition-intervention package utilization among pregnant women and lactating mothers in Rwanda: an exploratory qualitative study. Curr Dev Nutr. 2023;7(1):100018.
71. Shah N, Zaheer S, Safdar NF, Turk T, Hashmi S. Women's awareness, knowledge, attitudes, and behaviours towards nutrition and health in Pakistan: evaluation of kitchen gardens nutrition program. PLoS One. 2023;18(9):e0291245.
72. Olson R, Gavin-Smith B, Ferraboschi C, Kraemer K. Food fortification: the advantages, disadvantages and lessons from sight and life programs. Nutrients. 2021;13(4)
73. Das JK, Salam RA, Kumar R, Bhutta ZA. Micronutrient fortification of food and its impact on woman and child health: a systematic review. Syst Rev. 2013;2(1):67.
74. Suchdev PS, Peña-Rosas JP, De-Regil LM. Multiple micronutrient powders for home (point-of-use) fortification of foods in pregnant women. Cochrane Database Syst Rev. 2015;6
75. Kominiarek MA, Rajan P. Nutrition recommendations in pregnancy and lactation. Med Clin North Am. 2016;100(6):1199–215.
76. Piro SS, Ahmed HM. Impacts of antenatal nursing interventions on mothers' breastfeeding self-efficacy: an experimental study. BMC Pregnancy Childbirth. 2020;20(1):19.
77. Guenther T, Nsona H, Makuluni R, Chisema M, Jenda G, Chimbalanga E, et al. Home visits by community health workers for pregnant mothers and newborns: coverage plateau in Malawi. J Glob Health. 2019;9(1):010808.

78. Toolan M, Barnard K, Lynch M, Maharjan N, Thapa M, Rai N, et al. A systematic review and narrative synthesis of antenatal interventions to improve maternal and neonatal health in Nepal. AJOG Global Reports. 2022;2(1):100019.
79. McCauley H, Lowe K, Furtado N, Mangiaterra V, van den Broek N. Essential components of postnatal care—a systematic literature review and development of signal functions to guide monitoring and evaluation. BMC Pregnancy Childbirth. 2022;22(1):448.
80. Dietrich Leurer M, Misskey E. "Be positive as well as realistic": a qualitative description analysis of information gaps experienced by breastfeeding mothers. Int Breastfeed J. 2015;10(1):10.
81. Mruts KB, Tessema GA, Gebremedhin AT, Scott J, Pereira G. The effect of family planning counselling on postpartum modern contraceptive uptake in sub-Saharan Africa: a systematic review. Public Health. 2022;206:46–56.
82. Yonemoto N, Nagai S, Mori R. Schedules for home visits in the early postpartum period. Cochrane Database Syst Rev. 2021;7(7):Cd009326.
83. Anne C, Khalid O, Yagana G, Muhammad Chadi B, Amar A, Umaira A, et al. The impact of universal home visits with pregnant women and their spouses on maternal outcomes: a cluster randomised controlled trial in Bauchi State, Nigeria. BMJ Glob Health. 2019;4(1):e001172.
84. Doocy S, Busingye M, Lyles E, Colantouni E, Aidam B, Ebulu G, et al. Cash-based assistance and the nutrition status of pregnant and lactating women in the Somalia food crisis: a comparison of two transfer modalities. PLoS One. 2020;15(4):e0230989.
85. Mshanga N, Martin H, Petrucka P. Food-basket intervention to reduce micronutrient deficiencies among Maasai-pregnant women in Tanzania: a quasi-experimental study. J Hum Nutr Diet. 2019;32(5):625–34.
86. McFadden A, Green JM, Williams V, McLeish J, McCormick F, Fox-Rushby J, et al. Can food vouchers improve nutrition and reduce health inequalities in low-income mothers and young children: a multi-method evaluation of the experiences of beneficiaries and practitioners of the Healthy Start programme in England. BMC Public Health. 2014;14(1):148.
87. Razzazi A, Griffiths MD, Alimoradi Z. The effect of nutritional education based on the health action process approach (HAPA) on the pregnancy outcomes among malnourished pregnant mothers. BMC Pregnancy Childbirth. 2024;24(1):83.

Newborn Nutrition

Shabina Ariff, Sajid Soofi, Unzela Ghulam, and Aqsa Ishaq

1 Introduction

Neonatal nutrition refers to the unique dietary requirements and needs of neonates during the first 28 days of life. This is a crucial period for the development of the brain and the immune system and physical growth. The essential macronutrients (proteins, carbohydrates, and fats) and micronutrients critical for neonatal growth and development are present in human milk (HM) or infant formula [2]. Neonatal malnutrition is a serious public health problem that affects newborns globally, particularly in the low- and middle-income countries (LMICs) [3]. Poor nutrition in neonates can result in significant growth retardation, slowed cognitive development, increased susceptibility to infections, and even death during this vulnerable period. Socioeconomic disparities, maternal malnutrition, poor breastfeeding practices, and restricted access to quality health-care services are major factors that contribute to neonatal malnutrition [4].

Neonatal growth and development are greatly influenced by fetal nutrition [5]. Optimum fetal nutrition during pregnancy is ensured by adequate maternal nutrition. Micronutrients, lactoferrin, and essential fatty and amino acids are important nutrients for fetal programming and development. Optimal fetal development and growth depend largely on the mother's nutritional status and her well-being [6]. Many babies in LMICs suffer from in utero malnutrition, resulting in poor outcomes such as preterm deliveries and low birth weights (LBW), resulting in an immunocompromised

S. Ariff (✉)
Department of Pediatrics and Child Health, Aga Khan University, Karachi, Pakistan
e-mail: shabina.ariff@aku.edu

S. Soofi · U. Ghulam · A. Ishaq
Centre of Excellence in Women and Child Health, Aga Khan University, Karachi, Pakistan
e-mail: sajid.soofi@aku.edu; aqsa.ishaq@aku.edu

© The Author(s), under exclusive license to Springer Nature Switzerland AG 2025
Z. S. Lassi, R. A. Salam (eds.), *Nutrition Across Reproductive, Maternal, Neonatal, Child, and Adolescent Health Care*,
https://doi.org/10.1007/978-3-031-95721-5_9

state and further vulnerability. A birth weight of less than 2500 g (5.5 pounds) is considered as LBW [7], which may result from preterm birth (gestational age fewer than 37 weeks), intrauterine growth restriction (IUGR), or small for gestational age (SGA). Newborns with LBW and who are SGA are more likely to experience malnutrition, delayed growth, and increased susceptibility to illnesses [8]. Infants with LBW and who are SGA may require specialized nutrition interventions, such as specialized formulas or fortified human milk. A large burden of stunting in older children are a consequence of low birth weight and newborn malnutrition.

Preterm babies face an additional challenge to growth as they are born with low dietary reserves and require higher calories to maintain weight and growth trajectory. They must consume more protein and energy to support catch-up growth and remain healthy [9]. To promote optimal growth and neurodevelopment in preterm infants, specialized nutrition regimes, such as fortification of human milk [10], addition of specialized formulas in enteral feeds, and supplementation of micronutrients and vitamins, are needed.

The Barker's hypothesis of fetal programming suggests that intrauterine conditions determine the outcome of infants in utero and ex utero. The fetus responds to a compromised state such as malnutrition and adapts to the condition to survive (diverts nutrition to the vital organs of the body such as the heart and the brain). This cellular level of programming during embryonic or fetal life determines the physiological and metabolic responses that continue till adulthood [11].

In this chapter, we will delve into neonatal requirements, the problem of malnutrition, dietary intake, and essential laboratory measurements.

2 Neonatal Nutrition

Neonatal nutrition encompasses the unique dietary requirements and feeding practices that are tailored to meet the needs of newborn during the initial 28 days of life [12]. Adequate nutrition is vital for the growth, development, and well-being of newborns, as they have specific nutritional needs due to rapid growth, immature organ systems, and limited nutrient reserves [13]. Breast milk is widely known as the comprehensive and ideal source of nutrition, offering vital nutrients, bioactive substances, and protective elements that promote optimal growth and development [14]. In cases where breastfeeding is not possible, specialized formulas are formulated to provide the necessary nutrition. Optimal neonatal nutrition has many benefits in both the short and long terms, such as decreased susceptibility to infections, enhanced cognitive development, and the prevention of nutritional deficiencies. It plays a vital role in the optimal weight gain and growth trajectory of a newborn [15].

2.1 Situation Analysis of Nutrients in Newborns

According to the World Health Organization (WHO), nearly 45% of newborn mortality is attributed to malnutrition either directly or through indirect pathways [16].

Poor weight gain during the early newborn period and subsequent months predisposes infants to infections such as pneumonia, diarrhea, and sepsis, often resulting in adverse outcomes and deaths. In countries with the highest rates of malnutrition, the average life expectancy is reported to be 38 years, with a relatively good health. In contrast, in 24 of the wealthiest nations in the world, life expectancy exceeds 70 years, reflecting "optimal well-being." One in seven children is destined to die before their fifth birthday in countries with the worst hunger rates or food insecurity. Although information on dietary changes, nutritional status, or the number of malnourished people is monitored, the impact on overall mortality is less well recognized [17, 18].

Limited access to nutrient-rich foods, poverty, insufficient breast-feeding techniques, and maternal malnutrition are all factors that contribute to undernutrition. In contrast, overnutrition is also becoming a problem with infants consuming high-sugar, high-energy, and low-fat foods. Rapid infant weight gain from overnutrition increases the risk of later obesity, diabetes, and cardiovascular issues [19].

A multifaceted strategy is required to address neonatal malnutrition effectively. This strategy includes promoting healthy diets, supplementing maternal nutrition, supporting breastfeeding, ensuring food access, and implementing public health initiatives for undernutrition and overnutrition. Early detection and intervention are crucial for identifying at-risk newborns and optimizing their growth, development, and long-term health [20].

2.2   Neonatal Nutrition and Energy Requirements

The nutrition required to sustain and promote optimal growth, well-being, and nutrient balance is determined by the specific needs of a newborn, which change from neonatal to infant period. When studying early growth, standardized definitions are used. The infant's caloric intake is determined by the energy expenditure for normal physical activity, basic metabolic functions, and unexpectedly increased energy utilization for pathological conditions. A healthy infant should receive around 100 kcal/kg/day from birth to the age of 1 year. However, the caloric needs of newborns are higher, averaging 110–135 kcal/kg/day [2] because of their rapid growth.

A healthy infant uses around 40–60 kcal/kg/day for basal metabolic rate out of the total energy needed. Early infancy is a crucial time for thermoregulation, which demands a large quantity of energy. In smaller preterm infants with lower subcutaneous fat reserves, this energy consumption is much higher. Energy is also needed in large amounts for feeding, digestion, absorption, storage, and elimination—consumptions of up to 30–50 kcal/kg/day is not uncommon. Premature or ill infants often need even more energy to maintain sufficient growth. Infants' energy requirement decreases as they get older, with boys often needing more energy than girls due to higher weights [21].

The term "dietary reference intakes" is used to collectively describe nutritional demands objectively [22]. The term "estimated average requirements" (EAR) describes the minimal amount of a nutrient needed to satisfy the demands of 50% of the population. The recommended dietary allowances (RDA) are based on a 20% higher limit because the EAR only covers roughly half of the population. RDA stands for an adequate amount of average daily food intake, which at a given stage meets the nutrient needs of most of the healthy population. When there is lack of data to support the use of EAR or RDA, appropriate intake (AI) is the acceptable range of nutrient intake based on healthy populations. The greatest nutrient intake amounts that can be consumed without having negative consequences are known as tolerable upper intake levels upper limit (UL) [22].

3 Essential Components of Neonatal Nutrition

3.1 Breast Milk as a Comprehensive Nutrient for Newborns

The development of an infant's immune system and optimum growth are supported by the complex and dynamic fluid that is human milk. Human milk has a variable chemical composition that includes macro-, micro-, and bioactive nutrients, as well as living cells. Colostrum, the first fluid secreted by the breasts after giving birth, has a bright yellow color due to its high concentration of carotenoids. Initially, only a little amount of colostrum is produced, containing bioactive substances such as secretory IgA, leucocytes, lactoferrin, and epidermal growth factor [23]. Colostrum also contains higher levels of magnesium and sodium chloride and lower levels of potassium, lactose, and calcium compared to later milk. However, over time, lactose secretion increases efficiently and the sodium content in colostrum/milk decreases.

Transitional milk, which develops between 5 and 14 days after conception, has higher levels of fat, lactose, and calories while having lower levels of immunoglobulins and total proteins. Human milk is considered mature at 2–4 weeks, and its composition remains consistent for the following few months.

The composition of human milk may differ among populations, and the content of milk samples from the same woman can also vary greatly. The mother–infant pair successfully adapts to these variances, and most mothers and infants can nurse well and experience normal growth. Breast milk contains a variety of bioactive compounds, including lymphocytes, macrophages, and T cells, which play a significant role in the infant's host defense. Human milk also contains a variety of bioactive substances, including growth factors, immunoglobulins, cytokines, and other small molecules [23].

Breastfeeding is generally advisable, but there are specific medical conditions and maternal situations where it is not recommended. These include metabolic abnormalities in newborns, specific maternal medications, and select maternal illnesses. Maternal illnesses such as human T-cell lymphotropic virus (type 1 and type 2), untreated brucellosis, active pulmonary tuberculosis without 2 weeks of complete treatment, and active herpes simplex lesions on the breast serve as contraindications to breastfeeding. In developed nations, breastfeeding is not recommended for HIV-positive mothers. Infants diagnosed with the inborn metabolic error of

Table 1 Concentrations of selected nutrients in mature (2-week) human milk

Energy	66 ± 9 kcal
Protein	1.3 ± 0.2 g
Fat	3.0 ± 0.9 g
Lactose	6.2 ± 0.6 g
Calcium	28 ± 7 mg
Phosphorus	15 ± 4 mg
Sodium	18 ± 4 mg
Potassium	53 ± 4 mg
Chloride	42 ± 6 mg
Iron	0.03 ± 0.01 mg
Vitamin D	2.2 ± 0.4 IU/100 mL

Source: Kleinman R. Pediatric Nutrition Handbook. 7th edition. Elk Grove Village (IL): American Academy of Pediatrics; 2014; and Gidrewicz DA, Fenton TR. A systematic review and meta-analysis of the nutrient content of preterm and term breast milk. BMC Pediatric 2014;14(1):216
[a]All the concentrations are reflected per 100 ml of human milk mean are reflected ± SD

galactosemia should not be breastfed. While most maternal medications align with breastfeeding, certain medications, such as those involving antineoplastic drug therapy, are contraindicated. Due to the dynamic nature of medication information relevant to breastfeeding, it is advisable to consult the Drugs and Lactation Database (LacMed) before prescribing. LacMed is conveniently accessible from the US National Library of Medicine website [24] (Table 1).

3.1.1 Support and Promotion of Breastfeeding

The WHO recommends that nursing should be started within half an hour of birth and exclusive breastfeeding to be continued for the first 6 months [3]. The WHO, American Academy of Pediatrics (AAP), and Institute of Medicine all support continuing breastfeeding and recommend it for at least the first year of life. Breastfeeding should be done exclusively for about 6 months. If both the mother and the child agree, breastfeeding may continue toward the first year of life. It is crucial to note that the prescription of vitamin D and iron are included in the concept of exclusive breastfeeding [1].

In LMICs, immediate and early breastfeeding after delivery is linked to better newborn outcomes, including a decrease in neonatal mortality, the length of hospital stays for unwell infants, and infections [4, 25]. In comparison with mainly breastfed infants, partially breastfed infants are 4.8 times at a higher risk of death than non-breastfed infants under the age of 6 months, according to a meta-analysis of studies from LMIC settings [26].

Despite the known benefits of breastfeeding, only 42% of babies are nursed within the first hour of life globally [9]. Women in the postpartum period need special counselling and support to ensure early and adequate lactation under stressful conditions [5, 6]. The WHO strongly advises that maternity and newborn services should have adequate competent and trained staff to support lactation efforts, but

Table 2 The Ten Steps to Successful Breastfeeding

Every facility providing maternity services and care for newborn infants should:
1. Have a written breastfeeding policy that is consistently communicated to all health-care staff.
2. Train all health-care staffs in skills vital to implement this policy.
3. Inform all pregnant women about the advantages and management of breastfeeding.
4. Help mothers initiate breastfeeding within the first half-hour after giving birth.
5. Show mothers how to breastfeed and how to maintain lactation even if they should be separated from their infants.
6. Give newborn infants no drink or food other than breastmilk, unless medically indicated.
7. Practice rooming-in—allow infants and mothers to remain together—24 hours a day.
8. Encourage breastfeeding on demand.
9. Give no artificial pacifiers or treats (also called dummies or soothers) to breastfeeding infants.
10. Foster the establishment of breastfeeding support groups and refer mothers to them on discharge from the clinic or hospital.

implementation of zero separation is rare. [13] Breastfeeding is particularly challenging in neonatal intensive care units (NICUs) as in majority of countries NICUs are not designed to ensure zero separation of the mother and baby dyad. As a result, many of the sick babies in critical care unit do not have early initiation of breastfeeding. This poses the greatest challenge for sick newborns [10].

Worldwide, there are numerous community- and facility-level initiatives to support exclusive and early breastfeeding. The Baby Friendly Hospital Initiative (BFHI) was developed by WHO and UNICEF in 2009 to incorporate breastfeeding into maternity and infant care in hospitals. Hospitals must execute the "Ten Steps to Successful Breastfeeding" through this multilevel approach to become BFHIs, which includes having a breastfeeding policy, allowing rooming-in, and providing staff with proper training [13, 27]. Additionally, certain suggestions for extending BFHI to address the special requirements of small and ill neonates have been proposed [6, 28]. In addition, a comprehensive analysis of high-income nations has demonstrated that using lactation consultants for breastfeeding assistance and lactation education increases the rates of commencement, duration of any breastfeeding, and exclusive breastfeeding compared to standard practices [17]. Supporting breastfeeding mothers requires appropriate institutional policies and the expertise of health-care professionals. The WHO has outlined ten guidelines to ensure hospital support for breastfeeding [29] as demonstrated in Table 2.

All breastfeeding neonates should undergo a follow-up visit with their primary care physician within 48–72 hours post-hospital discharge or between Days 3 and 5. During this visit, the doctor should assess weight, ensuring a weight loss of no more than 7% and cessation of weight loss by Day 5. Feeding practices should be evaluated, and more frequent follow-up appointments should be scheduled if weight loss is a concern. The assessment of infants' urination patterns and hydration is crucial, addressing any additional concerns after observing for feeding [30].

Breastfeeding often leads to mastitis, engorgement, and nipple pain. Nipple soreness in the initial nursing days is common and can be addressed with proper positioning, ensuring the baby's ideal attachment and withdrawal after satisfaction. Seeking assistance from a breastfeeding specialist can enhance attachment and removal. Between Days 3 and 5, breast engorgement is typical, alleviated by post-feeding breast massages and more frequent nursing. Mastitis, characterized by a painful red, swollen breast area and fever, occurs in 10%–20% of women. Treatment involves regular milk removal and occasional antibiotics [1].

4 Supplementation of Nutrients for Nursing Babies

Despite being particularly well suited to promote optimal growth, human milk is deficient in iron and vitamin D. Therefore, the American Academy of Pediatrics (AAP) advises all breastfed newborns to be administered 400 IU/day of vitamin D supplementation. Beginning in the infant's first few days of life, vitamin D supplementation should continue until the child is weaned to at least 1 L/day, or 1 quart/day, of vitamin D-fortified formula or whole milk. Similarly, it recommends supplementing iron at 4 months of age, with an oral iron dose of 1–2 mg/kg/day up till the infant is on a weaning diet with adequate iron-rich food group [1].

Vitamin D plays a pivotal role in infant and maternal health, influencing various physiological processes crucial for optimal well-being. Research has indicated that adequate vitamin D is essential for proper bone development in infants, helping to prevent conditions such as rickets. Furthermore, maternal vitamin D status during pregnancy has been linked to several health outcomes. A study by Wagner et al. (2012) highlighted the importance of vitamin D in attaining optimal health for both the mother and the fetus, and maternal Vitamin D deficiency is documented to be associated with an increased risk of gestational diabetes, preeclampsia, and adverse neonatal outcomes [31].

Another significant contribution comes from the clinical practice guidelines of Holick et al. (2011), emphasizing the evaluation, treatment, and prevention of vitamin D deficiency, underscoring its critical role in maternal and infant health [32].

5 Indications for Formula Feeding

There is significant evidence on the protective and promotive role of breastfeeding ("Acta Paediatrica" Horta & Victora, 2013), against infections, allergies, and chronic diseases [33]. For mothers, breastfeeding promotes postpartum recovery and reduces the risk of health issues, as evidenced by research published in the "American Journal of Obstetrics and Gynecology" (Stuebe, Willett, & Michels, 2009). The unique composition of breast milk caters to the specific needs of the growing infant, fostering optimal health outcomes [34].

Although breastfeeding is favored for normal, healthy term infants, formula feeding can assist nutrition and growth in certain circumstances as shown in Fig. 1:

The level of 29 key nutrient regulations batch of infant formula must be verified by manufacturers, who are subject to US Food and Drug Administration (FDA)

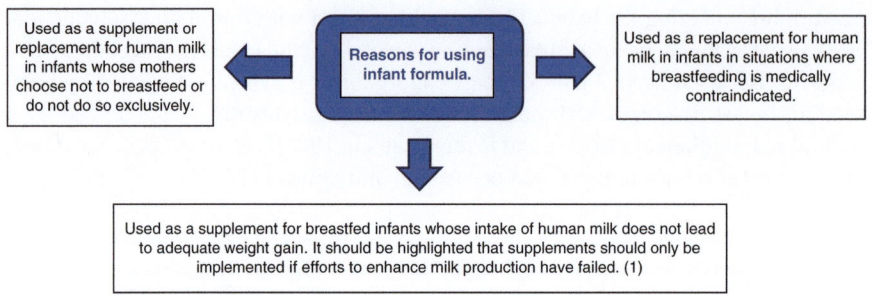

Fig. 1 Reasons for using infant formula

regulation. In the United States, commercially available infant formulae support the healthy development and normal growth of term newborns. Although the nutrient makeup of products from different manufacturers may vary a little, the products are considerably more similar than different. Given the previously mentioned variability of human milk, standard infant formula has 19–20 calories per ounce [24].

However, infant formula has a protein content that is almost 50% more than that of human milk (1.4 g/100 mL for infant formula) and about 3.6 g of fat per 100 mL, comparable to the quantity in human milk. Vegetable oil blends are the main source of this fat. Arachidonic acid and docosahexaenoic acid, two very long-chain polyunsaturated fatty acids, have been included in most infant formulae. Even though the long-term advantage of these additives appears to be negligible or nonexistent, these substances may aid in promoting brain and eye development. However, there are no safety issues with the docosahexaenoic acid and arachidonic acid additions to newborn formulae. Infant formula is identical to human milk in terms of content and carbohydrate levels (about 7.5 g/100 mL) [24].

Iron is commonly present in formula milk of infants, ideally at a level of 12 mg/L. Anemia and iron deficiency are prevented by this iron concentration. Due to the assumption that using higher-iron formulas causes gastrointestinal (GI) symptoms (colic and constipation), low-iron newborn formulae are still offered [24].

Human breast milk is widely acknowledged as the optimal choice for infant nourishment, providing a comprehensive and bioactive-rich diet. When breastfeeding is not feasible or preferred, infant formula serves as an alternative. Formula feeds have incorporated probiotics and prebiotics to enhance their biological functionality [35].

6 Role of Probiotics in Neonatal Nutrition

Probiotics play a crucial role in promoting gut health and immunological function in newborn nutrition (Table 3). These living bacteria contribute positively to the host's health when administered in adequate doses. As supplements, probiotics are commonly provided to newborns to support the development of a healthy gut microbiome [35].

Table 3 Key roles of probiotics

1. *Gut microbiota development*	Probiotics help newborns develop a healthy, diverse gut microbiome. For the growth of the immune system, nutrition absorption, and defense against hazardous pathogens, the gut must be early colonized by good bacteria. Probiotics can aid in the growth of good bacteria like lactobacilli and bifidobacteria while preventing the colonization of dangerous bacteria.
2. *Improved digestion and nutrient absorption*	Neonatal digestion and nutrient absorption can be improved with probiotics. They create enzymes that help break down complex carbs, proteins, and lipids so that they are easier to digest. Neonatal growth and development may benefit from this increased nutrient absorption.
3. *Immune system modulation*	The immunological response in newborns is regulated by the immunomodulatory actions of probiotics. They encourage the growth of an immune system that is balanced and boost the synthesis of immune cells. Preterm infants, who have underdeveloped immune systems and are more prone to infections, can benefit greatly from this.
4. *Reduction of infection risk*	It has been demonstrated that probiotics lower the risk of illnesses in newborns, particularly gastrointestinal and respiratory tract infections. Probiotics can aid in preventing the colonization and expansion of harmful bacteria, hence lowering the risk of illness by preserving healthy gut microbiota and boosting immune function.
5. *Prevention of necrotizing enterocolitis (NEC)*	NEC is a serious disorder that mainly affects premature infants and is characterized by intestinal inflammation and destruction. Probiotics, particularly certain strains of the bacteria Bifidobacterium and lactobacillus, have demonstrated encouraging benefits in reducing the incidence and severity of NEC. They support the firmness of the intestinal barrier, lessen inflammation, and regulate the immune system, all of which can help prevent NEC [35] The grade of evidence for the use of probiotics in the prevention of necrotizing enterocolitis (NEC) is generally considered moderate to high. Numerous systematic reviews and meta-analyses, including studies like the Cochrane review by AlFaleh and Anabrees in 2014, have demonstrated a significant reduction in the incidence of NEC in preterm infants with the administration of probiotics. However, it is essential to note that specific doses, strains, and protocols may differ, and ongoing research continues to refine recommendations and assess the long-term effects of probiotic use in this context [36]

7   Role of Lactoferrin

Human milk (HM) and the milk of other mammals include the bioactive protein lactoferrin, which offers several advantages, including anti-infective, immunological, and gastrointestinal benefits. By preventing sepsis and necrotizing enterocolitis in preterm infants and lowering the incidence of gastrointestinal and respiratory infections in early childhood, it contributes to neonatal and infant health [37].

HM contains a variety of bioactive proteins, with Lactoferrin being one of the most notable and accounting for about 20% of HM's total protein content. The initial milk produced after birth, colostrum, has the highest concentration of Lactoferrin and continues to be raised during the first month of breastfeeding. Lactoferrin concentrations in colostrum vary from 7 to 9 g/L, while those in mature milk range from 1 to 3 g/L. Mothers who gave preterm birth had higher Lactoferrin levels as compared to the mothers who gave birth at full term [37].

Due to its iron-binding properties and capacity to interact with a variety of chemicals and receptors, Lactoferrin is thought to have numerous roles. It has antibacterial effects on viruses, fungi, and bacteria. Because Lactoferrin binds to iron, it reduces the amount of free iron that is available, which helps to suppress bacterial development. Additionally, Lactoferrin can influence the immune system, encourage the creation of healthy gut bacteria, and support the growth and operation of the digestive system [37].

Clinical research indicates that adding Lactoferrin to preterm infants' meals, either by itself or in combination with probiotics, can considerably lower the risk of late-onset sepsis and necrotizing enterocolitis [37].

To determine the ideal Lactoferrin supplementation amount, timing, and potential long-term effects, additional research is necessary. Further research is also necessary into quality assurance procedures, the standardization of Lactoferrin preparations, and the influence of processing methods on Lactoferrin's characteristics [37]. Different types of macronutrients and micronutrients and their requirement and benefits for neonates have been mentioned in Table 4.

Table 4 Macronutrients and micronutrients and their requirements and benefits for neonates

Macronutrients	Requirements and Benefits for Neonates
Proteins	Neonates mainly consume whey or casein proteins. Contribute to tissue building, repair, and the regulation of bodily functions. Increased protein intake has been linked to improved weight and length among neonates and infants.
Lipids	Medium- and short-chain triglycerides (MCT) are easier to absorb. SMOF and Omegaven are specialized lipid emulsions. Essential fatty acids, such as omega-3 and omega-6, are important for cognitive and visual development. Omegaven, rich in omega 3, may reduce inflammation and hepatotoxicity.
Carbohydrates	Glucose is the primary brain fuel. 40–55% of daily calories come from carbs. Provides energy and supports brain development and mineral absorption.
Zinc	Essential for growth and enzyme function. Preterm infants need more zinc for rapid growth. Deficiency can cause various symptoms including dermatitis and anemia [38].
Selenium	Acts as an antioxidant, reducing the risk of various diseases. Important for enzyme function and cellular protection. In neonates with renal impairment, care is advised due to predominately renal excretion [38, 39].
Copper	Cofactor for numerous enzymes [20] Preterm infants may have lower storage and increased needs [40]. Deficiency may lead to iron insufficiency and anemia.
Manganese	Essential for enzyme function. Toxicity risk in preterm infants, especially with long-term parenteral nutrition (PN).

(continued)

Table 4 (continued)

Macronutrients	Requirements and Benefits for Neonates
Chromium	Necessary for insulin metabolism. Toxicity documented, especially in infants on long-term PN. Therefore, it is advised to decrease the dose but not completely stop chromium in children with renal insufficiency [38].
Iron	Vital for myoglobin and hemoglobin. Preterm infants may need supplementation for catch-up growth [38].
Hepcidin	Regulates iron metabolism. Imbalances can affect iron levels and susceptibility to infections [41].
Vitamin	*Fat-soluble vitamins (A, D, E, and K):* Essential for various physiological functions. Deficiency or toxicity can lead to specific health issues. Vitamin A (Retinol) is essential for the growth and development of the pulmonary epithelium, skin, eyes, and bones. In iron-induced hemolysis, vitamin E (tocopherol) plays an antioxidant role. Vitamin K plays a crucial role in coagulation and is therefore crucial in preventing hemorrhagic illness in newborns. Vitamin D and parathyroid hormones are important for the metabolism of calcium and phosphorus. Lack of vitamin D is linked to rickets, prematurity-related osteopenia, and developmental delays. *Water-soluble vitamins (B and C):* Need daily consumption to meet requirements [39].

8 Neonatal Nutrition in Special Circumstances

8.1 Nutrition in Sepsis

Preterm infants face an elevated risk of malnutrition due to low nutritional levels and underdeveloped gastrointestinal systems. Preterm infants with sepsis are particularly susceptible to bacterial translocation, heightening the risk of complications like necrotizing enterocolitis (NEC) and increased morbidity and mortality rates [42].

Managing preterm infants as immunosuppressed patients is vital for survival, necessitating prompt antibiotic therapy and supportive interventions. Sepsis exacerbates dietary challenges, leading to a hypercatabolic state, negative nitrogen balance, and malnutrition. Breast milk and early enteral nutrition are essential for preventing newborn sepsis and reducing infection risks. Enteral nutrition promotes short-chain fatty acid production, benefiting the intestinal epithelium, and enhances glucose tolerance through gluconeogenesis precursor and ketone body generation [42].

8.2 Preterm Nutrition

Prematurity refers to birth before 37 weeks of pregnancy. These babies are at high risk of morbidity and mortality. Both short- and long-term outcomes predominantly depend on the gestational age and weight at birth. Extreme preterm babies face significant challenges during the first few weeks of life ex utero and may succumb to complications such as NEC and sepsis.

Due to various complications, they have prolonged hospital stay and are at risk of cognitive or neurodevelopment delays. From 26 weeks of gestation onward, there is an increase in the complexity of neural connections and rapid development of oligodendrocytes, glial cells, and axons in white matter, which improves brain maturation. Interruptions and insults during this rapid period of nerve cell differentiation (NDV) because of preterm birth serve as major triggers to potential neurodevelopment delays later in life [43].

The advancements in modern technology and improved case management have led to increased survival rates among preterm infants. Consequently, it is imperative to prioritize ensuring sufficient nutritional supplementation during the rapid growth phase. This strategic focus is essential to minimize the negative effects associated with prematurity and safeguard against potential long-term complications.

Preterm infants frequently encounter malnutrition in their first few days of life (DoL). Insufficient nutrition with impaired body growth is linked to the development of cerebral palsy, poor psychomotor, and mental development. Hence, to reduce the suboptimal environment during rapid NDV, early optimal nutrition is essential [43].

Enteral feeding is the primary method of nutrition in preterm infants. However, early initiation of enteral feeds is dependent upon the extent of immaturity and the clinical condition of the vulnerable preterm baby.

Many of these preterm babies require a few hours to days for hemodynamic stability (due to thermoregulation, circulation, and respiratory compromise) and hence cannot be challenged with feeds. Therefore, parenteral nutrition (PN) is the mainstay of feeding in the first week of life. According to current recommendations, these infants should receive substantial protein and energy doses by PN shortly after delivery to prevent slowing of growth and associated long-term effects.

Concerning the optimal dietary intake for the long-term NDV of preterm neonates, there is a lack of research. Although some studies have suggested the benefits of increased protein intake in parenteral nutrition (PN) for NDV, the ideal calorie intake for preterm infants remains unknown [43].

Addressing their overall medical needs, optimizing nutrition aims to bridge this gap and enhance growth and health outcomes. During this critical period, nutrition must prioritize delivering the optimal protein and caloric content, along with appropriate amounts of each macronutrient, micronutrient, and electrolyte. Meeting the lifelong dietary needs of preterm children requires a multidisciplinary approach involving experts such as gastroenterologists, neonatologists, and dietitians [44].

Enteral feeds are initiated as soon as possible, gradually increased according to the assigned "feeding bundles" until full feeds are achieved. Colostrum is administered orally in numerous neonatal intensive care units (NICUs) around the world, acting as an oral immune treatment [45].

Freshly expressed colostrum is favored for colostrum care due to the breakdown of stem cells within approximately 6 hours. According to a Cochrane review, utilizing colostrum care has been shown to reduce the time required to achieve full enteral

Table 5 Differentiation of ingredients of breast milk and formula milk

	Breast Milk	Formula Milk
Carbohydrates	Primary lactose	Usually, lactose
Proteins	Whey and casein	Often cow's milk-based
Fats	Rich in Docosahexaenoic acid (DHA) and Arachidonic acid (AA)	Often supplemented
Micronutrients	Naturally occurring vitamins and minerals	Added vitamins and minerals

Table 6 Comparison of the caloric contents of different types of milk and milk fortifiers

Type	Calories per 100 mL
Breast milk	65–75 kcal [47]
Formula milk	65–70 kcal (standard)
Preterm milk	80–100 kcal
Term milk	65–75 kcal
Milk fortifiers	Variations by brand

feeds by half, with a mean reduction of 2.5 days [46]. No additional significant benefits or adverse outcomes were discerned. The studies included in the review were of low quality. Once the baby is stable and ready to feed, small volume of feeding is commenced with 10–15 ml/kg/day of human milk. This is referred to as "trophic feeds," for gut stimulation.

In the majority of NICUs, trophic feeding is started within the first 24 hours. The feeds are progressively increased by 10–30 ml/kg/day, and full feeds are reached approximately in 10–14 days. While there are no "one-size-fits-all" guidelines for feeding preterm newborns, the ideal period for establishing full enteral feeds is inversely correlated to the size of the infants, taking approximately 7–14 days in infants with birth weights of 750–1500 g [46].

Currently, unit-specific protocols apply to the use of donor breast milk. Breastmilk (either donor's or mother's milk) may be supplemented with human milk fortifiers (HMFs) to 24 calories/ounce (cal/oz), with some units practicing a gradual increase in fortification to 22 cal/oz. and then 24 cal/oz., once the newborn is receiving roughly 75–80 ml/kg/day. Standard infant formulae, which are modeled after breastmilk, contain 19 to 20 kcal per ounce [46]. The ingredients of breast milk and formula milk have been differentiated in Table 5. Moreover, a comparison of the caloric contents of different types of milk and milk fortifiers has been provided in Table 6.

8.2.1 Innovations in Preterm Nutrition
Innovations in preterm nutrition (Table 7) have been a crucial focus in neonatal care to address the unique nutritional needs of premature infants.

8.2.2 Role of Parenteral Nutrition in Preterm Neonates
Individuals unable to tolerate sufficient enteral feedings for various reasons must receive parenteral nutrition. When enteral feeds are introduced, intravenous nutrition is gradually tapered. The concentration of intravenous nutrition depends partly on the type of intravenous access. Parenteral nutrition comprises equal proportions

Table 7 Innovations in preterm nutrition

Human milk fortifiers (HMF)	Fortifying human milk with additional nutrients, such as proteins, minerals, and vitamins, helps meet the higher nutritional requirements of preterm infants. HMFs are designed to enhance the nutritional content of mother's milk, providing essential elements for optimal growth and development [48].
Donor human milk banks	For infants who cannot receive their mother's milk, donor human milk banks provide an alternative. Pasteurized donor milk is carefully screened, processed, and made available to preterm infants, offering the benefits of human milk when maternal milk is unavailable [49].
Exclusive human milk diets (EHMD)	EHMD involves feeding preterm infants only human milk, either mother's own milk or donor milk, without introducing formula. This approach has shown benefits in reducing the risk of complications such as necrotizing enterocolitis (NEC) and improving long-term outcomes [50].

of 30% fat (lipid formulations like intralipids, SMOF, or Omegaven), 15% protein (amino acids), and 55% carbs (dextrose). Dextrose administered intravenously is the most used form of carbohydrate. Except for extremely preterm infants, who may require a lower dextrose content, dextrose (10%) is typically used as the initial fluid. Dextrose concentrations are titrated based on the infant's requirements, serum glucose levels, and the rate of glucose infusion. A peripheral venous catheter can safely administer up to 12.5% dextrose, but larger concentrations require the insertion of a central venous access. Even in premature infants, parenteral amino acids can be administered as early as the first day of life. The importance of early protein consumption in infancy is increasingly recognized. The length at discharge in preterm newborns correlates with escalating protein supplements. Parenteral feeding necessitates routine lab testing [44].

9 Conclusion

Neonatal nutrition is optimal for fulfilling the unique dietary requirements of newborn infants during their first 28 days of life to support optimal growth, health, and development. Micronutrients such as iron, folate, vitamins A and D, zinc, and iodine play significant roles in various physiological processes that impact the overall health and well-being of neonates and infants. Micronutrient deficiencies can lead to adverse effects on fetal and neonatal health, including an increased risk of stillbirth, weakened immune response, and impaired cognitive development. Macronutrients, including fats, carbohydrates, and proteins, are essential for rapid growth and neurodevelopment in neonates.

Breast milk is considered the ideal choice for neonatal nutrition due to its essential nutrients, bioactive substances, and protective elements. Breastfeeding provides a unique combination of nutrients and offers numerous health, social, and economic benefits, including lower morbidity and mortality in infants. Lactoferrin, a protein found in human milk, has demonstrated clinical benefits in preterm and term infants. Supplementation with lactoferrin in infant formulas may be considered, but further research is needed to evaluate its efficacy and safety.

Overall, neonatal nutrition, including proper prenatal and postnatal nutrition, the adequate intake of micronutrients and macronutrients, and promotion of breastfeeding, plays an important role in ensuring the optimal growth, development, and health of newborn infants.

References

1. Kleinman RE, Greer FR. Nutrition AAoPCo. Pediatric nutrition. Elk Grove Village: American Academy of Pediatrics; 2014.
2. Agostoni C, Buonocore G, Carnielli VP, De Curtis M, Darmaun D, Decsi T, et al. Enteral nutrient supply for preterm infants: commentary from the European Society of Paediatric Gastroenterology, Hepatology and Nutrition Committee on Nutrition. J Pediatr Gastroenterol Nutr. 2010;50(1):85–91.
3. Yang W, Li X, Li Y, Zhang S, Liu L, Wang X, et al. Anemia, malnutrition and their correlations with socio-demographic characteristics and feeding practices among infants aged 0–18 months in rural areas of Shaanxi province in northwestern China: a cross-sectional study. BMC Public Health. 2012;12:1127.
4. Ali SS. A brief review of risk-factors for growth and developmental delay among preschool children in developing countries. Adv Biomed Res. 2013;2:91.
5. Hsu C-N, Tain Y-L. The good, the bad, and the ugly of pregnancy nutrients and developmental programming of adult disease. Nutrients. 2019;11(4):894.
6. Susan Kazen M. Nutrition Through the Lifecycle. 2021. Available from: https://pressbooks.pub/nutritionessentials/chapter/chapter-16-nutrition-through-the-lifecycle/.
7. Deshmukh J, Motghare D, Zodpey S, Wadhva S. Low birth weight and associated maternal factors in an urban area. Indian pediatr. 1998;35:33–6.
8. Wahyuningsih E. <1161-Article Text-6288-1-10-20,220,811.pdf>. Indonesian J Global Health Res. 2022;4.
9. Zhang X, Donnelly B, Thomas J, Sams L, O'Brien K, Taylor SN, et al. Growth in the high-risk newborn infant post-discharge: results from a neonatal intensive care unit nutrition follow-up clinic. Nutr Clin Pract. 2020;35(4):738–44.
10. Taylor SN, Martin CR. Evidence-based discharge nutrition to optimize preterm infant outcomes. Neoreviews. 2022;23(2):e108–e16.
11. de Boo HA, Harding JE. The developmental origins of adult disease (Barker) hypothesis. Aust N Z J Obstet Gynaecol. 2006;46(1):4–14.
12. Agostoni C, Buonocore G, Carnielli V, De Curtis M, Darmaun D, Decsi T, et al. Enteral nutrient supply for preterm infants: commentary from the European Society of Paediatric Gastroenterology, Hepatology and Nutrition Committee on Nutrition. J Pediatr Gastroenterol Nutr. 2010;50(1):85–91.
13. Savarino G, Corsello A, Corsello G. Macronutrient balance and micronutrient amounts through growth and development. Ital J Pediatr. 2021;47(1):109.
14. Bertino E, Giuliani F, Baricco M, Di Nicola P, Peila C, Vassia C, et al. Benefits of donor milk in the feeding of preterm infants. Early Hum Dev. 2013;89:S3–6.
15. Martin CR, Ling PR, Blackburn GL. Review of infant feeding: key features of breast milk and infant formula. Nutrients. 2016;8(5)
16. Malnutrition: World Health Organization. Available from: https://www.who.int/health-topics/malnutrition.
17. Sotiraki M, Malliou A, Tachirai N, Kellari N, Grammatikopoulou MG, Sergentanis TN, et al. Burden of childhood malnutrition: a roadmap of global and European policies promoting healthy nutrition for infants and young children. Children (Basel). 2022;9(8)
18. Djoumessi YF. The impact of malnutrition on infant mortality and life expectancy in Africa. Nutrition. 2022;103–104:111760.

19. Ke-You G, Da-Wei F. The magnitude and trends of under- and over-nutrition in Asian countries. Biomed Environ Sci. 2001;14(1–2):53–60.
20. Irshath AA, Raghuraman D, Rajan AP, Rajan AP. A focus on SDG target for the prevention of undernourishment. 2023.
21. Albelbeisi A, Shariff ZM, Mun CY, Abdul-Rahman H, Abed Y. Growth patterns of Palestinian children from birth to 24 months. East Mediterr Health J. 2018;24(3):302–10.
22. Intakes IoMSCotSEoDR. DRI Dietary Reference Intakes: applications in dietary assessment. 2000.
23. Ballard O, Morrow AL. Human milk composition: nutrients and bioactive factors. Pediatr Clin North Am. 2013;60(1):49–74.
24. Denne SC. Neonatal nutrition. Pediatr Clin. 2015;62(2):427–38.
25. Deshmukh JS, Motghare DD, Zodpey SP, Wadhva SK. Low birth weight and associated maternal factors in an urban area. Indian Pediatr. 1998;35(1):33–6.
26. Gato S, Biziyaremye F, Kirk CM, De Sousa CP, Mukuralinda A, Habineza H, et al. Promotion of early and exclusive breastfeeding in neonatal care units in rural Rwanda: a pre- and post-intervention study. Int Breastfeed J. 2022;17(1):12.
27. Bertino E, Giuliani F, Baricco M, Di Nicola P, Peila C, Vassia C, et al. Benefits of donor milk in the feeding of preterm infants. Early Hum Dev. 2013;89(Suppl 2):S3–6.
28. Martin CR, Ling P-R, Blackburn GL. Review of infant feeding: key features of breast milk and infant formula. Nutrients. 2016;8(5):279.
29. Organization WH. Evidence for the ten steps to successful breastfeeding. 1998.
30. Eidelman AI, Schanler RJ, Johnston M, Landers S, Noble L, et al. Breastfeeding and the use of human milk. Pediatrics. 2012;129(3):e827–e41.
31. Wagner CL, Taylor SN, Dawodu A, Johnson DD, Hollis BW. Vitamin D and its role during pregnancy in attaining optimal health of mother and fetus. Nutrients. 2012;4(3):208–30.
32. Holick MF, Binkley NC, Bischoff-Ferrari HA, Gordon CM, Hanley DA, Heaney RP, et al. Evaluation, treatment, and prevention of vitamin D deficiency: an Endocrine Society clinical practice guideline. J Clin Endocrinol Metab. 2011;96(7):1911–30.
33. Horta BL, Victora CG. Long-term effects of breastfeeding: a systematic review. Acta Paediatr. 2013.
34. Stuebe AM, Michels KB, Willett WC, Manson JE, Rexrode K, Rich-Edwards JW. Duration of lactation and incidence of myocardial infarction in middle to late adulthood. Am J Obstet Gynecol. 2009;200(2):138.e1–8.
35. Parracho H, McCartney AL, Gibson GR. Probiotics and prebiotics in infant nutrition. Proc Nutr Soc. 2007;66(3):405–11.
36. AlFaleh K, Anabrees J. Probiotics for prevention of necrotizing enterocolitis in preterm infants. Cochrane Database Syst Rev. 2014(4):CD005496.
37. Manzoni P, Dall'Agnola A, Tomé D, Kaufman DA, Tavella E, Pieretto M, et al. Role of lactoferrin in neonates and infants: an update. Am J Perinatol. 2018;35(6):561–565.
38. Zemrani B, McCallum Z, Bines JE. Trace element provision in parenteral nutrition in children: one size does not fit all. Nutrients. 2018;10(11)
39. Gathwala G, Aggarwal R. Selenium supplementation for the preterm Indian neonate. Indian J Public Health. 2016;60(2):142–4.
40. Devaguru A, Gada S, Potpalle D, Dinesh Eshwar M, Purwar D. The prevalence of low birth weight among newborn babies and its associated maternal risk factors: a hospital-based cross-sectional study. Cureus. 2023;15(5):e38587.
41. Koenig MD, Tussing-Humphreys L, Day J, Cadwell B, Nemeth E. Hepcidin and iron homeostasis during pregnancy. Nutrients. 2014;6(8):3062–83.
42. Freitas BAC, Leão RT, Gomes AP, Siqueira-Batista R. Nutritional therapy and neonatal sepsis. Revista Brasileira de Terapia Intensiva. 2011;23:492–8.
43. Terrin G, Boscarino G, Gasparini C, Di Chiara M, Faccioli F, Onestà E, et al. Energy-enhanced parenteral nutrition and neurodevelopment of preterm newborns: a cohort study. Nutrition. 2021;89:111219.

44. Skinner AM, Narchi H. Preterm nutrition and neurodevelopmental outcomes. World J Methodol. 2021;11(6):278–93.
45. Nasuf AWA, Ojha S, Dorling J. Oropharyngeal colostrum in preventing mortality and morbidity in preterm infants. Cochrane Database Syst Rev. 2018;9(9):Cd011921
46. Sharma D, Kaur A, Farahbakhsh N, Agarwal S. Role of oropharyngeal administration of colostrum in very low birth weight infants for reducing necrotizing enterocolitis: a randomized controlled trial. Am J Perinatol. 2020;37(7):716–21.
47. Kim SY, Yi DY. Components of human breast milk: from macronutrient to microbiome and microRNA. Clin Exp Pediatr. 2020;63(8):301–9.
48. Arslanoglu S, Boquien CY, King C, Lamireau D, Tonetto P, Barnett D, et al. Fortification of human milk for preterm infants: update and recommendations of the European Milk Bank Association (EMBA) Working Group on Human Milk Fortification. Front Pediatr. 2019;7:76.
49. Tyebally Fang M, Chatzixiros E, Grummer-Strawn L, Engmann C, Israel-Ballard K, Mansen K, et al. Developing global guidance on human milk banking. Bull World Health Organ. 2021;99(12):892–900.
50. Philip RK, Romeih E, Bailie E, Daly M, McGourty KD, Grabrucker AM, et al. Exclusive human milk diet for extremely premature infants: a novel fortification strategy that enhances the bioactive properties of fresh, frozen, and pasteurized milk specimens. Breastfeed Med. 2023;18(4):279–90.

Nutritional Intervention Among Children Under Five, School-Age Children, and Adolescents to Overcome Undernutrition

Aamer Imdad, Areeba Fatima, and Uzma Rani

1 Introduction

Malnutrition occurs when an individual's dietary intake is not balanced with the nutritional needs, leading to ill effects on health, well-being, and/or productivity, and it includes undernutrition, overnutrition, and micronutrient deficiencies [4, 5]. Undernutrition is a form of malnutrition characterized by an insufficient dietary intake to sustain good health in an individual. It can be broadly categorized into wasting, stunting, and underweight. Table 1 gives the definition of terms related to undernutrition. Wasting in a child indicates recent or severe weight loss and is defined as weight-for-height z-score (WHZ) or weight-for-length z-score (WLZ) more than 2 standard deviations (SD) below the median of the World Health Organization (WHO) Child Growth Standards (WHZ or WLZ < −2). Wasting could be moderate and severe based on WHZ or WLZ. The term 'severe wasting' is used interchangeably with severe acute malnutrition, protein-energy malnutrition, marasmus, and kwashiorkor. Even though all these terms indicate severe undernutrition, there are subtle differences, for example, the definition of severe acute malnutrition

---

A. Imdad (✉)
Department of Pediatrics, Division of Gastroenterology, Hepatology, Pancreatology and Nutrition, Stead Family Children's Hospital, University of Iowa, Iowa City, IA, USA
e-mail: aamer-imdad@uiowa.edu

A. Fatima
Dow Medical University, Karachi, Pakistan
e-mail: areeba.fatima@nixorcollege.edu.pk

U. Rani
Department of Pediatrics, Division of General Pediatrics, Stead Family Children's Hospital, University of Iowa, Iowa City, IA, USA
e-mail: uzma-rani@uiowa.edu

© The Author(s), under exclusive license to Springer Nature Switzerland AG 2025
Z. S. Lassi, R. A. Salam (eds.), *Nutrition Across Reproductive, Maternal, Neonatal, Child, and Adolescent Health Care*,
https://doi.org/10.1007/978-3-031-95721-5_10

Table 1 Definitions related to undernutrition

Term	Definition
Acute malnutrition [1]	WHZ or WLZ more than 2 SD below the median of the WHO child growth standards (WHZ or WLZ < −2) or having nutritional edema or MUAC <125 mm in children under 5 years of age.
Stunting [1]	HAZ more than two standard deviations (SD) below the median of the WHO child growth standards.
Wasting [1]	WHZ or WLZ more than 2 standard deviations (SD) below the median of the World Health Organization.
Moderate wasting [1]	WHZ or WLZ between −3 SD and less than −2 SD, or MUAC is between 115 mm and less than 125 mm in children 6–59 months of age.
Severe wasting [1]	WHZ or WLZ z-score less than −3 SD, or MUAC less than 115 mm in children 6–59 months of age.
Protein-energy malnutrition [2]	Condition in which the most salient elements are the depletion of body energy stores and tissue proteins.
Kwashiorkor [1]	Severe calorie and protein insufficiency that leads to characteristic bilateral pitting pedal edema and ascites.
Marasmus [3]	Manifestation of severe dietary malnutrition, which occurs because of a calorie deficiency.
Underweight [3]	WAZ more than 2 standard deviations (SD) below the median of the World Health Organization.
Nutritional oedema [1]	Bilateral pitting edema, which starts in the feet and can progress up to the legs and the rest of the body, including the face.
Micronutrient deficiency [3]	A deficiency of the essential vitamins and minerals, which are needed for physiological function and development.

Abbreviations: *HAZ* height-for-age z-scores, *MUAC* mid-upper arm circumference, *WAZ* weight-for-age z scores, *WHZ* weight-for-height z-score, *WLZ* weight-for-length z-score

also considers the nutritional edema and mid-upper arm circumference as part of the definition, while severe wasting is mainly defined based on weight for height/length.

Marasmus and kwashiorkor indicate severe undernutrition; however, the term kwashiorkor is often used when there is nutritional edema as part of the clinical manifestation of severe wasting [2, 3]. Stunting occurs due to chronic or recurring undernutrition and is defined as a height-for-age z-score (HAZ) more than two standard deviations (SD) below the median of the WHO Child Growth Standards (HAZ < −2). Stunting is associated with long-term morbidity, including risk of neurodevelopmental delays, decreased school performance, and adult productivity. Underweight children have low weight-for-age z scores (WAZ) and may have characteristics of wasting, stunting, or both [2, 4, 5].

Most of the definitions mentioned above are related to children 6–59 months of age, and there is a lack of consensus on the definition of undernutrition in infants less than 6 months of age. WHO recently reviewed the evidence related to the definition of wasting in infants less than 6 months of age, and Fig. 1 (adapted from the WHO guidelines on prevention and management of wasting and nutritional edema [1]) summarizes considerations about infants less than 6 months of age at risk of poor growth and development. The considerations about making an assessment about which infants are at increased risk of poor growth and development

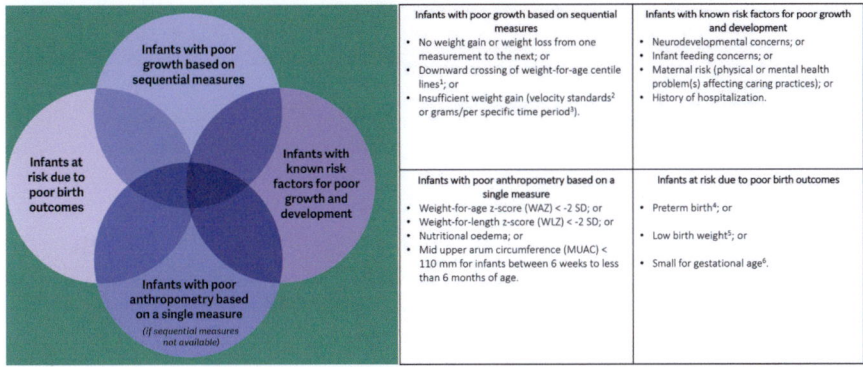

Fig. 1 Infants less than 6 months of age are at risk of poor growth and development
Footnotes: 1 ≥ 1 growth centile space if birth weight < ninth centile; ≥ 2 centile spaces if birth weight is 9th–91st centiles; ≥ 3 centile spaces if birth weight > 91st centile. 2 Less than 2 standard deviations (SD) below the median on the WHO growth velocity standards from one measurement to the next. 3 Approximately less than 500 g/month, or if measured weekly: birth to 3 months, approximately less than 150–200 g/week, and 3–6 months, approximately less than 100–150 g/week. 4 Defined as babies born alive before 37 weeks of pregnancy are completed. 5 Defined as birth weight < 2500 g (5.5 pounds). 6 Defined as infants below the tenth centile of birth weight for gestational age, based on a gender-specific reference population. Figure adopted from WHO guidelines on prevention and management of wasting and nutritional edema [1]

involve assessment based on anthropometric measures such as those defined for children 6–59 months of age and other considerations such as sequential measures (weight loss, no weight gain, crossing of weight for age centile lines, and insufficient weight gain), maternal and infants risk factors such as suboptimal maternal mental health and history of preterm birth, low birth weight, and small for gestational age, respectively [1].

2 Epidemiology of Undernutrition

According to the 2023 joint report by the United Nations International Children's Emergency Fund (UNICEF), the World Health Organization (WHO), and the World Bank group, stunting affected 148 million (22.3%) of all children under 5 years of age worldwide, and 45 million children under 5 years of age (6.8%) were afflicted by wasting [6]. Asia, followed closely by Africa, bears the greatest share of stunting and wasting (Fig. 2). Specifically, Asia accounts for 52% of the global burden of stunting and over 75% of the global burden of wasting. Within Asia, Central Asia, encompassing countries like India, Pakistan, and Afghanistan, carries the highest number of cases with stunting (7.7% of the global burden) and wasting (0.6% of the global burden). More than half of all children affected by stunting live in low and middle income countries (64%), followed by low-income (26%), upper-middle-income (8%), and high-income (2%). A similar trend is followed by wasting, which also affects lower- and middle-income countries the most (76%). Compared to

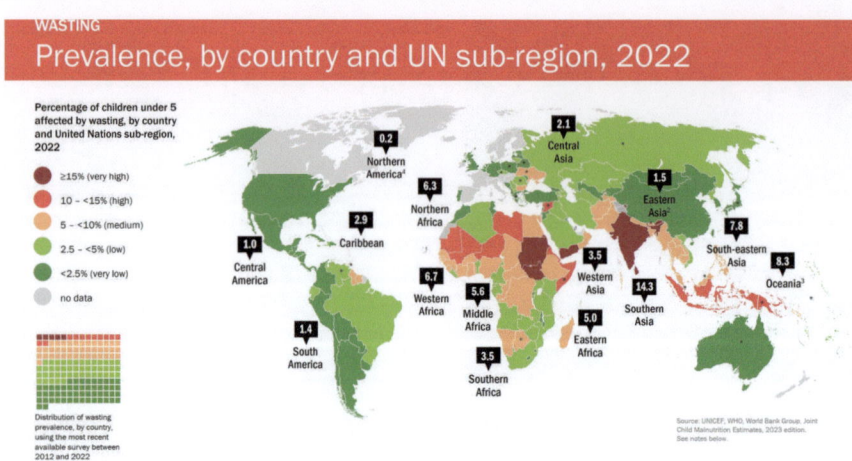

Fig. 2 Prevalence of children under 5 years of age affected by wasting, by country and United Nations subregion, 2022. (Source: UNICEF, WHO, World Bank Group, Joint Child Malnutrition Estimates, 2023 edition) [7]

2000, the prevalence of stunting has decreased from 33% to 22.3%; whereas wasting has only decreased slightly from 8.7% in 2000 to 6.8% in 2022 [6].

Historically, the epidemiology of undernutrition has been described in terms of wasting, stunting, and underweight. However, these conditions can coexist and are important considerations in terms of defining the severity of malnutrition and response to treatment. A study by Khara et al. included data from 84 countries from demographic and health surveys and multi-indicator cluster survey data sets and showed that the overall prevalence of concurrence of wasting and stunting was 3% [8]. The concurrence of wasting and stunting was higher in children 12–24 months of age, which was 4.2% compared to 3.2% in 24–36 months of age, 2.52% in 36–48 months of age, and 2.37% in 48–60 months of age. The estimates for the concurrence of wasting and stunting were higher in males at about 3.54% compared to females, where it was 2.46%. A study by Obeng-Amoako et al. included data from 24,829 children from nine countries who were being treated in outpatient settings for severe or moderate wasting and determined the prevalence of severe underweight (weight-for-age z-scores <3 for WHO growth standards) in this study population. The results showed that overall, 55% of the wasted children were also severely underweight [9]. About 42% of the moderately wasted children were severely underweight, and 64% of the severely wasted children were severely underweight. Children with concurrence of wasting and severe underweight had lower recovery rates at 28% and higher risk of mortality, 1.8%, compared to 9% and 0.7% in children who were wasted but not severely underweight, respectively. The author suggested that not only should severe underweight be a consideration in children with the treatment of severely wasted children, but also children with moderate wasting, as the children with moderate wasting and severe underweight are at higher risk of morbidity and mortality [9].

3 Etiology of Undernutrition

In 2020, UNICEF updated its conceptual framework for the determinants of maternal and child nutrition [7]. The framework addresses the multifaceted factors that impact nutrition at different societal levels, shedding light on the intricate and interconnected web of determinants that influence maternal and child health and nutrition. These determinants can be broadly categorized into immediate and underlying factors. The immediate determinants revolve around the availability of nourishing foods, promoting sound feeding practices, and delivering essential services. These foods include age-appropriate, nutrient-rich options, breastmilk, and complementary foods for infants, as well as access to safe drinking water and household food security. Feeding practices, food preparation, consumption habits, and hygiene also play pivotal roles in these immediate determinants [7].

Services are another crucial component, encompassing adequate nutrition, health care, sanitation, education, and social protection. These services are bolstered by environments that encourage healthy dietary choices and overall well-being. This holistic approach is aimed at preventing diseases and promoting good dietary habits and physical activity [7].

The effectiveness of these elements is closely intertwined with governance and political strategies that ensure the availability of necessary resources. Importantly, this framework underscores the importance of considering social, gender, and cultural norms in all strategies and policies. In conclusion, this framework is a valuable tool for improving maternal and child nutrition. It offers essential guidance for policymakers and public health authorities [7].

4 Nutritional Interventions for Undernourished Children

The treatment of undernutrition in children depends on the severity of undernutrition, related complications, and the age of the child. For children with severe wasting, the treatment consists of two phases: stabilization and rehabilitation. During the stabilization phase, children are treated for complications such as dehydration, electrolyte imbalance, infection, and other complications. Once the patient is stabilized, the rehabilitation phase begins, in which the catch-up growth is the main focus, supported by nutritional rehabilitation through protein and energy supplementation. We will discuss treatment considerations for wasting in infants less than 6 months and children aged 6–59 months separately [5].

4.1 Treatment of Wasting: Infants Less than 6 Months of Age

The World Health Organization recently issued its guidelines for the prevention and management of wasting and nutritional edema in infants and children under 5 years of age [1]. The current WHO guidelines are an update of the previous guideline published in 2013, where the focus was on the treatment of severe malnutrition in children 6–59 months of age only, and infants were not considered [5]. The most recent guidelines included eight statements about the diagnosis and management of undernutrition in infants less than 6 months of age (Table 2). Of these statements, four were good practice statements and the rest were guideline statements that included strength of recommendation and certainty of evidence (Table 3). Overall, the focus is to define the criteria for admission, discharge, and outpatient follow-up. The approach to management of infants at risk of poor growth and development is similar to older children in that to stabilizes the infant in case of complications due to undernutrition, and then focuses on nutritional rehabilitation. Nutritional rehabilitation mainly revolves around the success of breastfeeding and supplemental feeds in case the breastfeeding/breastmilk is not available. The supplemental feeds are given with infant formula F-75 or F-100. The composition of F-75 and F-100 is

Table 2 World Health Organization recommendations for treatment of wasting in infants less than 6 months of age [1]

Considerations for the treatment of wasting in infants less than 6 months of age	Recommendation
Admission criteria **Strength of recommendation:** Conditional **Certainty of evidence:** Low	*(a) Infants less than 6 months of age at risk of poor growth and development who have any of the following characteristics should be referred and admitted for inpatient care:* (i) one or more integrated management of childhood illness (IMCI) danger signs; (ii) Acute medical problems or conditions under severe classification as per IMCI; (iii) Edema (nutritional); and (iv) Recent weight loss. *(b) Infants less than 6 months of age at risk of poor growth and development who do not meet any of the criteria from part a should have an in-depth assessment to consider if they need inpatient admission or outpatient management based on clinical judgement if they have any of the following characteristics:* (i) medical problems that do not need immediate inpatient care, but do need further examination and investigation; (ii) Medical problems needing mid or long-term follow-up care and with a significant association; (iii) Specific anthropometric criteria from the list of criteria used to identify infants at risk of poor growth and development: WAZ < −2 SD, WLZ < −2 SD, and MUAC <110 mm for infants between 6 weeks and less than 6 months of age, failure to gain weight based on two consecutive measurements; (iv) Ineffective breastfeeding or perceived breastmilk insufficiency; (v) feeding concerns for non-breastfed infants; and (vi) Any maternal-related or social issue needing more detailed assessment or intensive support. *(c) Infants less than 6 months of age at risk of poor growth and development who have all of the following characteristics should be enrolled and managed as outpatients:* (i) no danger signs or any of the criteria from part a needing inpatient admission and (ii) No criteria needed for in-depth assessment.

(continued)

Table 2 (continued)

Considerations for the treatment of wasting in infants less than 6 months of age	Recommendation
Discharge criteria **Strength of recommendation:** Strong **Certainty of evidence:** Moderate	*(a) Infants less than 6 months of age at risk of poor growth and development who are admitted for inpatient care can be transferred to outpatient care when:* (i) there have been no danger signs for at least 48 h before transfer time; (ii) All acute medical problems are resolved; (iii) Nutritional edema is resolving; (iv) The infant has good appetite; (v) documented weight gain for at least 2–3 days is satisfactory on either exclusive breastfeeding or replacement feeding; (vi) All attempts have been made to refer the infants with medical problems needing mid or long-term follow-up care and with a significant association with nutritional status to appropriate care/support services and/or the limits of inpatient care have been reached; (vii) The infant has been checked for immunizations and other routine interventions delivered or plans made for follow-up; and (viii) The mothers/caregivers are linked with needed follow-up care and support.
Outpatient management **Strength of recommendation:** Conditional **Certainty of evidence:** Very low	*(a) Infants less than 6 months of age at risk of poor growth and development can have a reduced frequency of outpatient visits when they:* (i) are breastfeeding effectively or feeding well with replacement feeds; and (ii) Have sustained weight gain for at least two consecutive weekly visits. *(b) Infants less than 6 months of age at risk of poor growth and development should be assessed (including assessment of their anthropometry) once they reach 6 months of age to determine if they need ongoing follow-up or referral to services for infants 6 months of age and older (including for nutritional treatment/supplementation) as appropriate according to their clinical and nutritional status.*
Approach to treatment: Management of breastfeeding/lactation difficulties and supplemental feeds with formula milk **Strength of recommendation:** Strong **Certainty of evidence:** Very low	*Infants who are less than 6 months of age with severe wasting and/or nutritional edema who are admitted for inpatient care:* (a) infants should be breastfed where possible, and the mothers or female caregivers should be supported to breastfeed them. If an infant is not breastfed, support should be given to the mother or female caregiver to re-lactate. If this is not possible, wet nursing should be encouraged; (b) should also be provided a supplementary feed: Expressed breast milk should be given, and where this is not possible, commercial (generic) infant formula or F-75 or diluted F-100 may be given, either alone or as the supplementary feed together with breast milk; for infants with edema, commercial (generic) infant formula or F-75 should be given as a supplement to breast milk. (c) Should not be given full-strength F-100 if they are clinically unstable and/or have diarrhea or dehydration and/or nutritional edema; and (d) should, if there is no realistic prospect of being breastfed, be given appropriate and adequate replacement feeds such as commercial (generic) infant formula, with relevant support to enable safe preparation and use, including at home when transferred from inpatient care.

Table 3 Composition of F-75 and F-100 formula

Constituent	Amount per 100 mL	
	F-75	F-100
Energy	75 kcal (315 kJ)	100 kcal (420 kJ)
Protein	0.9 g	2.9 g
Lactose	1.3 g	4.2 g
Potassium	3.6 mmol	5.9 mmol
Sodium	0.6 mmol	1.9 mmol
Magnesium	0.43 mmol	0.73 mmol
Zinc	2.0 mg	2.3 mg
Copper	0.25 mg	0.25 mg
Percentages of energy from		
Protein	5%	12%
Fat	32%	53%
Osmolarity	333 mOsm/L	419 mOsm/L

Adopted from WHO management of severe malnutrition [10]

given in Table 3. The F-75 formula is mainly used during the stabilization phase, followed by F-100. In case the F-75 or F-100 formula is not available, commercial generic infant formula can be used. The good practice statements include suggested guidance on diagnosis and management not covered in the guideline statements. The overall key message was that the criteria to diagnose wasting in this age-group are not well established and that treatment strategies should not only focus on the infant's health but also consider maternal physical and mental health [1].

4.2 Treatment of Wasting: Children 6–59 Months of Age

The approach to the treatment of wasting in children 6–59 months of age starts with the initial determination of the severity of wasting and the presence of complications. If the child has severe wasting and has complications based on the presence of signs and symptoms listed in the Integrated Management of Childhood Illnesses (IMCI), that patient qualifies for inpatient management for initial stabilization. Children who have severe wasting but do not have any complications can be managed as an outpatients. We will discuss the inpatient management of severe wasting first.

The inpatient treatment plan for severe malnutrition and wasting includes initial stabilization phase to address issues such as hypoglycemia, hypothermia, dehydration, and infection (Table 4) [2, 4, 5]. After the initial stabilization phase, patients are provided with a specialized liquid formula known as F-75. This formula is carefully calibrated to meet the unique nutritional needs of patients at this stage. Subsequently, a rehabilitation phase focuses on achieving steady weight gain, whereby formula F-100 is introduced through a carefully designed feeding regimen. Both of these formulas are adjusted to the specific requirements of each patient (Table 3).

Table 4 Initial stabilization of a child with severe wasting

Initial stabilization	Treatment
Hypoglycemia (defined as blood glucose <3 mmol/L (54 mg/dL)	If the child is conscious, administer 50 mL of 10% glucose or sucrose solution orally or by NG tube, followed by feeding as soon as possible. If the child is unconscious, administer 10% glucose or sucrose solution, 5 mL/kg IV or by NG tube, if IV is not possible. If oral, IV, or NG administration is not possible; administer one teaspoon of moistened sugar with one to two drops of water sublingually. Repeat every 20 min.
Hypothermia (defined as body temperature <35.5 °C (96 °F)	A warm child with a heated blanket or placed under an incandescent lamp. If these options are unavailable, the child can be warmed by close contact with the caregiver's body.
Infection	All hospitalized children are given ampicillin (50 mg/kg intramuscularly or IV every 6 h + gentamicin (7.5 mg/kg intramuscularly or IV once daily). For children who look particularly ill or in areas of antibiotic resistance, ceftriaxone (50 mg/kg intramuscularly or IV once daily) can be used instead. Prolonged diarrhea: Administer metronidazole (10–12 mg/kg orally every 8 h). Children should be tested for HIV as soon as possible. If not already treated with antiretroviral (ARV) drugs, these should be started as soon as possible. Doses of ARV should be the same as those without malnutrition. In areas of endemic malaria, some practitioners recommend antimalarial drugs for all children with malnutrition (artemisinin-based combination therapy).
High fevers (38.5–39 °C or higher [>102 °F])	Antipyretics (acetaminophen/paracetamol, ibuprofen, etc.) can be used to treat fever, but should be reserved for high fevers. Small risk of renal toxicity (ibuprofen) or hepatic toxicity (acetaminophen) when using these medications, especially in children with kwashiorkor. Aspirin (acetylsalicylic acid) should never be used in malnourished children.
Dehydration	Treat with oral rehydration. The child should drink rehydration solution for malnutrition (ReSoMal) by mouth; an NG tube can also be used. 70–100 mL/kg body weight of ReSoMal solution should be an adequate volume to restore hydration. Initial bolus: No more than 15 mL/kg over 1 h. A second bolus can be given if the child is not ready to hydrate by mouth. Caution should be taken with the IV route and monitored for signs of improvement (decrease in pulse and respiration rates).

Adopted from the WHO guidance on management of severe acute malnutrition [4, 5]
Abbreviations: *IV* Intravenous, *NG* Nasogastric tube

Patients admitted to inpatient care may transition to outpatient care when specific criteria are met. Firstly, they must exhibit no danger signs for a period of at least 24–48 h prior to the transfer. Additionally, the medical conditions that led to their admission should have improved to the extent that inpatient care is deemed no longer necessary. For children admitted with wasting, it is crucial that there is no ongoing weight loss, and particularly that they have not experienced nutritional edema. Any existing nutritional edema should have improved and no longer be categorized as severe (grade +++). Furthermore, the patient should demonstrate a healthy appetite. Lastly, all reasonable attempts should have been made to refer children with medical concerns requiring mid or long-term follow-up care, especially those significantly associated with their nutritional status, to appropriate care and support services [2, 4].

4.3 Outpatient Management of Severe Acute Malnutrition

The outpatient treatment of uncomplicated severe malnutrition involves administering ready-to-use therapeutic food (RUTF) at a rate of 150–185 kilocalories per kcal/kg per day [1]. RUTFs are dehydrated nutrition supplements designed to be easily administered in community settings, with minimal risk of contamination. Most commonly, RUTFs are oil-based pastes or spreads, and they can now be produced locally using basic technologies. These products have a high energy density of 5.5 kilocalories per gram and are composed of peanuts, milk powder, sugar, oil, and a mix of essential micronutrients. They can be stored without refrigeration in simple packaging for several months, are consumed raw, and their low water content prevents bacterial growth [11].

A Cochrane review evaluated the use of ready-to-use therapeutic foods for home-based nutritional rehabilitation and severe acute malnutrition in children from 6 to 59 months of age. The review included 15 studies consisting of 7976 participants, with most of the studies being conducted in Africa and Southeast Asia [11]. The meta-analysis of seven studies consisting of 2261 children in which RUTF was compared to alternative dietary strategies showed that RUTF improved the recovery rates by 33%; however, the evidence was not conclusive on the risk of relapse and mortality. When data were meta-analyzed from eight studies consisting of 5502 children, where WHO-based RUTF was compared with alternative formulations of RUTF, there was little to no difference in rates of recovery, mortality, and weight gain, however, the relapse rates were lower in the standard RUTF compared to the alternative formulations of RUTF. Overall, ready-to-use therapeutic foods have improved the outcomes in children with severe acute uncomplicated malnutrition and are recommended for outpatient nutritional rehabilitation of children in the most recent WHO guidelines [1].

4.4 Treatment of Moderate Wasting

The treatment of moderate wasting is mostly done in outpatient settings, with the focus on nutritional rehabilitation and prevention of exacerbation of episodes to severe wasting. The approach to the treatment of moderate wasting includes promotion of breast-feeding (for infants), introduction of appropriate complementary foods, treatment of the underlying condition, and use of supplemental foods. Table 5

Table 5 Definition of terms for supplementary foods for moderate wasting [12]

Lipid-based nutrient supplements (LNS)	These are ready-to-use foods consisting of lipid-based pastes (typically including ground peanuts) with added micronutrients that do not require refrigeration or preparation.
Fortified blended flours (FBFs)	"Combinations of partially precooked and milled cereals, soya, beans, pulses fortified with micronutrients. Improved fortified blended foods refer to products with added sugar, oil, and/or milk over and above what was in the original specifications for these products." the examples include super cereal (with added sugar but without milk) and super cereal plus (with added milk and sugar).
Corn–soy blend (CSB)	These are a type of FBF that does not contain milk and has lower concentrations of some micronutrients than enhanced FBFs. These are not as commonly used as they were in the past.
Ready-to-use supplementary foods (RUSF)	Fortified lipid-based paste/spread used for the supplementation of children with moderate wasting. These are RUTFs that have been adapted for use in the management of moderate wasting and should not be used for the nutritional treatment of severe wasting and/or nutritional edema.

gives the description of the most used supplementary foods for the treatment of moderate wasting. A recent systematic review evaluated the nutritional interventions for the treatment of moderate wasting in outpatient settings and included 17 randomized controlled trials. The results showed that lipid-based nutrient supplements lead to better recovery rates compared to fortified blended foods in terms of rates of recovery and changes in anthropometric outcomes. However, when the lipid-based nutrient supplements were compared to enhanced fortified blended foods, there was no difference in these outcomes [12]. The most recent WHO guidelines recommend specially formulated foods (SFFs) with counseling for children with moderate wasting. Among the specially formulated foods, lipid-based nutrient supplements were preferred, and when these supplements were not available, fortified blended foods with added sugar, oil, and/or milk were preferred compared to fortified blended foods with no added sugar, oil, and/or milk [1].

Lipid-based nutrient supplements (LNS) designed for preventing wasting or stunting are given in much smaller amounts (20–50 g/day), making them more concentrated in micronutrients and cost-effective. These products encompass essential nutrients such as micronutrients, essential fatty acids, and modest protein content, allowing for greater dietary variety. Commonly used ingredients in these products include peanut paste, vegetable oil, sugar, skimmed milk powder, and a pre-blended assortment of essential vitamins and minerals [13].

The current standard ration provided in emergency settings, consisting of cereals, pulses, fortified blended food (FBF), oil, and sugar, inadequately caters to the nutritional needs of vulnerable groups like infants, young children, and pregnant and lactating women (PLW). These groups exhibit heightened nutrient requirements for growth and development, which prove challenging to meet with limited food diversity and sources of micronutrients. Even with the inclusion of breast milk for children aged 6–24 months, the standard ration supplies less than 75% of the recommended intake for crucial micronutrients like calcium, iron, zinc, B vitamins, and fat-soluble vitamins. Relying solely on micronutrient supplements is insufficient, as there are also deficiencies in macronutrients. The FBF, originally intended for feeding children, may not adequately address the nutrient needs of infants and young children due to factors like poor mineral bioavailability. Implementing lipid-based nutrient supplements (LNS) for point-of-use fortification could effectively cater to individual nutrient requirements [13, 14].

According to the World Health Organization (WHO), in high-risk contexts characterized by recent or ongoing humanitarian crises, infants and children suffering from moderate wasting can also be treated as severe wasting. This entails the provision of specially formulated foods (SFFs) alongside counseling and the preparation of home-cooked meals for both the affected child and their families. This outpatient treatment approach is essential for managing moderate wasting in settings with limited resources. High-risk contexts are marked by factors such as elevated rates of food insecurity, inadequate water quality and sanitation, low socioeconomic status, and a significant incidence of wasting and nutritional edema, which may be seasonal [15].

4.5 Prevention of Wasting in Children Aged 6–59 Months

As noted in the conceptual framework for undernutrition by UNICEF, etiology of malnutrition involves multiple factors, and prevention of undernutrition requires a multisectoral and multisystemic approach [1, 7, 16]. The preventive approach includes interventions like food security, safe water, sanitation, and hygiene, and social protection services. The prevention of malnutrition starts with the health of the mother at the time of conception, healthy pregnancy and birth, and breastfeeding and appropriate complementary feeding during infancy and continuation of a diverse healthy diet during early childhood and adolescence, who will grow to be healthy mothers and fathers, thus a life cycle approach. American Academy of Pediatrics, World Health Organization, and Dietary Guidelines for Americans recommend exclusive breastfeeding for the first 6 months of life followed by appropriate, nutrient dense, diverse solid feet starting at 6 months of age with continuation of breastfeeding up to 2 years of age as desired by the baby and the mother [17–19]. Maternal education about appropriate complementary feeds has been shown to improve the growth of children [20]. In addition to education, supplementary feeding might be helpful in certain situations.

Supplementary feeding for infants entails introducing slightly denser and more diverse food options that can be moved to the back of the mouth using the tongue. This introduction typically begins around the age of 4–5 months, with small portions of semisolid food being offered at a time. It is common for infants to initially experience some difficulty in swallowing thicker foods, but this is considered a normal part of their development. As time progresses, both the quantity and frequency of supplementary feedings can be gradually increased. Supplementary feeding plays a crucial role in providing infants with vital nutrients, including essential vitamins, iron, and protein. It also introduces them to a variety of tastes and textures, which contributes to their overall development, particularly in cases where breastfeeding may not be possible due to medical reasons. Supplementary food should be culturally appropriate, easily accessible, and appealing in taste. In instances where fortified blended foods are unavailable, high-energy biscuits, particularly for pregnant women, can serve as an alternative. It is crucial to emphasize that supplementary feeding serves to complement regular meals and should not serve as a replacement for them. There are various types of supplementary feeding programs outlined as follows: Blanket supplementary feeding: This involves providing temporary assistance to high-risk groups, including the elderly, pregnant and breastfeeding women, young children, and individuals at risk of HIV/AIDS during emergencies [15, 21]. Its primary aim is to prevent a decline in nutritional health. Targeted supplementary feeding: This type of feeding is administered based on specific criteria, such as mid-upper arm circumference or weight-for-height measurements. It is directed toward elderly individuals, pregnant women, lactating women, and children aged from 6 months to 5 years who are acutely malnourished. Supplementary feeding linked to therapeutic feeding: This is provided to moderately malnourished children who have completed therapeutic feeding but still require additional support. In the most recent WHO guidelines, in areas with high food insecurity, specially formulated foods including medium quantity lipid-based nutrient supplements or small quantity lipid-based nutrient supplements can be considered for prevention of wasting and nutritional edema in children from 6 to 23 months of age [1]. The approach should focus on children living in the most vulnerable household through a targeted approach, however, when targeting is not possible, the supplementary food should be provided to all household through a blanket approach for infants and children from 6 to 23 months of age in addition to continuing the efforts to enable access to adequate home diets for the whole family [1].

5 Micronutrient Supplementation

Micronutrients refer to vital vitamins and minerals acquired from one's diet, necessary for day-to-day cellular operations. Micronutrient malnutrition (MNM), denoting the deficiency of these crucial elements, remains a prevalent issue in today's low and middle income countries (LMICs), particularly among infants and children. In these contexts, MNM can manifest in two ways: either from inadequate nutrient intake due to limited consumption of foods or a lack of dietary variety, or from hindered nutrient absorption due to infections, inflammation, or chronic illnesses, or even a combination of both [22, 23].

5.1 Vitamin A Supplementation

According to the World Health Organization, 190 million children are vitamin A deficient around the globe, with a majority of them living in low and middle income countries. Vitamin A deficiency (VAD) is a risk factor for infections such as diarrhea, pneumonia, and measles and can lead to death. Vitamin A deficiency is the most common cause of blindness due to a nutritional deficiency in the world [24].

A Cochrane review that assessed the effect of vitamin A supplementation for prevention of morbidity and mortality in children included 47 randomized trials that represented data from more than 100,000 children from low- and middle-income countries. The results of the meta-analysis showed that vitamin A supplementation reduced the risk of all-cause mortality and mortality due to diarrhea by 12% in the vitamin A supplemented group compared to the control; however, there was little to no difference in mortality due to measles, respiratory disease, and meningitis. Vitamin A supplementation reduced the risk of morbidity due to diarrhea, measles, and blindness, and vitamin A supplementation was associated with a small increased risk of vomiting within 48 h of supplementation [25].

Vitamin A supplementation programs have been one of the most effective nutrition interventions to reduce mortality and morbidity in children [26]. A recent analysis of dietary diversity of children from 51 low and middle income countries showed that very few children in low and middle income countries have diverse and adequate diets that would fulfill the recommended dietary allowance (RDA) for vitamin A intake [27]. Vitamin A supplementation has contributed significantly to improving the intake of vitamin A in children in low and middle income countries [26, 27]. Vitamin A supplementation programs also help deliver other interventions such as vaccinations and detecting severe acute malnutrition [26]. Vitamin A supplementation however is a temporary measure and there is a need to advocate for policies that would help eliminate the micronutrient deficiencies with strategies to increase the dietary diversity of foods, large-scale intervention such as food fortification and encouragement of crops with high content of vitamin A, as well as additional societal measure that help reduce poverty, inequities, and social injustice, which are the key determinants of undernutrition in much of the developing word.

5.2 Zinc Supplementation

Zinc is a crucial element in biological processes, playing pivotal roles in cell growth, differentiation, and metabolism. Insufficient levels of this micronutrient hinder childhood growth and weaken the body's ability to fend off infections, significantly contributing to health challenges and mortality rates among young children [28]. While severe zinc deficiency is uncommon in humans, milder forms may be prevalent, particularly in communities where there is limited intake of zinc-rich animal-derived foods and high consumption of phytate-rich foods, which impede zinc absorption. Identifying mild to moderate deficiency can be challenging, as symptoms like heightened vulnerability to infections and stunted growth are also indicative of other nutrient deficiencies and common childhood ailments [29–31].

The global prevalence of zinc deficiency is estimated at 9%, and about 2800 deaths are attributed to zinc deficiency according to the Global Burden of Disease 2019 [16]. The efficacy of zinc supplementation was evaluated in the recent Cochrane review that included 98 randomized controlled trials with 221,495 eligible participants, with 89 of the included studies conducted in low- and middle-income countries [29]. Even though the inclusion criteria for the Cochrane review were from 6 months to 12 years of age, most of the studies included participants less than 5 years of age. The most common form of supplementation was syrup, supplemented as zinc sulfate. The most common dose was 10–15 mg daily. The median duration of follow-up and included studies was 26 weeks. The results from pooled analysis showed high certainty evidence that zinc supplementation had little to no effect on all-cause mortality (RR: 0.93, 95% confidence interval, 0.84–1.03). Zinc supplementation also did not have a significant effect on mortality due to diarrhea (RR: 0.95, 95% confidence interval, 0.69–1.31) and lower respiratory tract infection (RR: 0.86, 95% confidence interval, 0.64–1.15). Preventive zinc supplementation, however, led to the reduction in all-cause diarrhea (RR: 0.91, 95% confidence interval, 0.90–0.93), but did not affect morbidity due to lower respiratory tract infection (RR: 1.0, 95% confidence interval, 0.96–1.08). There was a moderate certainty of evidence that zinc implementation improves height compared to control (SMD: 0.12, 95% confidence interval, 0.9–0.14). This effect size was, however, small and may not be clinically important. Zinc Supplementation was associated with an increase in the number of participants with vomiting (RR: 1.29, 95% confidence interval, 1.14–1.46) and had a negative effect on copper levels, and co-supplementation with iron decreased the efficacy of zinc supplementation. The World Health Organization currently does not have a recommendation for routine zinc supplementation for children. While considered safe, the necessity for daily administration poses programmatic challenges, including procurement, distribution, and adherence [32].

Zinc supplementation was studied for the treatment of diarrhea, which showed a reduction in duration of acute diarrhea by 0.5 days and a reduction in duration of persistent diarrhea by 0.68 days. Similar to preventive zinc supplementation, the therapeutic zinc supplementation during acute diarrhea led to increased risk of vomiting in the intervention group compared to the control [33].

5.3 Iodine Supplementation

Iodine deficiency is a major health concern in many countries, and it is estimated that about 1.9 billion people worldwide are affected by iodine-deficient disorders [34]. Iodine deficiency is associated with preventable deficits of central nervous system development and impairment of cognitive function, as well as highlighting problems [35, 36]. The most effective way to supplement iodine is through the ionization of the salt; however, more recently, other strategies such as fortification of food and condiments with iodine have been studied. A recent Cochrane review evaluated such strategies and included 11 studies consisting of 4317 participants [34]. Seven of these studies were conducted among school-aged children. The iodine fortification compared to control increased urinary iodine concentration, however, there was uncertain evidence on quieter prevalence, physical development, and growth outcomes. Currently, the World Health Organization recommends universal salt iodization and considers it a safe, cost-effective, and sustainable strategy to eliminate iron deficiency [36].

5.4 Micronutrient Powdered Supplements

Due to the coexistence of multiple micronutrient deficiencies, home fortification with micronutrients has been studied in children less than 2 years of age. A Cochrane review recently evaluated the efficacy of fortification with multiple micronutrients for children less than 2 years of age and included 29 studies consisting of 33,147 children. All the studies were conducted in low and middle income countries. The home fortification with multiple micronutrient powder reduces the risk of anemia by 18% in infants and young children compared to placebo and iron deficiency by 53%. There was, however, no effect on weight-for-age when the micronutrient powders were compared to daily item supplementation. However, there were fewer episodes of diarrhea compared to iron supplementation. The Cochrane concluded that the multiple micronutrient powder is efficacious for children aged 6–23 months living in settings with widespread problems of multiple micronutrient deficiencies [37].

5.5 Probiotics Supplementation

Probiotics are defined as live microorganisms that, when administered in adequate amounts, confer a health benefit to the host. Probiotic supplementation has been proposed as a therapeutic intervention for undernourished children; however, there is limited evidence for the efficacy of the use of probiotics in the treatment of undernutrition. A recent systematic review and meta-analysis assessed the efficacy of probiotics supplementation for undernourished children and included nine randomized controlled trials with 5295 children included in the review [38]. Data from seven of the included studies showed that their probiotics supplementation and little to no effect on weight-for-age and height-for-age [38]. Another systematic review assessed the probiotic supplementation for promotion of growth in otherwise healthy children, and probiotic supplementation had little to no effect on weight and height gain in high-income countries, however, there was a small effect on weight-for-age and height-for-age in studies from low and middle income countries. The evidence for these analyses was of low certainty [39]. Lancet nutrition series 2021 discusses the probiotic supplementation for children, however, no recommendation was made for the prevention or treatment of malnutrition in children [16]. This is an emerging area, and several trials are ongoing to assess the potential benefit of probiotic supplementation for the prevention and treatment of malnutrition [38, 39].

5.6 Adolescence Nutrition

About 17.6% of the world's total population (an estimated 1.8 billion people) consists of young people between the ages of 10 and 24 years. Most of this young population lives in low and middle income countries [40, 41]. The preadolescent and adolescent period is a transitional period in which there are unique physical, emotional, and nutritional changes compared to early childhood or adulthood. For example, the energy expenditure to support growth during this period is more than infancy. Also, the micronutrient requirements such as calcium, phosphorus, and iron are different than childhood and, even though the nutritional status during early childhood impacts the onset of puberty, adiposity, and growth, the nutrition during the adolescence period also has a determining effect on body composition, immune system development, and neurodevelopment [42]. Adolescent health is dependent on health during infancy and early childhood, and suboptimal health during the adolescent period might affect the reproductive age, including suboptimal outcomes of pregnancy and birth (Fig. 3).

Even though there are unique features and requirements of adolescence, there has been limited attention to adolescent health globally. There are significant disparities in adolescent health between high-income countries compared to lower- and middle-income countries. It is noted that the infant and child nutrition indicators have improved over the last five decades, however, the same improvement has not been seen for nutrition of adolescents. Prevalence of severe underweight is highest in South Asia, where about one in five girls between the ages of 5 and 19 years is severely underweight. It is also noted that overweight and obesity are emerging problems relating to poor nutrition among adolescents in developing countries [40–42].

Limited data are available to assess the impact of nutritional and micronutrient supplementation on adolescence. Iron supplementation and multiple micronutrient supplementation have been shown to improve the iron status in adolescent girls. Calcium supplementation showed an increase in bone mineral density. However, there was no improvement in linear growth [43]. Other nutritional interventions such as protein energy supplementation, have also been studied, however, the results are not conclusive, and more research is needed to define optimal nutritional interventions for adolescents [44].

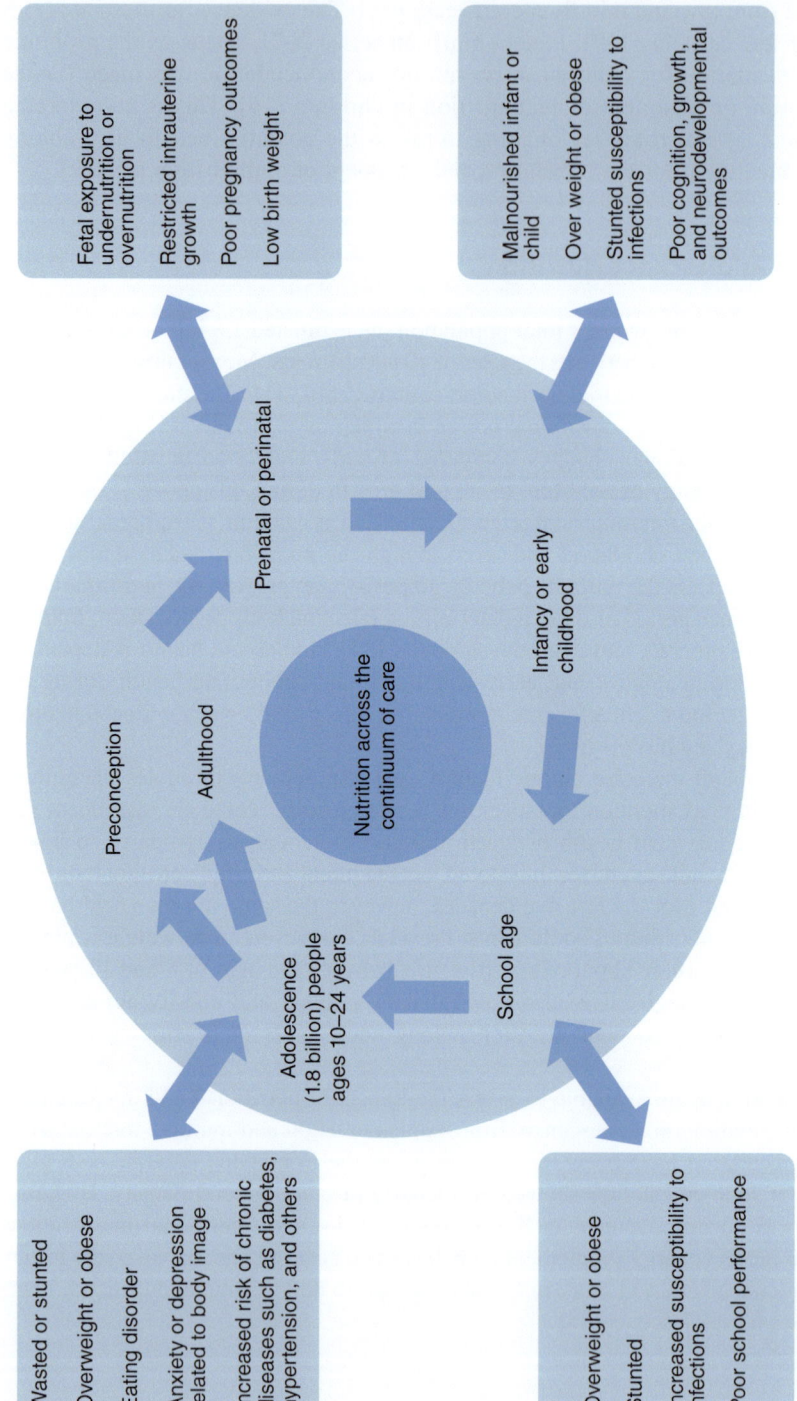

Fig. 3 Nutrition and related risk factors across the continuum of care. (Adopted from Lassi et al. [43])

6 Conclusions

Even though the rates of childhood undernutrition have decreased over the last two decades, millions of children are still undernourished and are at increased risk of morbidity and mortality. The approach to tackle childhood undernutrition needs to consider a life cycle approach with healthy mothers giving birth to healthy infants who grow to be healthy children and adolescents and enter the reproductive age in the best possible health. This approach needs an enabling environment at the individual and society levels with adequate access to appropriate food, hygiene, and sanitation, education, economic and political stability and social justice, and avoidance of conflict. Unfortunately, more resources are being spent on wars and conflicts, and the potential of next generations is getting lost in the midst of lost peace.

References

1. WHO. WHO guideline on the prevention and management of wasting and nutritional oedema (acute malnutrition) in infants and children under 5 years. 2023. Available at https://app.magicapp.org/#/guideline/noPQkE. Last accessed 17 Jan 2024.
2. Bhutta ZA, Berkley JA, Bandsma RHJ, Kerac M, Trehan I, Briend A. Severe childhood malnutrition. Nat Rev Dis Primers. 2017;3:17067.
3. Titi-Lartey OA, Gupta V. Marasmus. In: StatPearls [Internet]. Treasure Island (FL): StatPearls Publishing; 2023 Jan-. Available from: https://www.ncbi.nlm.nih.gov/books/NBK559224/. 2023.
4. WHO. Pocket book of hospital care for children: Second edition, Guidelines for the management of common childhood illnesses, release January 1, 2013. Available at https://www.who.int/publications/i/item/978-92-4-154837-3. Accessed 2 May 2022. 2013.
5. WHO. World Health Organization. Guideline: updates on the management of severe acute malnutrition in infants and children, release August, 2013. Available at https://www.who.int/publications/i/item/9789241506328. Accessed 22 Jan 2024. 2013 [Available from: https://www.who.int/publications/i/item/9789241506328].
6. United Nations Children's Fund (UNICEF), World Health Organization (WHO), International Bank for Reconstruction and Development/The World Bank. Levels and trends in child malnutrition: UNICEF/WHO/World Bank Group Joint Child Malnutrition Estimates: key findings of the 2023 edition. New York: UNICEF and WHO; 2023. Available at https://data.unicef.org/topic/nutrition/malnutrition/. Accessed 17 Jan 2024.
7. The United Nations Children's Fund (UNICEF). Conceptual Framework on Maternal and Child Nutrition, release 2020. Available at https://www.unicef.org/documents/conceptual-framework-nutrition. Accessed 15 Sept 2022.
8. Khara T, Mwangome M, Ngari M, Dolan C. Children concurrently wasted and stunted: a meta-analysis of prevalence data of children 6–59 months from 84 countries. Matern Child Nutr. 2018;14(2):e12516.
9. Odei Obeng-Amoako GA, Stobaugh H, Wrottesley SV, Khara T, Binns P, Trehan I, et al. How do children with severe underweight and wasting respond to treatment? A pooled secondary data analysis to inform future intervention studies. Matern Child Nutr. 2023;19(1):e13434.
10. WHO. Management of severe malnutrition: a manual for physicians and other senior health workers. World Health Organization, Geneva; 1999. Available online at https://www.who.int/publications/i/item/9241545119. Last accessed on 26 Jan 2024.

11. Schoonees A, Lombard MJ, Musekiwa A, Nel E, Volmink J. Ready-to-use therapeutic food (RUTF) for home-based nutritional rehabilitation of severe acute malnutrition in children from six months to five years of age. Cochrane Database Syst Rev. 2019;5(5):CD009000.
12. Cichon B, Das JK, Salam RA, Padhani ZA, Stobaugh HC, Mughal M, et al. Effectiveness of dietary management for moderate wasting among children >6 months of age-a systematic review and meta-analysis exploring different types, quantities, and durations. Nutrients. 2023;15(5)
13. Dewey KG, Arimond M. Lipid-based nutrient supplements: how can they combat child malnutrition? PLoS Med. 2012;9(9):e1001314.
14. Chaparro CM, Dewey KG. Use of lipid-based nutrient supplements (LNS) to improve the nutrient adequacy of general food distribution rations for vulnerable sub-groups in emergency settings. Matern Child Nutr. 2010;6(Suppl 1):1–69.
15. WHO. Supplementary foods for the management of moderate acute malnutrition in children aged 6–59 months. 2023. Available at https://www.who.int/tools/elena/interventions/food-children-mam. Last accessed 13 Jan 2024.
16. Keats EC, Das JK, Salam RA, Lassi ZS, Imdad A, Black RE, et al. Effective interventions to address maternal and child malnutrition: an update of the evidence. Lancet Child Adolesc Health. 2021;5(5):367–84.
17. U.S. Department of Agriculture and U.S. Department of Health and Human Services. Dietary Guidelines for Americans, 2020–2025. 9th Edition. December 2020. Available at DietaryGuidelines.gov. last accessed 19 Dec 2023 [9th Edition].
18. Meek JY, Noble L, Section on B. Policy statement: breastfeeding and the use of human Milk. Pediatrics. 2022;150(1)
19. WHO. WHO guideline for complementary feeding of infants and young children 6-23 months of age. Geneva: WHO Guidelines Approved by the Guidelines Review Committee; 2023.
20. Imdad A, Yakoob MY, Bhutta ZA. Impact of maternal education about complementary feeding and provision of complementary foods on child growth in developing countries. BMC Public Health. 2011;11(Suppl 3):S25.
21. Humanitarian Global. Supplementary feeding for infants. Humanitarian Global. Available at: https://humanitarianglobal.com/supplementary-feeding-for-infants/.
22. Imdad A, Bhutta ZA. Intervention strategies to address multiple micronutrient deficiencies in pregnancy and early childhood. Nestle Nutr Inst Workshop Ser. 2012;70:61–73.
23. Imdad A, Bhutta ZA. Global micronutrient deficiencies in childhood and impact on growth and survival: challenges and opportunities. Nestle Nutr Inst Workshop Ser. 2012;70:1–10.
24. WHO. Global prevalence of vitamin A deficiency in populations at risk 1995–2005. WHO Global database on vitamin A deficiency. Geneva: World Health Organization; 2009. Available at https://iris.who.int/bitstream/handle/10665/44110/9789241598019_eng.pdf?sequence=1. Last accessed 17 Jan 2024.
25. Imdad A, Mayo-Wilson E, Haykal MR, Regan A, Sidhu J, Smith A, et al. Vitamin A supplementation for preventing morbidity and mortality in children from six months to five years of age. Cochrane Database Syst Rev. 2022;3(3):CD008524.
26. Thorne-Lyman AL, Parajuli K, Paudyal N, Chitekwe S, Shrestha R, Manandhar DL, et al. To see, hear, and live: 25 years of the vitamin A programme in Nepal. Matern Child Nutr. 2022;18(Suppl 1):e12954.
27. Karlsson O, Kim R, Hasman A, Subramanian SV. Consumption of vitamin-A-rich foods and vitamin a supplementation for children under two years old in 51 low- and middle-income countries. Nutrients. 2021;14(1)
28. Kewcharoenwong C, Schuster GU, Wessells KR, Hinnouho GM, Barffour MA, Kounnavong S, et al. Daily preventive zinc supplementation decreases lymphocyte and eosinophil concentrations in rural Laotian children from communities with a high prevalence of zinc deficiency: results of a randomized controlled trial. J Nutr. 2020;150(8):2204–13.
29. Imdad A, Rogner J, Sherwani RN, Sidhu J, Regan A, Haykal MR, et al. Zinc supplementation for preventing mortality, morbidity, and growth failure in children aged 6 months to 12 years. Cochrane Database Syst Rev. 2023;3(3):CD009384.

30. Hess SY. National risk of zinc deficiency as estimated by National Surveys. Food Nutr Bull. 2017;38(1):3–17.
31. Hess SY, Wessells KR, Haile D, Rogers LM, Tan X, Barros JG, et al. Comparison of published estimates of the national prevalence of iron, vitamin a, and zinc deficiency and sources of inconsistencies. Adv Nutr. 2023;14(6):1466–78.
32. Imdad A, Bhutta ZA. Effect of preventive zinc supplementation on linear growth in children under 5 years of age in developing countries: a meta-analysis of studies for input to the lives saved tool. BMC Public Health. 2011;11(Suppl 3):S22.
33. Lazzerini M, Wanzira H. Oral zinc for treating diarrhoea in children. Cochrane Database Syst Rev. 2016;12:CD005436.
34. Santos JAR, Christoforou A, Trieu K, McKenzie BL, Downs S, Billot L, et al. Iodine fortification of foods and condiments, other than salt, for preventing iodine deficiency disorders. Cochrane Database Syst Rev. 2019;2(2):CD010734.
35. Victora CG, Christian P, Vidaletti LP, Gatica-Dominguez G, Menon P, Black RE. Revisiting maternal and child undernutrition in low-income and middle-income countries: variable progress towards an unfinished agenda. Lancet. 2021;397(10282):1388–99.
36. WHO. Assessment of iodine deficiency disorders and monitoring their elimination. 2007. Available at https://iris.who.int/bitstream/handle/10665/43781/9789241595827_eng.pdf;sequence=1. Last accessed 23 Jan 2024.
37. Suchdev PS, Jefferds MED, Ota E, da Silva LK, De-Regil LM. Home fortification of foods with multiple micronutrient powders for health and nutrition in children under two years of age. Cochrane Database Syst Rev. 2020;2(2):CD008959.
38. Imdad A, Pandit NG, Ehrlich JM, Catania J, Zaman M, Smith A, et al. Probiotic supplementation for promotion of growth in undernourished children: a systematic review and meta-analysis. J Pediatr Gastroenterol Nutr. 2023;77(6):e84–92.
39. Catania J, Pandit NG, Ehrlich JM, Zaman M, Stone E, Franceschi C, et al. Probiotic supplementation for promotion of growth in children: a systematic review and meta-analysis. Nutrients. 2021;14(1)
40. UNFPA. United Nations Population Fund; Adolescent and Youth Demographics: a brief. 2012. https://www.unfpa.org/resources/adolescent-and-youth-demographicsa-brief-overview.
41. Population Reference Bureau. Focus on youth most populous countries (Millions) 2017 China India United States Indonesia Brazil Pakistan Nigeria Bangladesh Russia Mexico. 2017. https://www.prb.org/resources/2017-world-population-data-sheet-with-focus-on-youth/. Last accessed 23 Jan 2024.
42. Feskens EJM, Bailey R, Bhutta Z, Biesalski HK, Eicher-Miller H, Kramer K, et al. Women's health: optimal nutrition throughout the lifecycle. Eur J Nutr. 2022;61(Suppl 1):1–23.
43. Lassi Z, Moin A, Bhutta Z. Nutrition in middle childhood and adolescence. In: DAP B, Silva ND, Horton S, et al., editors. Child and adolescent health and development. 3rd ed. Washington, DC: The International Bank for Reconstruction and Development/The World Bank; 2017. Chapter 11. Available from: https://www.ncbi.nlm.nih.gov/books/NBK525242/. Last accessed 23 Jan 2024.
44. Soliman AT, Alaaraj N, Noor H, Alyafei F, Ahmed S, Shaat M, et al. Review nutritional interventions during adolescence and their possible effects. Acta Biomed. 2022;93(1):e2022087.

Nutritional Interventions Among Children and Adolescents to Prevent/ Treat Overweight/Obesity

Doris González-Fernández, Paulo Augusto Neves, and Zulfiqar A. Bhutta

> **Key Messages**
> - Obesity trends are rising worldwide, especially in low- and middle-income countries. The multicausality of obesity involves aspects during pregnancy and early childhood, including social, family, and community factors that promote the intake of foods and beverages that are high in calories, energy-dense, but low in nutrients, as well as sedentary lifestyles.
> - Earliest interventions have shown best results. Interventions during pregnancy and early childhood show that the promotion of exclusive breastfeeding may reduce the risk of overweight and obesity during childhood, but the evidence is limited for the use of low-protein formula.
> - Interventions in preschool children that achieved significant improvements in reducing overweight and obesity, usually combined the promotion of a healthy diet with physical exercise, lasted at least 1 year, had long-term follow-ups, used a personalized and culturally adapted approach, and were implemented in home settings. Results of school- and health facility–based interventions were mixed.
> - Among children and adolescents, the combination of interventions was more effective in tackling the growing pandemic of excessive weight gain in individuals in this age-group.
>
> (continued)

D. González-Fernández · P. A. Neves
Centre for Global Child Health, Hospital for Sick Children, Toronto, ON, Canada
e-mail: doris.gonzalez@sickkids.ca; paulo.neves@sickkids.ca

Z. A. Bhutta (✉)
Centre for Global Child Health, Hospital for Sick Children, Toronto, ON, Canada

Centre of Excellence in Women and Child Health, Aga Khan University, Karachi, Pakistan
e-mail: zulfiqar.bhutta@sickkids.ca

- Interventions targeting overweight and obesity require the combination of healthy diet and physical activity, having a long-term follow-up, being context-specific and culturally appropriate, and considering various environmental factors that influence lifestyle choices, like schools, households, and marketing of ultra-processed foods targeted at this population.

1 Introduction

Overweight and obesity are defined as abnormal or excessive fat accumulation that may impair health [1]. Currently, there are no unified criteria for the classification of overweight and obesity among children and adolescents. The three most used international classification systems are the World Health Organization (WHO) Child Growth Standards for children under 5 years of age and growth reference data for children and adolescents (5–19 years) [1]; the US Centers for Disease Control and Prevention (CDC) that created standards using data from US national health examination surveys [2]; and the International Obesity Task Force [3], which is based on data from Brazil, China, the United States, the United Kingdom, Holland, and Singapore [4].

According to the WHO Child Growth Standards, overweight and obesity correspond to weight-for-height >2 standard deviations (SD) and >3 SD above the median, respectively, in children under 5 years; and in children aged 5–19 years overweight is defined as body mass index (BMI)/age >1 SD, and obesity is defined as BMI >2 SD [1]. The use of BMI as an obesity measure has several limitations, including possible bias when using self-reported weight and height and the fact that it does not directly measure adiposity, leading to under- or over-estimating individuals with excess body fat, particularly in certain racial or ethnic groups and in children born small for gestational age [5].

Irrespective of the classification used, the prevalence of overweight and obesity in children and adolescents has increased worldwide. It is estimated that 206 million children and adolescents between 5 and 19 years will live with obesity in 2025, increasing to 254 million in 2030. The rapid increase of obesity in this age-group is expected to occur mostly in low- and middle-income countries (LMICs) [6], considering that trends of mean BMI reached a plateau in high-income countries (HIC) [7]. The regions of the world with the largest increments in the age-standardized BMI for individuals 5–19 years between 1975 and 2016 were Polynesia and Micronesia, Southern Africa, Middle East and North Africa, and Latin America and the Caribbean [7]. The age-standardized prevalence of obesity rose globally, from 0.7% to 5.6% in girls and 0.9% to 7.8% in boys, in the same period [7]. Currently, Asia (17%), Africa (10.2%), followed by Latin America and the Caribbean (4.2%), Europe (2.6%), and Oceania (0.2%) are the regions with the highest prevalence of overweight among children in 2022 [8]. Using data from the NCD Risk Factor Collaboration [9], we show an increased trend in the prevalence of overweight (Fig. 1) and obesity (Fig. 2) between 1990 and 2016 among boys and girls aged 5–19 years in LMICs.

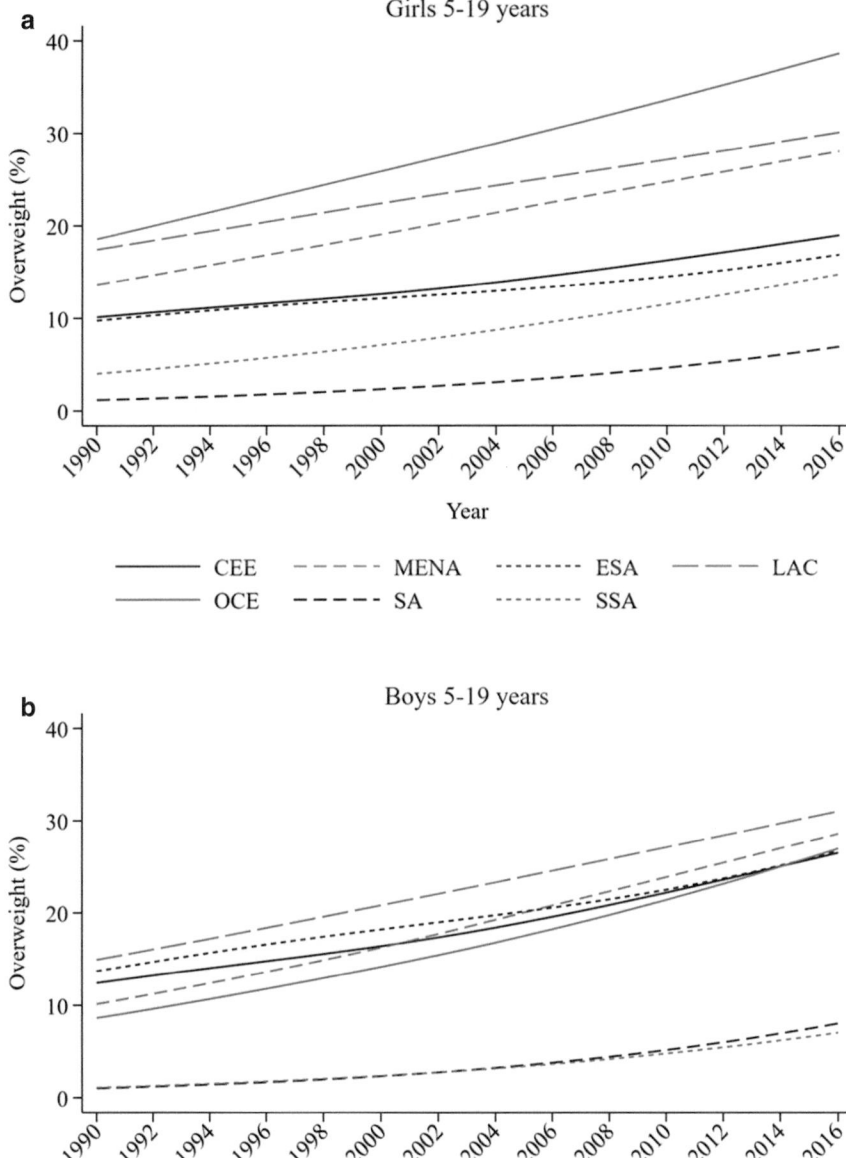

Fig. 1 (**a**) Trends in the prevalence of overweight per region in low- and middle-income countries between 1990 and 2016 among girls aged 5–19 years. (**b**) Trends in the prevalence of overweight per region in low- and middle-income countries between 1990 and 2016 among boys aged 5–19 years. (Data source. NCD Risk Factor Collaboration. *CEE* Central and Eastern Europe, *MENA* Central Asia and North Africa-Middle East, *ESA* East and South East Asia, *LAC* Latin America and Caribbean, *OCE* Oceania, *SA* South Asia, *SSA* Sub-Saharan Africa)

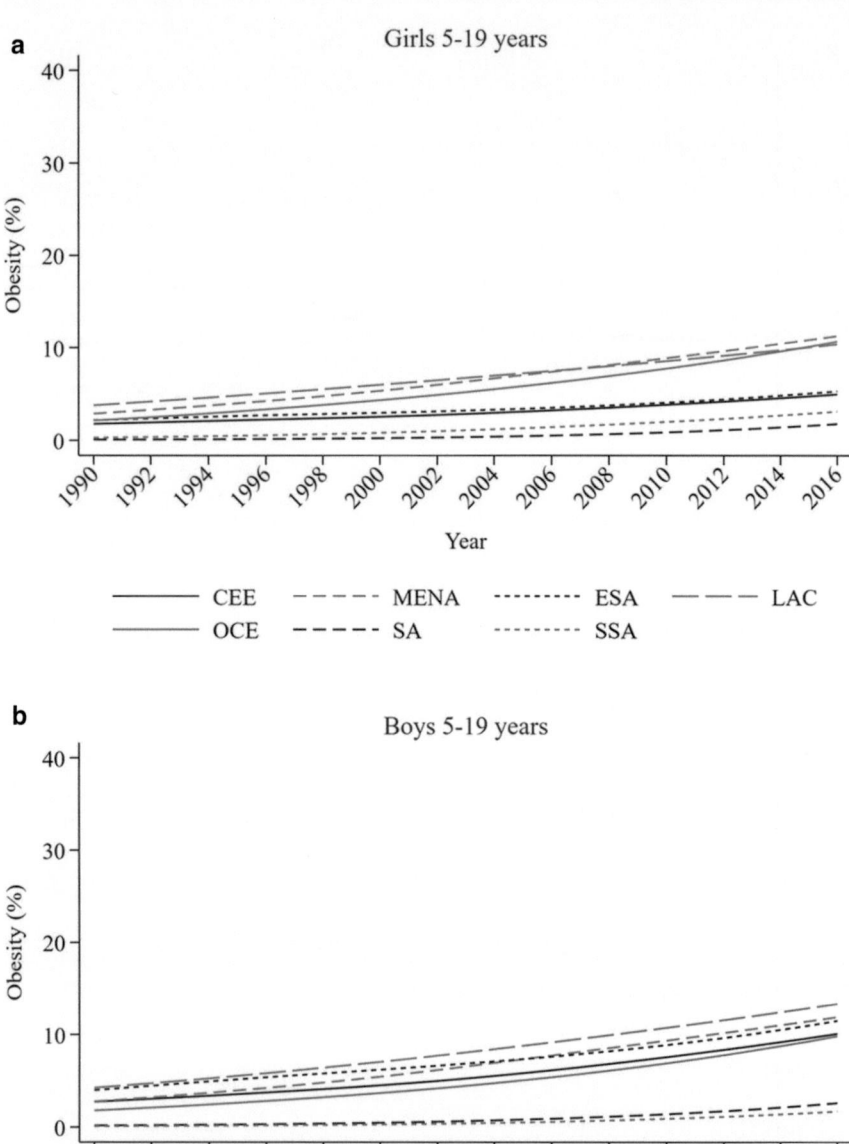

Fig. 2 (**a**) Trends in the prevalence of obesity per region in low- and middle-income countries between 1990 and 2016 among girls aged 5–19 years. (**b**) Trends in the prevalence of obesity per region in low- and middle-income countries between 1990 and 2016 among boys aged 5–19 years. (Data source. NCD Risk Factor Collaboration. *CEE* Central and Eastern Europe, *MENA* Central Asia and North Africa-Middle East, *ESA* East and South East Asia, *LAC* Latin America and Caribbean, *OCE* Oceania, *SA* South Asia, *SSA* Sub-Saharan Africa)

Obesity is a complex problem, involving the gut microbiome, the intrauterine environment, and low birth weight (LBW), where rapid changes in weight during infancy can lead to excessive adiposity and increased risk of metabolic disorders [10]. An "obesogenic environment" comprising social, family, community, and environmental factors that promote the intake of foods and beverages that are high in calories, energy-dense, but low in nutrients, as well as sedentary lifestyles, is a key driver of the increasing world trends in obesity [11].

Obesity in young individuals negatively impacts the productivity and the economy of families, communities, and countries. Medical costs are higher among obese children, and caregivers could be less productive at work because of caring for the sick children [12, 13]. In the United States, lifetime medical costs were estimated to be $25 billion higher compared to individuals who maintained a healthy weight during childhood and adulthood [14]. A recent meta-analysis estimated the increases in health costs associated with obesity in childhood worldwide, where obesity increased nonhospital health care costs by $68.2 per capita annually, outpatient visit costs by $20.9 per capita per visit, and the annual prescribed medication costs per capita by $64.7 [12]. Another study forecasted that the adolescent overweight rate between 1971 and 2000 would result in excess annual direct medical costs of $13.6 billion and annual indirect medical costs of lost productivity of $49.0 billion in 2050 [15].

In this chapter, we present evidence on the consequences of obesity throughout the lifecycle, obesity-related risk factors, and interventions addressing childhood and adolescent overweight and obesity.

2 Lifelong Consequences Associated with Obesity

Obesity in childhood and adolescence is a major challenge for children and their parents as it affects personal, societal, and economical aspects of life [12]. The current global escalation in overweight and obesity rates among children and adolescents is critical considering the long-term detrimental effects on health and well-being [16–18]. The increased adiposity alters metabolism, which affects regulation of diverse functions in the body, hence increasing the risk of adverse health outcomes throughout life and reducing life expectancy [16]. Additionally, the complex pathophysiology of obesity not only negatively impacts metabolic parameters but also influences psychological and economic factors and the community at large [17, 19]. The lifelong effects of obesity in childhood and adolescence are still understudied [20], especially in LMICs, where the long-term impact of obesity could be even worse owing to the lack of appropriate policies and poor health systems to cope with the consequences of noncommunicable diseases [21].

2.1 Mental Health

Body image, especially body weight, is a strong constituent of self-image in adolescence, and deviation from normal weight is often subjected to discrimination and stigmatization [22], which may have severe long-term implications for emotional and physical health and performance [23]. A European study found that adolescent obesity was associated with anxiety/depression (odds ratio (OR): 1.8, 95% confidence interval (CI): 1.3, 2.5) and withdrawal/depression (OR: 1.6; 95% CI: 1.02–2.5) [22]. Other psychological disturbances associated with body image dissatisfaction and the desire to be in an acceptable body shape can lead to self-guided dieting to extremes of pathologic conditions like bulimia nervosa, binge-eating disorder, and anorexia [16].

2.2 Metabolic and Cardiovascular Events

The increased adiposity expressed by higher BMI in young individuals has been associated with the early onset of diabetes in mid-adulthood [16, 20]. Insulin resistance is commonly observed in obese children [24], higher BMI in adolescents has been associated with higher glycated hemoglobin [25], and there is evidence demonstrating the importance of high BMI in children and adolescents as an independent risk factor for type 2 diabetes in mid-life [20, 26, 27].

There is robust evidence on the causal relationship between obesity in people younger than 19 years and increased risk of other cardiovascular outcomes, such as hypertension, stroke, and other fatal and nonfatal events among young adults [28]. A recent prospective cohort study found that youths between 3 and 19 years with high BMI showed elevated risk of adverse cardiovascular outcomes, such as high systolic blood pressure and triglyceride concentrations, from 35 years onward [29]. Some evidence supports the hypothesis that cardiovascular events in adulthood are more likely to occur when the individual is obese from childhood to adulthood [30]. In Taiwan, children with persistent obesity until early adulthood had higher odds of early onset of hypertension compared to obese children with normal BMI in adulthood [31]. Such early life adverse events are of great significance considering the association between higher all-cause mortality and BMI >25 kg/m^2 [32, 33].

2.3 Infections

Obese individuals are more susceptible to infectious diseases including respiratory, urinary, cutaneous, and surgical site infections, favored by impairment of innate and adaptive immune responses, and indirectly, by inapt respiratory mechanics, skin and subcutaneous tissue homeostasis, and obesity-related comorbidities [34]. The impacts of obesity on immunity have been highlighted by the increased severity of pneumonia and acute respiratory distress syndrome as causes of death from COVID infection [35]. It has been proposed that the increased risk for the severity of COVID infection in children may be related to micronutrient deficiencies and gut dysbiosis status [36]. Of note, the pediatric SARS-CoV-2 multisystem inflammatory syndrome, which causes significant morbidity (fever, gastrointestinal and cardiocirculatory manifestations, shock, and need of intensive care treatment) has been found to be associated with obesity as the only significant comorbidity [37]. Another evidence suggests that a high BMI in adolescents increases the risk of death by infectious diseases, especially among men [38].

2.4 Chronic Diseases

The World Cancer Research Fund recognizes that obesity is a significant risk factor for at least 13 different types of cancer [39]. Current evidence suggests that one of the potential mechanisms behind the association between obesity and cancer is the chronic inflammation derived from adipokines from adipose tissue [40]. Studies that followed up participants since childhood aiming at investigating the relationship between increased adiposity and cancer risk in adult life are scant. The Boyd Orr study with 50-year follow-up provided evidence that the relationship between high BMI and cancer risk is dependent on the age when obesity started. They reported that obesity in late childhood (8–14 years) was associated with cancer in adulthood (OR: 1.2, 95% CI: 1.05–1.4), but such association was not observed for obesity in younger children (2–8 years) [41].

Nonalcoholic fatty liver disease (NAFLD) is the most common liver disease in the pediatric population, and although considered as relatively benign, it can evolve into severe hepatic conditions, like fibrosis and cirrhosis [42]. This is probably because NAFLD is associated with obesity and its consequences, such as metabolic syndrome and insulin resistance [43]. Likewise for cancer, longitudinal investigations linking obesity, NAFLD, and other consequences are scarce for children and adolescents. One study reported that NAFLD in children and young people is associated with long-term mortality in a Swedish population (hazard ratio (HR): 5.9, 95% CI: 3.8–9.2) [44].

Novel evidence has suggested that obesity at younger ages impacts other diseases. One study found an association between obesity in adolescents and kidney-related mortality in adulthood compared to normal-weight individuals (HR: 8.4; 95% CI: 5.1–13.8) [38]. In women, polycystic ovary syndrome (PCOS) is a recognized risk factor for hyperandrogenism, anovulation, infertility, and adverse cardiometabolic and/or psychological outcomes [45]. Obesity has been documented in 30–80% of PCOS cases [46], and obese girls are considered to have a higher risk of PCOS [45], as childhood body size has been independently associated with higher odds of PCOS after adjusting for adult body size (OR: 2.6, 95% CI: 1.6–4.2) [46].

3   Risk and Protective Factors

Obesity has intergenerational impacts on health that have been elucidated by genetic and epigenetic studies. There is evidence of the important contribution of environmental factors such as an energy-dense diet combined with low energy expenditure [47, 48].

Maternal pre-pregnancy BMI and excessive gestational weight gain have been associated with birth weight >4 kg (macrosomia), which implies a higher risk of obesity later in life [49]. In developed settings, LBW is also associated with postnatal catch-up growth and greater abdominal fat, and despite the association between LBW and lower BMI in developing countries, studies have shown that LBW children have higher body fat mass and lower lean body mass in adulthood [54]. Observational studies have demonstrated that maternal obesity increases the likelihood of offspring developing obesity-related diseases such as coronary heart disease, stroke, type 2 diabetes, asthma, and neurodevelopmental disorders [50].

Obesity in childhood is primed by early exposures in life, where rapid weight gain (RWG), defined as ≥ 0.67 SD between two time points during the first 2 years of life, is a known risk factor for later obesity [51]. There is strong evidence from studies in HIC and LMIC that RWG during infancy is independently associated with later obesity, a finding that has been reproduced in term and preterm, normal, or LBW infants, as well as those breastfed or fed with formula [51, 52]. This association has been most recently challenged by evidence from a large German study, where obesity in 2–6 years of life rather than during infancy predicted adolescent obesity [53], showing that consequences of rapid infant growth may differ among populations.

Given that the amount of protein in breastmilk (around 1.03 g/100 mL) is lower than the one available in infant formula (1.3–1.9 g/100 mL), it has been considered that a higher content of protein in formula could increase the odds of RWG [54]. In a review including research from HICs, only one study over 12 showed an association of low-protein formula feeding with lower BMI at 6 years [55], but a study using discrete event simulation data generated from children born from overweight/obese Mexican women predicted that individuals who received low-protein infant formula (1.65 g/100 kcal, 62.8 kcal/dL) would have 10.5% reduction in the likelihood of developing obesity [56].

Current clinical recommendations for infants born preterm include the administration of high-protein formula, which has been shown to improve neurodevelopment [57]. In contrast, there is a debate for administration of high-protein formula in term infants born small-for-gestational-age from developed countries and in LBW infants from developing settings, given the cardiovascular risk later in life associated with RWG [52]. It has also been observed that formula-fed infants have higher energy intakes than breastfed infants, in part related to parental practices of mixing formula with cereal or increased density during formula preparation above manufacturer's recommendations, which have been associated with excess weight gain [54].

Beyond nutrition, the composition of breast milk or formula determines nutrient availability to gut microbiota in the infant, and the protective role of breastfeeding may be mediated by the presence of prebiotics, oligosaccharides, and antibodies, which can selectively modulate bacterial abundance, establishing long-term effects on gut microbiota [58]. Early feeding components determine the infant microbiome conferring either lifelong protection against obesity or irreversible establishment of microbial dysbiosis that may lead to overweight and its consequences later in life [58]. In fact, human milk differs between mothers depending on their weight status, allergic conditions, and birth mode and may in turn impact on infant microbiome and later health, therefore, obese lactating mothers may theoretically transfer "unhealthy" microbiota through breastmilk and increasing the risk of obesity in their infants [58–60], but to date, specific gut bacterial species related to the intergenerational transmission of obesity have not been identified [61].

Dietary factors contributing to obesity risk in children and adolescents include specific "unhealthy" eating patterns such as early introduction of sugar-sweetened beverages (SSB), skipping breakfast and meal spacing, portion sizes, and glycemic content of foods. The strongest evidence on dietary factors influencing obesity in this age-group is the intake of empty calories (high calories but low micronutrient content), SSBs, and the increased availability of these foods [6, 62]. Early introduction of (SSB) is of special concern in the complementary feeding period. A review of studies dating from 1980 to 2016 showed that in three out of eight studies from the US, early introduction (<12 months of age) of SSB was associated with increased risk of obesity in childhood [63]. A recent systematic review and meta-analysis of observational studies found that higher intake of refined grains [OR: 1.28, 95% CI: 1.05–1.56, $n = 3$], SSB [OR: 1.20, 95% CI: 1.09–1.33, $n = 26$], fast food [OR: 1.17, 95% CI: 1.07–1.28, $n = 24$], and meat [OR: 1.02, 95% CI: 1.01–1.03, $n = 7$] increased the odds of overweight/obesity [64].

Diet and lifestyle transitions between childhood and adolescence are important in the prevention of obesity. An important axis on obesity research during childhood and adolescence is the possible impact of SSB on the current obesity pandemic, which has been attributed to a decreased satiety with calorie intake from fluids, which promotes an incomplete compensation for energy in liquid form [65]. Factors influencing the consumption of SSB in children include the socio-economic environment and parental behaviors [66]. Consumption of SSB during childhood has been linked to obesity and cardiovascular risk later in life. For example, a Mexican study reported that increasing cumulative SSB intake during the preschool period was associated with an increased likelihood of obesity in 8–14-year-old children [67].

A complex myriad of other factors has been found to be responsible for the increased prevalence of obesity in childhood and adolescent ages. Family environment, including habits of physical activity (PA), screen use, and sleep, availability of community facilities for social support (childcare and schools), and green spaces, as well as larger socio-political context including food availability and marketing, transport systems, are all capable of influence individual's

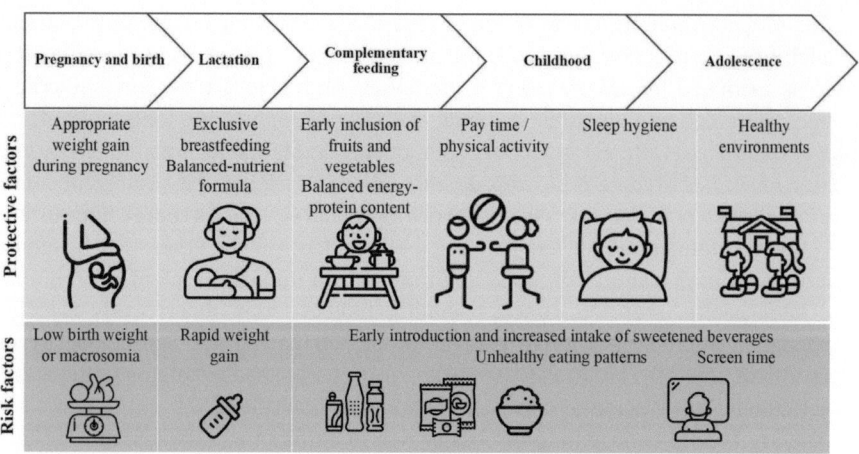

Fig. 3 Risk and protective factors for obesity from pregnancy to adolescence

behavior that modulates weight [6]. Children spend most of their time at school, and although schools provide a context to promote healthy eating behaviors and PA, more than 20% of young children are already at risk for overweight or overweight when entering school, therefore other demographic characteristics, health facilities, communities, and families need to be targeted for addressing the problem of child obesity [68].

PA, in particular moderate and vigorous exercise, is a main determinant of an individual's health as it modulates energy expenditure, controls appetite, improves mental health, and reduces cardiometabolic risks [69]. PA has beneficial effects on cardiovascular parameters and modulates inflammation through the reduction of visceral fat mass and its pro-inflammatory adipokines [70]. On the other hand, sedentary behaviors have been associated with higher fat mass and cardiometabolic risk in children and adolescents. For example, prolonged screen time can lead to erratic eating habits that can consequently lead to increased weight, and in obese children and adolescents, it has been associated with increased BMI, high blood pressure, and altered biomarkers of cardiovascular risk, independent of PA [69]. It is known that environmental and individual factors may prevent children and adolescents to engage in PA, with the most important barriers being gender, age, ethnicity, and self-concept, followed by the environmental support (family, friends, teachers). Important facilitators for PA are the accessibility to facilities and safe neighborhoods [71]. Therefore, multisectoral approaches are needed to be taken into account when designing interventions for reducing child obesity. Figure 3 shows a summary of risk and protective factors to be considered for designing interventions to prevent child and adolescent obesity.

4 Novel Strategies and Interventions to Prevent and Treat Obesity Among Children and Adolescents

4.1 Care During Pregnancy

The first 1000 years of life, from conception to 2 years, is recognized as a critical period of development and provides a window for preventing obesity later in life [72]. Interventions to prevent obesity targeting obese pregnant women have shown that diet, in particular reducing glycemic index, can help reduce excessive gestational weight gain (GWG), infant adiposity, and large-for-gestational age [73]. It has been shown that providing prenatal and postpartum nutrition counseling and parental support groups in low-income Hispanic mothers reduced mean weight-for-age trajectories in their children up to 2 years of age, but failed to achieve differences compared with controls at age three [74]. Moreover, increased protein intake during pregnancy has been shown to increase lean body mass (but not fat mass) in children at 6 years of age, whereas the intake of saturated fat, sugar, low n-3, and high n-6 poly-unsaturated fatty acids during pregnancy has been associated with higher childhood body fat [73].

The combination of diet, exercise, and behavioral change interventions has shown to be effective in decreasing the likelihood of weight gain above recommendations, but the evidence on improving neonatal complications such as macrosomia and respiratory distress, is limited [75]. Since majority of the evidence on the benefit of reducing GWG comes from observational studies, there is a need for randomized-controlled trials intending to decrease child obesity targeting the pre-pregnancy and pregnancy stages.

4.2 Early Interventions During Infancy

As per the Lancet Breastfeeding series published in 2016, breastfeeding showed a pooled reduction in the prevalence of overweight and obesity of 13% (95% CI: 6–19) in a sample of 1500 participants from 23 high-quality studies, after controlling for socioeconomic status, maternal BMI and perinatal morbidity [76]. Based on data from HICs, there is consensus on the beneficial effect of breastfeeding on healthy growth velocity and reduced risk of obesity, compared to accelerated growth and risk of obesity with formula feeding [77, 78]. A large cohort study in Ireland found 38% and 51% reduction in risk of obesity at 9 years of age with breastfeeding duration of 13–25 weeks and >26 weeks, respectively [79]. Moreover, the Canadian CHILD cohort study that followed 2553 children for 12 months, showed that breastfeeding was inversely associated with weight gain velocity, BMI, and overweight risk, whereas breastfeeding cessation before 6 months was associated with a twofold increase in rapid weight gain, a 0.44 SD increase in BMI, and a threefold increased risk of overweight, compared with exclusive breastfeeding for 6 months [80]. Few studies suggest that these associations might be similar in LMICs.

A multinational study with 4740 children from 12 HICs and 12 LMICs found that breastfeeding decreased the odds of BMI >2 SD at the age of 9–11 years [81].

On the other hand, the possible increased risk of obesity in infants who had received formula feeding has received less attention. Data from the Special Supplemental Nutrition Program for Women, Infants and Children (WIC) in the US, found an association between the intake of lactose-reduced infant formula replaced by corn syrup solids with 10% higher obesity risk at 2 years of age (Risk Ratio (RR): 1.1; 95% CI: 1.02–1.2) and 4 years of age (RR: 1.1; 95% CI: 1.01–1.1), after controlling for covariates [82].

Probiotics, added to infant formula, simulate the beneficial effect of maternal microbiota transfer through breast milk. Reviewed by Koleva et al. [59], supplementation with *Lactobacillus paracasei ssp.* of children from 4 to 6 months of age did not change BMI z-scores at 13 months of age or at their follow-up at 7 years of age [83], but another study that supplemented pregnant mothers with *Lacticaseibacillus rhamnosus* 4 weeks before delivery until 6 months post-partum, found reduced excessive weight gain in offspring during their first 2 years of life [84]. Despite promising results, the evidence supporting the use of probiotics for prevention of child obesity is insufficient, while further research is still needed to better elucidate the type and dosage of helpful strains as well as possible interactions with diet and environmental factors.

4.3 Interventions to Reduce Obesity in Preschool Children

A recent review of the literature between 2015 and 2018 including 16 randomized controlled trials in preschool children [85] found that diet or PA alone was not effective in reducing anthropometric measurements, but interventions that combined diet and PA reduced BMI with a mean difference (MD) of -0.07 kg/m^2, 95% CI: -0.14 to -0.01, and BMI z-scores with MD: -0.11, 95% CI: -0.21 to 0.01.

A systematic review of evidence published from 2010 to 2020 [86] evaluated diet and/or PA and/or behavior interventions to reduce obesity in preschool children. This review found that interventions delivered at school/childcare settings achieved a reduction of anthropometric measurements (BMI or derived measurements or body fat) if lasted at least 1 year, intervened for at least 6 months, and had long follow-up periods (until 2 years of age). Long-home interventions (lasting 4–6 months to 1 year) also showed to be effective. Among the five community-based studies included in the review, only one led to reduction in anthropometric measurements after 12 months, by providing personalized and culturally adapted nutrition and exercise education for mothers and children, together with coping skills training [87]. Among hospital/clinic interventions, two reported changes in anthropometric measurements; low intensity, low adherence, short-term follow-up, and inclusion of nonobese children were described as possible reasons for nonsignificant changes in anthropometric outcomes [88]. Providing personalized advice on diet and PA to obese children through mixing home visits and group-based clinic sessions decreased BMI z-scores and BMI percentile, and led to an improvement in dietary intake [89], but e-health interventions did not show any changes in anthropometry [86].

4.4 Interventions to Reduce Obesity in School-Age Children and Adolescents

Dietary interventions in children often consist of individual educational approaches, which, when not accompanied by environmental and behavioral choices, fail to show significant outcomes [90]. The review by Bleich et al. [91] synthesized evidence published between 2013 and 2017 and included 56 studies. 41 of them delivered interventions in school/after-school settings, 7 in community settings, and 2 in home settings. Most studies combined interventions for children and adolescents and were done in school settings. Commonalities among 24 school-based randomized controlled trials with successful results (reduction in BMI or BMI z-scores) included a combined diet/PA approach with the involvement of the home setting and an implementation time of at least 1 school year. One of the studies done in the United States, achieved lower BMI z-scores (difference $-0.06, p = 0.005$), decreased odds of overweight (OR = 0.71, $p = 0.004$) in children from communities that received improved walkability of routes to school, combined with improved quality of school food, education on healthy eating and PA, and newsletters to parents and community members with information about restaurants offering healthy food options [92].

Another quasi-experimental study targeting children of Mexican origin in the US that combined workshops on nutrition and PA for parents; nutrition and enhanced PA for children; and a monthly voucher for fruits and vegetables, reported mixed results at 2 years, including a decrease in BMI (ß-coefficient = $-1.94, p = 0.05$) and waist circumference (ß-coefficient = $-5.2, p = 0.04$) in obese boys. A follow-up assessment of the same cohort after 3 years of the intervention found an improvement in BMI in obese boys and girls, and also in normal-weight boys >6 years [93].

SSBs are a possible target for public health strategies in settings with high prevalence of obesity in children, and interventions promoting SSB excise taxation, policies on reduction in their sugar content, restriction on price promotion, and television advertising have been proposed [94]. Current WHO recommendation is to reduce free sugars throughout the life course, and in adults and children, to reduce the intake of free sugars to less than 10% of total energy intake [95].

Interventions that have been evaluated to prevent or manage weight gain among adolescents include behavioral interventions, pharmacotherapy, and bariatric surgery [91, 96]. In a recent Cochrane review of trials conducted in Argentina, Brazil, and China, Brown and colleagues found mixed or null results in reducing adolescent obesity in school-based interventions using PA and diet [85]. This review also found that there is very low certainty that PA interventions could reduce BMI and BMI z-scores among individuals between 13 and 18 years; even when combined with diet, the level of certainty is still low for BMI (MD: −0.02 kg/m^2, 95% CI: −0.10 to 0.05) and BMI z-scores (MD: 0.01, 95% CI: −0.05 to 0.07) [85]. Similar findings were reported in a review restricted to African studies where authors identified narrow and low-quality evidence of effectiveness of behavioral interventions on weight, BMI or body composition, and also limited effects of changes in dietary behavior on obesity outcomes [97]. The mixed effect of school-based and behavioral interventions in LMIC studies can be associated with the lack of consensus about the minimum duration needed for an intervention to be in practice to show effective results. In addition, an international consensus has not been reached on successful reduction in obesity among children and adolescents after the implementation of an intervention [98, 99].

Lastly, various individual and environmental factors might influence the uptake and success of lifestyle and behavioral interventions among adolescents [100]. Behavioral support interventions, including setting goals, environment modification, and self-monitoring aiming to produce changes in dietary habits, sedentary behaviors, and sleep hygiene have demonstrated modest but long-lasting reductions in anthropometry measurements and cardiometabolic indicators, and psychological interventions are often incorporated into the behavioral management of obesity to reduce barriers for change, usually targeting distorted body image, negative mood, and stimulus control [6].

At the clinical level, pharmacologic interventions have been proposed for obese adolescents who responded sub-optimally to lifestyle interventions, even though their use has been argued due to the modest effect and observed side effects [96]. Adolescents with severe obesity and associated comorbidities are candidates for bariatric surgery, which has shown long-term effects in weight loss and reducing health complications. Nonetheless, these practices although useful on an individual basis, have no effectiveness at population level and might not be affordable or available for most populations in LMICs [96].

5 Conclusion

Strategies to tackle the growing obesity epidemic among individuals younger than 19 years must recognize its complicated and multifactorial etiology [96]. However, most of the research on programs and prevention of obesity in the pediatric and adolescent population comes from high-income settings [85, 97]. The available evidence from LMICs on the prevention/reduction of obesity focuses mostly on school-based interventions and lifestyle changes.

The burden associated with overweight and obesity in young individuals will likely increase the health, social, and economic disparities within and between countries. The number of children and adolescents affected by overweight in marginalized communities in developed settings and in LMICs is increasing rapidly compared to high-income contexts, resulting in most countries failing to achieve the child malnutrition SDG target [8]. This alarming scenario calls for special attention when designing interventions and policies tailored to specific groups to address inequalities in reducing overweight and obesity in young individuals.

Current evidence shows that multidisciplinary approaches (diet, exercise, and behavioral interventions), including multiple settings (homes, schools, and communities), are recommended by most of the reviews, and we observed the need of an intergenerational approach starting with interventions during pregnancy and early childhood, to prevent the burden and consequences of overweight and obesity in children and adolescents.

References

1. WHO. Obesity and overweight. World Health Organization; 2021. Available from: https://www.who.int/news-room/fact-sheets/detail/obesity-and-overweight.
2. Kuczmarski RJ, Ogden CL, Guo SS, Grummer-Strawn LM, Flegal KM, Mei Z, et al. CDC growth charts for the United States: methods and development. Vital Health Stat. 2000;11(2002(246)):1–190.
3. Llorca-Colomer F, Murillo-Llorente MT, Legidos-García ME, Palau-Ferré A, Pérez-Bermejo M. Differences in classification standards for the prevalence of overweight and obesity in children. A systematic review and meta-analysis. Clin Epidemiol. 2022;14:1031–52.
4. Cole TJ, Lobstein T. Extended international (IOTF) body mass index cut-offs for thinness, overweight and obesity. Pediatr Obes. 2012;7(4):284–94.
5. Oken E. Maternal and child obesity: the causal link. Obstet Gynecol Clin N Am. 2009;36(2):361 77, ix x.
6. Jebeile H, Kelly AS, O'Malley G, Baur LA. Obesity in children and adolescents: epidemiology, causes, assessment, and management. Lancet Diabetes Endocrinol. 2022;10(5):351–65.
7. NCD Risk Factor Collaboration (NCD-RisC). Worldwide trends in body-mass index, underweight, overweight, and obesity from 1975 to 2016: a pooled analysis of 2416 population-based measurement studies in 128·9 million children, adolescents, and adults. Lancet. 2017;390(10113):2627–42.
8. UNICEF, WHO, Bank TW. Joint Child Malnutrition estimates (JME) – Levels and Trends – 2023. UNICEF; 2023. Available from: https://data.unicef.org/resources/jme-report-2023/.
9. NCD Risk Factor Collaboration (NCD-RisC). Height and body-mass index trajectories of school-aged children and adolescents from 1985 to 2019 in 200 countries and territories: a pooled analysis of 2181 population-based studies with 65 million participants. Lancet. 2020;396(10261):1511–24.
10. Menendez A, Wanczyk H, Walker J, Zhou B, Santos M, Finck C. Obesity and adipose tissue dysfunction: from pediatrics to adults. Genes (Basel). 2022;13(10)
11. Di Cesare M, Sorić M, Bovet P, Miranda JJ, Bhutta Z, Stevens GA, et al. The epidemiological burden of obesity in childhood: a worldwide epidemic requiring urgent action. BMC Med. 2019;17(1):212.
12. Ling J, Chen S, Zahry NR, Kao TA. Economic burden of childhood overweight and obesity: a systematic review and meta-analysis. Obes Rev. 2023;24(2):e13535.
13. Pelone F, Specchia ML, Veneziano MA, Capizzi S, Bucci S, Mancuso A, et al. Economic impact of childhood obesity on health systems: a systematic review. Obes Rev. 2012;13(5):431–40.
14. Levitt DE, Jackson AW, Morrow JR. An analysis of the medical costs of obesity for fifth graders in California and Texas. Int J Exerc Sci. 2016;9(1):26–33.
15. Lightwood J, Bibbins-Domingo K, Coxson P, Wang YC, Williams L, Goldman L. Forecasting the future economic burden of current adolescent overweight: an estimate of the coronary heart disease policy model. Am J Public Health. 2009;99(12):2230–7.

16. Kansra AR, Lakkunarajah S, Jay MS. Childhood and adolescent obesity: a review. Front Pediatr. 2020;8:581461.
17. Black RE, Victora CG, Walker SP, Bhutta ZA, Christian P, de Onis M, et al. Maternal and child undernutrition and overweight in low-income and middle-income countries. Lancet. 2013;382(9890):427–51.
18. Baek Y, Owen AJ, Fisher J, Tran T, Ademi Z. Lifetime impact of being underweight or overweight/obese during childhood in Vietnam. BMC Public Health. 2022;22(1):645.
19. Ng M, Fleming T, Robinson M, Thomson B, Graetz N, Margono C, et al. Global, regional, and national prevalence of overweight and obesity in children and adults during 1980–2013: a systematic analysis for the global burden of disease study 2013. Lancet. 2014;384(9945):766–81.
20. Horesh A, Tsur AM, Bardugo A, Twig G. Adolescent and childhood obesity and excess morbidity and mortality in young adulthood-a systematic review. Curr Obes Rep. 2021;10(3):301–10.
21. Niessen LW, Mohan D, Akuoku JK, Mirelman AJ, Ahmed S, Koehlmoos TP, et al. Tackling socioeconomic inequalities and non-communicable diseases in low-income and middle-income countries under the sustainable development agenda. Lancet. 2018;391(10134):2036–46.
22. Drosopoulou G, Sergentanis TN, Mastorakos G, Vlachopapadopoulou E, Michalacos S, Tzvara C, et al. Psychosocial health of adolescents in relation to underweight, overweight/obese status: the EU NET ADB survey. Eur J Pub Health. 2021;31(2):379–84.
23. Rankin J, Matthews L, Cobley S, Han A, Sanders R, Wiltshire HD, et al. Psychological consequences of childhood obesity: psychiatric comorbidity and prevention. Adolesc Health Med Ther. 2016;7:125–46.
24. Lee YS. Consequences of childhood obesity. Ann Acad Med Singap. 2009;38(1):75–7.
25. Skinner AC, Perrin EM, Moss LA, Skelton JA. Cardiometabolic risks and severity of obesity in children and young adults. N Engl J Med. 2015;373(14):1307–17.
26. Magnussen CG, Koskinen J, Chen W, Thomson R, Schmidt MD, Srinivasan SR, et al. Pediatric metabolic syndrome predicts adulthood metabolic syndrome, subclinical atherosclerosis, and type 2 diabetes mellitus but is no better than body mass index alone: the Bogalusa heart study and the cardiovascular risk in young Finns study. Circulation. 2010;122(16):1604–11.
27. Twig G, Tirosh A, Leiba A, Levine H, Ben-Ami Shor D, Derazne E, et al. BMI at age 17 years and diabetes mortality in midlife: a nationwide cohort of 2.3 million adolescents. Diabetes Care. 2016;39(11):1996–2003.
28. Sommer A, Twig G. The impact of childhood and adolescent obesity on cardiovascular risk in adulthood: a systematic review. Curr Diab Rep. 2018;18(10):91.
29. Jacobs DR Jr, Woo JG, Sinaiko AR, Daniels SR, Ikonen J, Juonala M, et al. Childhood cardiovascular risk factors and adult cardiovascular events. N Engl J Med. 2022;386(20):1877–88.
30. Zhang T, Zhang H, Li Y, Li S, Fernandez C, Bazzano L, et al. Long-term impact of temporal sequence from childhood obesity to hyperinsulinemia on adult metabolic syndrome and diabetes: the Bogalusa heart study. Sci Rep. 2017;7:43422.
31. Su TC, Liao CC, Chien KL, Hsu SH, Sung FC. An overweight or obese status in childhood predicts subclinical atherosclerosis and prehypertension/hypertension in young adults. J Atheroscler Thromb. 2014;21(11):1170–82.
32. Aune D, Sen A, Prasad M, Norat T, Janszky I, Tonstad S, et al. BMI and all cause mortality: systematic review and non-linear dose-response meta-analysis of 230 cohort studies with 3.74 million deaths among 30.3 million participants. BMJ. 2016;353:i2156.
33. Bjørge T, Engeland A, Tverdal A, Smith GD. Body mass index in adolescence in relation to cause-specific mortality: a follow-up of 230,000 Norwegian adolescents. Am J Epidemiol. 2008;168(1):30–7.

34. Pugliese G, Liccardi A, Graziadio C, Barrea L, Muscogiuri G, Colao A. Obesity and infectious diseases: pathophysiology and epidemiology of a double pandemic condition. Int J Obes. 2022;46(3):449–65.
35. Maurya R, Sebastian P, Namdeo M, Devender M, Gertler A. COVID-19 severity in obesity: leptin and inflammatory cytokine interplay in the link between high morbidity and mortality. Front Immunol. 2021;12:649359.
36. D'Auria E, Calcaterra V, Verduci E, Ghezzi M, Lamberti R, Vizzuso S, et al. Immunonutrition and SARS-CoV-2 infection in children with obesity. Nutrients. 2022;14(9)
37. Hoste L, Van Paemel R, Haerynck F. Multisystem inflammatory syndrome in children related to COVID-19: a systematic review. Eur J Pediatr. 2021;180(7):2019–34.
38. Twig G, Geva N, Levine H, Derazne E, Goldberger N, Haklai Z, et al. Body mass index and infectious disease mortality in midlife in a cohort of 2.3 million adolescents. Int J Obes. 2018;42(4):801–7.
39. World Cancer Research Fund (WCRF). Obesity, weight and cancer risk [Internet]. London: WCRF; 2023. Available from: https://www.wcrf-uk.org/uk/preventing-cancer/what-can-increase-your-risk-cancer/obesity-weight-and-cancer-risk.
40. Weihe P, Spielmann J, Kielstein H, Henning-Klusmann J, Weihrauch-Blüher S. Childhood obesity and cancer risk in adulthood. Curr Obes Rep. 2020;9(3):204–12.
41. Jeffreys M, Smith GD, Martin RM, Frankel S, Gunnell D. Childhood body mass index and later cancer risk: a 50-year follow-up of the Boyd Orr study. Int J Cancer. 2004;112(2):348–51.
42. Chalasani N, Younossi Z, Lavine JE, Charlton M, Cusi K, Rinella M, et al. The diagnosis and management of nonalcoholic fatty liver disease: practice guidance from the American Association for the Study of Liver Diseases. Hepatology. 2018;67(1):328–57.
43. Faienza MF, Chiarito M, Molina-Molina E, Shanmugam H, Lammert F, Krawczyk M, et al. Childhood obesity, cardiovascular and liver health: a growing epidemic with age. World J Pediatr. 2020;16(5):438–45.
44. Simon TG, Roelstraete B, Hartjes K, Shah U, Khalili H, Arnell H, et al. Non-alcoholic fatty liver disease in children and young adults is associated with increased long-term mortality. J Hepatol. 2021;75(5):1034–41.
45. Koivuaho E, Laru J, Ojaniemi M, Puukka K, Kettunen J, Tapanainen JS, et al. Age at adiposity rebound in childhood is associated with PCOS diagnosis and obesity in adulthood-longitudinal analysis of BMI data from birth to age 46 in cases of PCOS. Int J Obes. 2019;43(7):1370–9.
46. Dobbie LJ, Pittam B, Zhao SS, Alam U, Hydes TJ, Barber TM, et al. Childhood, adolescent, and adulthood adiposity are associated with risk of PCOS: a Mendelian randomization study with meta-analysis. Hum Reprod. 2023;38(6):1168–82.
47. Reichetzeder C. Overweight and obesity in pregnancy: their impact on epigenetics. Eur J Clin Nutr. 2021;75(12):1710–22.
48. Trang K, Grant SFA. Genetics and epigenetics in the obesity phenotyping scenario. Rev Endocr Metab Disord. 2023;24(5):775–93.
49. Lanigan J. Prevention of overweight and obesity in early life. Proc Nutr Soc. 2018;77(3):247–56.
50. Godfrey KM, Reynolds RM, Prescott SL, Nyirenda M, Jaddoe VW, Eriksson JG, et al. Influence of maternal obesity on the long-term health of offspring. Lancet Diabetes Endocrinol. 2017;5(1):53–64.
51. Fangupo L, Daniels L, Taylor R, Glover M, Taungapeau F, Sa'u S, et al. The care of infants with rapid weight gain: should we be doing more? J Paediatr Child Health. 2022;58(12):2143–9.
52. Singhal A. Long-term adverse effects of early growth acceleration or catch-up growth. Ann Nutr Metab. 2017;70(3):236–40.
53. Arisaka O, Ichikawa G, Koyama S, Sairenchi T. Childhood obesity: rapid weight gain in early childhood and subsequent cardiometabolic risk. Clin Pediatr Endocrinol. 2020;29(4):135–42.

54. Appleton J, Russell CG, Laws R, Fowler C, Campbell K, Denney-Wilson E. Infant formula feeding practices associated with rapid weight gain: a systematic review. Matern Child Nutr. 2018;14(3):e12602.
55. Patro-Gołąb B, Zalewski BM, Kouwenhoven SM, Karaś J, Koletzko B, Bernard van Goudoever J, et al. Protein concentration in milk formula, growth, and later risk of obesity: a systematic review. J Nutr. 2016;146(3):551–64.
56. Marsh K, Möller J, Basarir H, Orfanos P, Detzel P. The economic impact of lower protein infant formula for the children of overweight and obese mothers. Nutrients. 2016;8(1)
57. Isaacs EB, Morley R, Lucas A. Early diet and general cognitive outcome at adolescence in children born at or below 30 weeks gestation. J Pediatr. 2009;155(2):229–34.
58. Mohammadkhah AI, Simpson EB, Patterson SG, Ferguson JF. Development of the gut microbiome in children, and lifetime implications for obesity and cardiometabolic disease. Children (Basel). 2018;5(12)
59. Koleva PT, Bridgman SL, Kozyrskyj AL. The infant gut microbiome: evidence for obesity risk and dietary intervention. Nutrients. 2015;7(4):2237–60.
60. Kozyrskyj AL, Kalu R, Koleva PT, Bridgman SL. Fetal programming of overweight through the microbiome: boys are disproportionately affected. J Dev Orig Health Dis. 2016;7(1):25–34.
61. Tang M, Marroquin E. The role of the gut microbiome in the intergenerational transmission of the obesity phenotype: a narrative review. Front Med (Lausanne). 2022;9:1057424.
62. Singhal A. Obesity in toddlers and young children: causes and consequences. Nestle Nutr Inst Workshop Ser. 2020;95:41–51.
63. English LK, Obbagy JE, Wong YP, Butte NF, Dewey KG, Fox MK, et al. Timing of introduction of complementary foods and beverages and growth, size, and body composition: a systematic review. Am J Clin Nutr. 2019;109(Suppl_7):935s–55s.
64. Jakobsen DD, Brader L, Bruun JM. Association between food, beverages and overweight/obesity in children and adolescents-a systematic review and meta-analysis of observational studies. Nutrients. 2023;15(3)
65. Kunzová M, Maranhao Neto GA, González-Rivas JP. Sugar-sweetened beverages and childhood abnormal adiposity in The Czech Republic – narrative literature review. Cent Eur J Public Health. 2023;31(1):30–7.
66. Calcaterra V, Cena H, Magenes VC, Vincenti A, Comola G, Beretta A, et al. Sugar-sweetened beverages and metabolic risk in children and adolescents with obesity: a narrative review. Nutrients. 2023;15(3)
67. Cantoral A, Téllez-Rojo MM, Ettinger AS, Hu H, Hernández-Ávila M, Peterson K. Early introduction and cumulative consumption of sugar-sweetened beverages during the preschool period and risk of obesity at 8–14 years of age. Pediatr Obes. 2016;11(1):68–74.
68. Birch LL, Ventura AK. Preventing childhood obesity: what works? Int J Obes. 2009;33(Suppl 1):S74–81.
69. Julian V, Ring-Dimitriou S, Wyszyńska J, Mazur A, Matlosz P, Frelut ML, et al. There is a clinical need to consider the physical activity: sedentary pattern in children with obesity – position paper of the European Childhood Obesity Group. Ann Nutr Metab. 2022;78(4):236–41.
70. Calcaterra V, Vandoni M, Rossi V, Berardo C, Grazi R, Cordaro E, et al. Use of physical activity and exercise to reduce inflammation in children and adolescents with obesity. Int J Environ Res Public Health. 2022;19(11)
71. Hu D, Zhou S, Crowley-McHattan ZJ, Liu Z. Factors that influence participation in physical activity in school-aged children and adolescents: a systematic review from the social ecological model perspective. Int J Environ Res Public Health. 2021;18(6)
72. Rossiter C, Cheng H, Appleton J, Campbell KJ, Denney-Wilson E. Addressing obesity in the first 1000 days in high risk infants: systematic review. Matern Child Nutr. 2021;17(3):e13178.
73. Iglesia Altaba I, Larqué E, Mesa MD, Blanco-Carnero JE, Gomez-Llorente C, Rodríguez-Martínez G, et al. Early nutrition and later excess adiposity during childhood: a narrative review. Horm Res Paediatr. 2022;95(2):112–9.

74. Messito MJ, Mendelsohn AL, Katzow MW, Scott MA, Vandyousefi S, Gross RS. Prenatal and pediatric primary care-based child obesity prevention program: a randomized trial. Pediatrics. 2020;146(4):e20200709.
75. Farpour-Lambert NJ, Ells LJ, Martinez de Tejada B, Scott C. Obesity and weight gain in pregnancy and postpartum: an evidence review of lifestyle interventions to inform maternal and child health policies. Front Endocrinol (Lausanne). 2018;9:546.
76. Victora CG, Bahl R, Barros AJ, França GV, Horton S, Krasevec J, et al. Breastfeeding in the 21st century: epidemiology, mechanisms, and lifelong effect. Lancet. 2016;387(10017):475–90.
77. Owen CG, Martin RM, Whincup PH, Smith GD, Cook DG. Effect of infant feeding on the risk of obesity across the life course: a quantitative review of published evidence. Pediatrics. 2005;115(5):1367–77.
78. Qiao J, Dai LJ, Zhang Q, Ouyang YQ. A meta-analysis of the association between breastfeeding and early childhood obesity. J Pediatr Nurs. 2020;53:57–66.
79. McCrory C, Layte R. Breastfeeding and risk of overweight and obesity at nine-years of age. Soc Sci Med. 2012;75(2):323–30.
80. Azad MB, Vehling L, Chan D, Klopp A, Nickel NC, McGavock JM, et al. Infant feeding and weight gain: separating breast milk from breastfeeding and formula from food. Pediatrics. 2018;142(4)
81. Ma J, Qiao Y, Zhao P, Li W, Katzmarzyk PT, Chaput JP, et al. Breastfeeding and childhood obesity: a 12-country study. Matern Child Nutr. 2020;16(3):e12984.
82. Anderson CE, Whaley SE, Goran MI. Lactose-reduced infant formula with corn syrup solids and obesity risk among participants in the special supplemental nutrition program for women, infants, and children (WIC). Am J Clin Nutr. 2022;116(4):1002–9.
83. Karlsson Videhult F, Öhlund I, Stenlund H, Hernell O, West CE. Probiotics during weaning: a follow-up study on effects on body composition and metabolic markers at school age. Eur J Nutr. 2015;54(3):355–63.
84. Luoto R, Kalliomäki M, Laitinen K, Isolauri E. The impact of perinatal probiotic intervention on the development of overweight and obesity: follow-up study from birth to 10 years. Int J Obes. 2010;34(10):1531–7.
85. Brown T, Moore TH, Hooper L, Gao Y, Zayegh A, Ijaz S, et al. Interventions for preventing obesity in children. Cochrane Database Syst Rev. 2019;7(7):Cd001871.
86. Flynn AC, Suleiman F, Windsor-Aubrey H, Wolfe I, O'Keeffe M, Poston L, et al. Preventing and treating childhood overweight and obesity in children up to 5 years old: a systematic review by intervention setting. Matern Child Nutr. 2022;18(3):e13354.
87. Berry D, Colindres M, Lugo-Sanchez L, Sanchez M, Neal M, Smith-Miller C. Adapting, feasibility testing, and pilot testing a weight management intervention for recently immigrated Spanish-speaking women and their 2- to 4-year-old children. Hispanic Health Care Int. 2011;9:186–93.
88. Martínez-Andrade GO, Cespedes EM, Rifas-Shiman SL, Romero-Quechol G, González-Unzaga MA, Benítez-Trejo MA, et al. Feasibility and impact of Creciendo Sanos, a clinic-based pilot intervention to prevent obesity among preschool children in Mexico City. BMC Pediatr. 2014;14:77.
89. Stark LJ, Spear S, Boles R, Kuhl E, Ratcliff M, Scharf C, et al. A pilot randomized controlled trial of a clinic and home-based behavioral intervention to decrease obesity in preschoolers. Obesity (Silver Spring). 2011;19(1):134–41.
90. Pereira AR, Oliveira A. Dietary interventions to prevent childhood obesity: a literature review. Nutrients. 2021;13(10)
91. Bleich SN, Vercammen KA, Zatz LY, Frelier JM, Ebbeling CB, Peeters A. Interventions to prevent global childhood overweight and obesity: a systematic review. Lancet Diabetes Endocrinol. 2018;6(4):332–46.
92. Economos CD, Hyatt RR, Must A, Goldberg JP, Kuder J, Naumova EN, et al. Shape up Somerville two-year results: a community-based environmental change intervention sustains weight reduction in children. Prev Med. 2013;57(4):322–7.

93. Sadeghi B, Kaiser LL, Hanbury MM, Tseregounis IE, Shaikh U, Gomez-Camacho R, et al. A three-year multifaceted intervention to prevent obesity in children of Mexican-heritage. BMC Public Health. 2019;19(1):582.
94. Onyimadu O, Violato M, Astbury NM, Hüls H, Heath L, Shipley A, et al. A systematic review of economic evaluations of interventions targeting childhood overweight and obesity. Obes Rev. 2023;24(9):e13597.
95. WHO. Guideline: sugars intake for adults and children [Internet]. Geneva: WHO; 2015. Available from: https://www.who.int/publications/i/item/9789241549028.
96. Cardel MI, Atkinson MA, Taveras EM, Holm JC, Kelly AS. Obesity treatment among adolescents: a review of current evidence and future directions. JAMA Pediatr. 2020;174(6):609–17.
97. Klingberg S, Draper CE, Micklesfield LK, Benjamin-Neelon SE, van Sluijs EMF. Childhood obesity prevention in Africa: a systematic review of intervention effectiveness and implementation. Int J Environ Res Public Health. 2019;16(7)
98. Gross AC, Kaizer AM, Kelly AS, Rudser KD, Ryder JR, Borzutzky CR, et al. Long and short of it: early response predicts longer-term outcomes in pediatric weight management. Obesity (Silver Spring). 2019;27(2):272–9.
99. Steinbeck KS, Lister NB, Gow ML, Baur LA. Treatment of adolescent obesity. Nat Rev Endocrinol. 2018;14(6):331–44.
100. Salam RA, Padhani ZA, Das JK, Shaikh AY, Hoodbhoy Z, Jeelani SM, et al. Effects of lifestyle modification interventions to prevent and manage child and adolescent obesity: a systematic review and meta-analysis. Nutrients. 2020;12(8)

Non-health Sectoral Interventions

Educational Settings and Nutrition Promotion: Practices and Policy

Shelina Bhamani, Zahra Ladhani, Zaibunissa Karim, and Sameeta Chunara

1 Nutrition: A Life-Span Approach

Fetal development and infancy indicate a significant and rapid progression in the growth, development, and maturation of organs and systems. The nutritional intake of mothers during pregnancy and infants during their first year plays a crucial role because variations in the quality or quantity of nutrients can have lasting and influential impacts on development [1]. There is a strong link between various factors from the environment, biological, and social context on overall health and wellbeing. Early nutrition has a profound impact in shaping health and setting trajectories for lifelong wellbeing [2]. Undernutrition during infancy and childhood has a negative impact on children's cognitive development. However, the extent to which this impact lasts throughout adolescence, adulthood, and old age remains unclear. The link between nutrition in early and later life emphasizes the need of addressing nutritional needs throughout a lifecycle to support optimal health and development at all stages [2]. Each stage has specific needs, requirements, and food diversity, ranging from maternal nutrition, exclusive breastfeeding, balanced adequate diet for school-going children and teenagers, energy-rich foods for adults, and high protein diet for the elderly.

Nutrition education plays a crucial role in the development of individuals and communities. It helps improve healthy eating practices and increases awareness regarding proper nutrition to systematically improve the quality of life for future generations [3]. Educational efforts on nutrition and communication strategies for

S. Bhamani (✉) · Z. Karim · S. Chunara
Aga Khan University, Karachi, Pakistan
e-mail: shelina.bhamani@aku.edu

Z. Ladhani
Freelance Health Consultant, Islamabad, Pakistan

behavior change can enhance the knowledge, practices, and health outcomes related to infant and child nutrition. Nutrition education and counseling facilitates improvement in nutritional status and has been utilized to enhance maternal nutrition during pregnancy. Education is a crucial component in empowering individuals to drive the change toward a healthier lifestyle. Based on an understanding of the significance of education in fostering proper nutrition, policymakers, educators, and healthcare professionals can unite to design and implement successful interventions that address the complex challenges of nutrition-related issues. To understand the full impact of nutrition, the different stages of human development ranging from prenatal or conception time, infancy and early childhood, middle childhood, adolescence, early to middle adulthood, and late adulthood must be thoroughly examined [5, 6].

2 Nutrition Education and Behavior Change

Various studies have reported the positive influence of nutrition education in changing an individual's behavior to choose healthy nutritious foods, seek a balanced lifestyle, and make smart dietary choices [7, 8]. Interventions targeting behavior change provide mothers with pertinent information, foster shifts in their feeding practices, and enable them to tackle poor diets and insufficient food consumption [9]. Essential information for mothers involves appropriate knowledge on the types of foods to include, correct methods of food preparation in suitable quantities and combinations, and ensuring a safe and hygienic approach that fosters the healthy growth and development of children. Celis-Morales et al. (2017) investigated the theory that offering personalized nutrition guidance based on individual diet and lifestyle encourages more substantial, suitable, and enduring changes in dietary behavior. The promotion of behavior change communication interventions is crucial for delivering relevant information to mothers, and thereby influence their feeding habits. Consequently, empowering women, particularly mothers, with nutrition knowledge and skills can facilitate positively impacting child nutritional outcomes [10].

Nutrition education can foster a positive attitude and relationship with food, body image, and overall well-being. Education has a profound role in promoting adequate nutrition among mothers and children as it empowers them to make healthier food choices and encourages them to care for their overall health and well-being. Girard and Olude (2012) reported that nutrition education and counseling among pregnant women demonstrated significant benefits. It contributed to increased gestational weight gain and birthweight, alongside a reduction in late pregnancy anemia and preterm delivery. Notably, it demonstrated greater effectiveness when complemented by nutrition support, such as food, micronutrient supplements, or nutrition safety nets [4].

A comprehensive curriculum for children that incorporates nutritional health and well-being can facilitate the making of educated nutritional decisions [11]. Children can learn about the effects of nutrients on the body, read food labels to understand the nutritional value of what they eat, and be encouraged to include nutritious food in their meals [12]. Research, including longitudinal studies, has indicated that good nutrition can aid in the improvement of students' cognitive function and academic performance [13]. Consequently, children can become advocates for healthier school environments and influence their families' and community's eating habits [14, 16].

Nutrition education can affect all aspects of human life [17]. It can aid students in understanding the social and cultural influences of nutrition and food choices and thus respecting the diversity of cultures and food habits [18].

3   Strategies to Promote Nutrition Using Educational Platforms

The nutrition can be notably improved by employing multi-strategy interventions including nutrition education or counseling, particularly when nutrition education is grounded in theory and administered collaboratively via school staff, parents, and families. Such interventions, encompassing modifications to the school food environment, have demonstrated significant effects on anthropometric measures and dietary intake [19]. A comprehensive approach to promoting nutrition education includes an integrated curriculum coupled with learning experiences. The implementation of a comprehensive strategy to promote nutrition education requires a commitment from the entire school community and beyond.

- *Interdisciplinary Approach to Teaching Nutrition:* Nutrition education should not be limited to the science curriculum and for the purpose of assessment of learning. There is a need for an integrated curriculum that teaches holistic skills, attitudes, and habits in understanding and perceiving the value of nutrition on overall health and well-being. For example, during the science block, students can learn about the nutritional value of food items, read about the cultural differences in food preferences across the world, and make a shopping list of unprocessed food items that they can buy on their next visit to the supermarket [20].
- *Hands-on Learning Experiences:* To develop skills and habits, students require practical, hands-on experiences that can be powerful learning tools. Cooking classes, school gardens, and field trips to local farms or farmers' markets can all provide opportunities for students to engage with nutrition in a tangible way [21].
- *Healthy Meals in School Canteens:* The school environment should reflect upon nutritional principles taught in the classroom, This includes providing healthy meals in the cafeteria, ensuring access to fresh drinking water, and limiting unhealthy options such as bakery items, fried foods, carbonated drinks and beverages, and high-calorie snacks [22]. School meals can potentially cater to inequities as schools can offer subsidized meal program where, regardless of the socioeconomic background, students can access nutritious food.
- *Physical Education (PE) Classes:* Along with regular sports and physical activities, PE classes in schools can provide valuable insights into managing a healthy mind and body. Schools should provide regular PE classes and further encourage students to participate in physical activities. Regular physical activity is important for maintaining good health and complements nutrition education.

- *Integrating Technology:* Digital platforms, educational apps, and online resources can render nutrition education more interactive and engaging. In addition, they can reach students outside of the classroom [23].
- *Teacher Training for Support:* Teachers must be trained to deliver the integrated curriculum, provide relevant information to the students, and engage them in meaningful learning. They should be able to appropriately answer questions and encourage discussion in class and beyond regarding the care required for a healthy mind and body.
- *Parental Engagement and Involvement:* Schools should provide nutrition education materials for parents and even host informational workshops. As the primary caregivers of their children, the role of parents is vital for reinforcing healthy habits at home. Parents belonging to the healthcare sector could visit frequently by setting up health camps, giving talks on nutrition, and supporting teachers in effectively delivering classroom content on nutrition education. Schools can involve parents in nutrition education initiatives, such as workshops or cooking classes for parents, advisory on healthy lifestyles, meal planning, and community gardening initiatives [15].
- *Student Mentoring Programs:* Peer-led initiatives can facilitate the effective development of knowledge, skills, and understanding of nutrition. Older students can be trained to educate their younger peers regarding nutrition. Further, students can work on group projects to promote healthy eating within the school.
- *Holistic Teaching and Learning Environment:* The school staff and facilities should appropriately uphold the school's position on promoting nutrition. Teachers must function as a role model for promoting effective behaviors; for example, eating wholesome snacks and natural drinks. The school environment should advocate healthy eating habits; for example, providing fresh produce in school canteens, creating school gardens for planting vegetables, and facilitating consistent uptake of nutrition education and physical education.

4   Universal Models of Nutrition Education Promotion

- *Save the Children's School Health and Nutrition (SHN):* The SHN program tackles prevalent health issues among school-age children that can affect their learning. This program operates in 30 countries, and includes health education and health services such as deworming, micronutrient supplementation, and improved sanitation facilities. Through this program, students are taught to adopt healthier daily habits for general health, nutrition, hygiene, and communicable disease prevention such as AIDS/HIV. Furthermore, it contributes to quality education globally, aligning with the efforts being exerted to achieve global educational and sustainable development goals [23].
- *The Food Literacy Model (FLM):* The FLM framework helps individuals understand and improve their interactions with food. The program develops food literacy based on three progressive levels. The basic level, also known as the

operational dimension, is focused on a student's direct interactions with food; for example, understanding personal food preferences, accessibility to various types of food, fundamental knowledge of food origins, and the nutritional and sensory properties of food in relation to personal health. The intermediate level involves the student learning about the cultural dimensions of food. Further, it includes exploring their interactions with other people in their immediate environment and the influence of these interactions on food-related decisions; for example, the reasoning behind a person preferring to be a vegetarian. In addition, the level includes understanding family food preferences, the person influencing food decisions at home and school, and the manner in which food is accessed under both home and community settings (including gardens, supermarkets, farmers' markets, etc.). Finally, the advanced level (also referred to as the critical dimension) is focused on the student's interaction with the wider social environment. The student is taught how to make ethical food decisions based on by social factors, including media, culture, technology, and sustainability considerations [24].

- *Farm-to-Schools Model:* This model directly connects farms to schools to facilitate the delivery of fresh, healthy food in schools. Moreover, students can visit these supply farms for hands-on learning activities, such as school gardening, farm visits, and cooking classes. Several other models are used worldwide. Most such models have been developed by non-governmental organizations (NGO) as per the requirement; however, state-level policy-based interventions will be more effective and can leverage NGO initiatives as well [25]. For example, certain countries provide school meal program as a matter of state policy. This ensures that no child is left behind and every family is equally benefitted from the state-wide interventions.

5 Implementation Challenges for Nutrition Education Programs

The implementation of nutrition education is plagued by several challenges that must be addressed to facilitate its effective integration into the education system. One significant hurdle is the limited resources available to several schools, encompassing financial constraints, time limitations, and a shortage of adequately trained staff. Further, access and equity issues also contribute to the disparity in nutrition education availability, with socioeconomic differences resulting in uneven access to nutritious foods and reliable nutrition information. Moreover, the integration of nutrition education into an already packed school curriculum is difficult, particularly when faced with a lack of trained teachers and resources. The impact of industry marketing further complicates matters. This because conflicting messages from the promotion of unhealthy foods and drinks may undermine the effectiveness of nutrition education. In addition, ensuring cultural sensitivity within the nutrition education curriculum is challenging in diverse societies owing to factors such as religious preferences in food and lifestyle choices. Overcoming these challenges requires the implementation of innovative strategies that can better serve the population and promote a comprehensive and culturally relevant approach to nutrition education [26–28].

6 Future Direction

Considering future directions for nutrition education, there exist several key ideas that can ensure its success. The first is the need for robust policy support, involving increased funding, state-wide policy interventions, mandatory curriculum inclusion, and comprehensive teacher training to ensure successful implementation in schools and other settings. Further, a collaborative approach that involves coordination among states, NGOs, public health programs, advocacy groups, and policymakers is essential. This approach must integrate nutrition education into various subjects and foster interdisciplinary learning, potentially partnering with local food producers or community health initiatives. In addition, family and community engagement are critical, emphasizing the importance of raising awareness among parents and the broader community to reinforce the messages delivered under school-based nutrition education.

Technology can help advance nutrition education. Personalized nutrition education, tailored to an individual's unique dietary needs, preferences, and health status, can be integrated into national health and education systems. Mobile apps and wearable technology offer real-time information by tracking dietary intake and health metrics. Further, social media platforms and online communities can promote public health campaigns, general awareness, and community support. In addition, the incorporation of game design elements into nutrition education can enhance engagement and potentially facilitate better retention of information and behavior change. Meanwhile, addressing digital disparities and ensuring the safety and reliability of online content remain critical considerations [29, 30]. However, challenges such as unequal access to the internet and digital devices, quality control of online content, and privacy concerns limit the reach of online nutrition education programs. Finally, ongoing research, monitoring, and evaluation programs are crucial for assessing the effectiveness of interventions, identifying best practices, and continuously improving nutrition education programs at both the school and national levels.

7 Policy Recommendations

Evidence suggests that connecting nutrition and education not only alleviates short-term hunger but also positively impacts school enrollment, attendance, and cognition of children. Considering the strong role of the education sector in the prevention of all forms of malnutrition, engaging policymakers and informing practices through further evidence is extremely important [31]. Policymakers can play multiple roles in promoting nutrition within the education sector. Certain examples include: establishment and enforcement of nutritional guidelines that can address issues such as reducing added sugars, limiting sodium intake, and increasing the availability of fruits, vegetables, and whole grains. Policymakers can regulate the marketing of unhealthy foods and beverages in schools and can implement restrictions on the advertising, sponsorship, and promotion of sugary snacks, sugary drinks, and unhealthy fast food within school premises. This would help create an environment that supports healthy food choices. Another important role of policymakers is engagement with parents, teachers, school administrators, health professionals, and community organizations to develop and implement effective nutrition policies. Further, collaboration and partnerships help ensure that the policies are comprehensive, well-supported, and sustainable. Finally, policymakers must establish mechanisms for monitoring and evaluating the effectiveness of nutrition policies in schools. Regular assessment facilitates adjustments, identifies successful practices, and ensures accountability [32].

Education systems at the national levels can facilitate the delivery of strategies and interventions to promote nutrition. Teachers, school staff, students, parents, caterers, food vendors, and farmers can all help in promoting positive nutritional behavior. In schools, nutrition education should ensure that children and families learn to make adequate food choices. Schools should promote healthy food environments, with access to nutritious foods and safe and palatable drinking water, and zero tolerance for junk food and beverages. In certain cases, school feeding programs may be required for vulnerable children [32, 33]. Globally, there are several school-based nutrition programs, considering that the preexisting infrastructure of the educational system can often offer a cost-effective route for the delivery of simple health interventions and health promotion.

8 Conclusion

Nutrition and education are interconnected and are vital for the promotion of individual and community well-being. The relationship between education and nutrition comprises two specific components: the impact of education on nutrition and that of nutrition on educational outcomes. Nutrition education programs provide students with essential information regarding the importance of a balanced diet, nutrient requirements, food preparation, and the consequences of unhealthy eating habits. By equipping students with this knowledge, education empowers them to make informed decisions about their diets, thereby leading to improved nutritional choices and healthier lifestyles. Adequate healthy nutrition is crucial for physical, mental, and immunity health, and each stage of human life span development has specific needs, amount requirements, and food diversity requirements. Nutrition is a critical part of the health, growth, and development of human life, with each stage of the development process having specific needs, amount requirements, and food diversity requirements. Good maternal nutrition, exclusive breastfeeding, a balanced adequate diet for school-going and teenagers, energy-rich foods for adults, and a high protein diet for elderly individuals are essential. Nutritional fragility in vulnerable elderly individuals can cause sudden weight loss, loss of muscle mass and strength, and physiologic reserves, leading to disability. Many elderly people encounter nutritional challenges owing to socioeconomic constraints, lack of family attention, and physical limitations. The lack of adequate food and moderating factors such as food scarcity, clean water, poverty, inflation, high prices of food items, socioeconomic status, and children comparing with each other with limited resources, have long-lasting impacts on human health. Furthermore, nutrition has a profound impact on the educational outcomes. As reported previously, proper nutrition is crucial for cognitive development, learning, and academic performance. The adequate intake of key nutrients, such as vitamins, minerals, and omega-3 fatty acids, supports brain function, memory, attention, and concentration. Nutrition is essential part of healthy living and educational institutions act as a hub to promote nutrition education. The awareness in the school years can set trajectory of a healthy lifestyle for future. It can help decrease the burden of non-communicable diseases. Nutrition is one of the most under rated ways to improve the quality of life. It is beneficial to implement appropriate policies and practices to ensure that children receive the required nutrition that can lead to success in education. Educational institutions, educators, careproviders and parents must advocate for promotion of nutrition education.

- Make nutrition education as a separate mandatory elective in all schools and educational institution. Display health promotive messages related to food, nutrients, and healthy lifestyle across different spaces within the school boundary and beyond.
- Offer annual nutrition checkups for early screening of any red flags like malnutrition, stunting and anemia. Provide referrals to parents to ensure the identified risks are addressed well on time.
- Equitize knowledge for the communities that do not have access to the nutrition education by using a wide range of platforms engaging schools like having a radio show hosted by the school for community health and focus nutrition messages via it, school scout youth groups which could go to underserved communities for campaigns, school based pictorial newsletters promoting awareness for health food intake, and children theatre for community education on health, obesity, substance abuse etc. There may be several challenges in creating such solutions to these problems including equity, resources, and integration. However, we should all work proactively to spread the knowledge of nutrition to better the lives of many populations.
- Nutrition is a way to improve the quality of life. It is beneficial to implement appropriate policies and practices to ensure that children receive the required nutrition education that can lead to success in education.

References

1. Langley-Evans SC. Nutrition in early life and the programming of adult disease: a review. J Hum Nutr Diet. 2015;28:1–14.
2. Halfon N, Forrest CB, Lerner RM, Faustman EM. Handbook of life course health development. 2018.

3. Sakthivel SJ, Hay P, Mannan H. A scoping review on the association between night eating syndrome and physical health, health-related quality of life, sleep and weight status in adults. Nutrients. 2023;15(12):2791.
4. Girard AW, Olude O. Nutrition education and counselling provided during pregnancy: effects on maternal, neonatal and child health outcomes. Paediatr Perinat Epidemiol. 2012;26:191–204.
5. Murimi MW, Moyeda-Carabaza AF, Nguyen B, Saha S, Amin R, Njike V. Factors that contribute to effective nutrition education interventions in children: a systematic review. Nutr Rev. 2018;76(8):553–80.
6. Balasundaram P, Avulakunta ID. Human Growth and Development. 2023 Mar 8. In: StatPearls [Internet]. Treasure Island (FL): StatPearls Publishing; 2025. PMID: 33620844.
7. Yang SC, Luo YF, Chiang C-H. Electronic health literacy and dietary behaviors in Taiwanese college students: cross-sectional study. J Med Internet Res. 2019;21(11):e13140.
8. Gold A, Larson M, Simpson J, Strang M. Classroom nutrition education combined with USDA'S fruit and vegetable snack program improves children's fruit and vegetable intake. J Nutr Educ Behav. 2015;47(4):S78.
9. Timlin D, McCormack JM, Kerr M, Keaver L, Simpson EE. Are dietary interventions with a behaviour change theoretical framework effective in changing dietary patterns? A systematic review. BMC Public Health. 2020;20:1–18.
10. Celis-Morales C, Livingstone KM, Marsaux CF, Macready AL, Fallaize R, O'Donovan CB, et al. Effect of personalized nutrition on health-related behaviour change: evidence from the Food4Me European randomized controlled trial. Int J Epidemiol. 2017;46(2):578–88.
11. Kumar B, Shrotriya VP, Srivastava PM, Mahmood SE, Srivastava A. Nutritional status of school-age children-a scenario of urban slums in India. Arch Public Health. 2012;70:8.
12. Baranowski T, Ryan C, Hoyos-Cespedes A, Lu AS. Nutrition education and dietary behavior change games: a scoping review. Games Health J. 2019;8(3):153–76.
13. Cohen JF, Hecht AA, McLoughlin GM, Turner L, Schwartz MB. Universal school meals and associations with student participation, attendance, academic performance, diet quality, food security, and body mass index: a systematic review. Nutrients. 2021;13(3):911.
14. Grantham-McGregor SM, Fernald LC, Kagawa RM, Walker S. Effects of integrated child development and nutrition interventions on child development and nutritional status. Ann N Y Acad Sci. 2014;1308(1):11–32.
15. Larson N, Ward DS, Neelon SB, Story M. What role can child-care settings play in obesity prevention? A review of the evidence and call for research efforts. J Am Diet Assoc. 2011;111(9):1343–62.
16. Tonetti L, Fabbri M, Filardi M, Martoni M, Natale V. The association between higher body mass index and poor school performance in high school students. Pediatr Obes. 2016;11(6):e27–e9.
17. Carraway-Stage V, Henson SR, Dipper A, Spangler H, Ash SL, Goodell LS. Understanding the state of nutrition education in the Head Start classroom: a qualitative approach. Am J Health Educ. 2014;45(1):52–62.
18. Critch JN. School nutrition: support for providing healthy food and beverage choices in schools. Paediatr Child Health. 2020;25(1):33–8.
19. Meiklejohn S, Ryan L, Palermo C. A systematic review of the impact of multi-strategy nutrition education programs on health and nutrition of adolescents. J Nutr Educ Behav. 2016;48(9):631–46. e1
20. Oostindjer M, Aschemann-Witzel J, Wang Q, Skuland SE, Egelandsdal B, Amdam GV, et al. Are school meals a viable and sustainable tool to improve the healthiness and sustainability of children's diet and food consumption? A cross-national comparative perspective. Crit Rev Food Sci Nutr. 2017;57(18):3942–58.
21. Graziose MM, Koch PA, Wang YC, Gray HL, Contento IR. Cost-effectiveness of a nutrition education curriculum intervention in elementary schools. J Nutr Educ Behav. 2017;49(8):684–91. e1.

22. Forrestal S, Potamites E, Guthrie J, Paxton N. Associations among food security, school meal participation, and students' diet quality in the first school nutrition and meal cost study. Nutrients. 2021;13(2):307.
23. Chau MM, Burgermaster M, Mamykina L. The use of social media in nutrition interventions for adolescents and young adults—a systematic review. Int J Med Inform. 2018;120:77–91.
24. Perry EA, Thomas H, Samra HR, Edmonstone S, Davidson L, Faulkner A, et al. Identifying attributes of food literacy: a scoping review. Public Health Nutr. 2017;20(13):2406–15.
25. Harrison K, Bost KK, McBride BA, Donovan SM, Grigsby-Toussaint DS, Kim J, et al. Toward a developmental conceptualization of contributors to overweight and obesity in childhood: the Six-Cs model. Child Dev Perspect. 2011;5(1):50–8.
26. Truman E, Elliott C. Barriers to food literacy: a conceptual model to explore factors inhibiting proficiency. J Nutr Educ Behav. 2019;51(1):107–11.
27. Fulkerson JA, Kubik MY, Rydell S, Boutelle KN, Garwick A, Story M, et al. Focus groups with working parents of school-aged children: what's needed to improve family meals? J Nutr Educ Behav. 2011;43(3):189–93.
28. Hall E, Chai W, Albrecht JA. A qualitative phenomenological exploration of teachers' experience with nutrition education. Am J Health Educ. 2016;47(3):136–48.
29. Tian J, Bryksa BC, Yada RY. Feeding the world into the future–food and nutrition security: the role of food science and technology. Front Life Sci. 2016;9(3):155–66.
30. Olson CM. Behavioral nutrition interventions using e-and m-health communication technologies: a narrative review. Annu Rev Nutr. 2016;36:647–64.
31. Bhutta ZA, Das JK, Rizvi A, Gaffey MF, Walker N, Horton S, et al. Evidence-based interventions for improvement of maternal and child nutrition: what can be done and at what cost? Lancet. 2013;382(9890):452–77.
32. Lepre B, Trigueiro H, Johnsen JT, Khalid AA, Ball L, Ray S. Global architecture for the nutrition training of health professionals: a scoping review and blueprint for next steps. BMJ Nutr Prev Health. 2022;5(1):106.
33. Cusick SE, Georgieff MK. The role of nutrition in brain development: the golden opportunity of the "first 1000 days". J Pediatr. 2016;175:16–21.

The Complementary Role of Social Protection Programs in Tackling Malnutrition

Wafa Aftab

Undernutrition among children and women of reproductive age has substantially decreased globally in the last few decades. The prevalence of stunting among children younger than 5 years of age reduced from 32.5% to 21.9% between 2000 and 2017 worldwide [1]. Wasting in this age group decreased from 10% in 2005 to 7.3% in 2017 [1]. Among women of reproductive age, the prevalence of low body mass index (BMI) fell from 14.6% to 9.7% from 1975 to 2014 [2]. While this is a welcome trend, there is still significant progress to be made in low- and middle-income contexts, particularly in low-income countries (LICs) [1]. According to the World Health Organization (WHO), the United Nations Children's Fund (UNICEF), and the World Bank's 2021 Joint Child Malnutrition Estimates [3], in 2020, globally, there were still 149.2 million children under the age of 5 years who were stunted and 45.4 million who were wasted. The report shows that the problem is particularly severe in LICs; the number of children with stunting is declining in all regions of the world except in Africa, and more than half of all children globally affected by stunting live in South Asia.

While many low- and middle-income countries (LMICs) are still grappling with the problem of undernutrition, they are facing a concomitant rise in overnutrition marked by increasing prevalence of overweight and obesity. According to the WHO/UNICEF 2021 report, there were 38.9 million overweight children under the age of 5 years globally, of whom 48% lived in Asia and 27% in Africa. Some children suffer from more than one form of malnutrition, e.g., stunting and overweight or stunting and wasting—there are no reliable global estimates for such instances of compound malnutrition. These estimates indicate that to achieve these

---

W. Aftab (✉)
Department of Community Health Sciences, Aga Khan University, Karachi, Pakistan
e-mail: wafa.aftab@aku.edu

© The Author(s), under exclusive license to Springer Nature Switzerland AG 2025
Z. S. Lassi, R. A. Salam (eds.), *Nutrition Across Reproductive, Maternal, Neonatal, Child, and Adolescent Health Care*,
https://doi.org/10.1007/978-3-031-95721-5_13

nutrition-related goals by 2030, the reduction in stunting and wasting will have to be accelerated, and the trends of increasing overweight will have to be reversed.

Improvement in these trends is vital because a high prevalence of under- and overnutrition has severe consequences for children's health, their ability to reach their full potential, and societies as a whole. Wasting predisposes children to an increased risk of death, and stunting can represent irreversible physical and cognitive damage that impacts not only the affected children throughout their lifetime but can also transcend generations. Overweight children are at higher risk of developing diet-related noncommunicable diseases in later life that can cause ill-health as well as premature adult death. These nutrition-related effects imply a severe impact on societies that would not be able to benefit from the full potential of these children's abilities and would suffer severe social and economic consequences as a result, creating cycles of poor nutrition and underdevelopment that need to be tackled on both health and socioeconomic fronts.

In tackling these problems, attention should be paid to direct health measures that can be delivered through the health system as well as measures that can be taken outside the health system by complementary action in other social sectors. Particularly for those households affected by poverty, structural inequalities, or acute humanitarian crises, the role of social protection mechanisms—whether in the form of direct food assistance or other measures such as food vouchers or cash transfers—can be vital in preventing short- and long-term effects of poor nutrition.

1 The RMNCH Continuum of Care and Nutrition Interventions in the Health Sector

The Reproductive, Maternal, Newborn, and Child Health continuum of care (RMNCH CoC) represents a comprehensive approach to maternal and child healthcare, emphasizing the interconnectedness of services across various stages of life. The continuum deals with service delivery across three main dimensions of care: (i) the life cycle of the individual from adolescence and pregnancy to childhood; (ii) different levels of care in the health system from community to health facilities; and (iii) different types of health services from prevention and promotion to curative and palliative care. The continuum connects these dimensions of care through functional linkages [4, 5].

Integrating nutrition interventions in this continuum is an effective strategy to improve the reach and quality of critical interventions and reap benefits that accrue throughout the different life stages of women and children. Adequate nutrition provided through prenatal care counseling and supplementation programs reduces risks for mothers and newborns by providing essential nutrients for a healthy pregnancy and fetal development. Effective postnatal care that supports breastfeeding and nutritional support enhances infant health by providing vital nutrients and antibodies for growth and immunity. Interventions that support healthy nutrition throughout childhood, such as breastfeeding promotion, appropriate complementary feeding practices, and micronutrient supplementation, prevent macro- and micronutrient deficiencies that could compromise a child's physical or cognitive development.

Community-based educational interventions promoting a balanced diet could counter both under- and overnutrition.

Current evidence suggests that if well-organized healthcare platforms could provide key evidence-based maternal and child health interventions, almost 25% of maternal and neonatal deaths and stillbirths could be avoided [6]. Nevertheless, many studies show that access to these services is inadequate in LMICs, and various studies show significant gaps in coverage and quality of services for antenatal care, family planning, and obstetric services across the RMNCH continuum of care [7].

Interventions to address maternal and child nutrition are highly cost-effective and produce disproportionate benefits for individuals and societies compared to the investments they incur. Bhutta et al. (2013) show that in 34 countries that have 90% of the world's children with stunting, the deaths of children under 5 years of age can be reduced by 15% if the population can get access to ten evidence-based nutrition interventions at 90% coverage [8]. They estimated that the investment needed to get these benefits across the 34 countries for all ten interventions was int$9.6 annually.

To get the most benefit out of these investments, the interventions have to be delivered in ways that are not only effective but also provide cost-efficient delivery. Delivering key evidence-based services using the RMNCH continuum of care is a highly efficient way of delivering these services. Black et al. (2016) report global estimates of the cost-effectiveness of delivering critical maternal and child health services, including nutrition services, using the RMNCH CoC approach [9]. They find that delivering reproductive, pregnancy, and childhood services, including key nutrition services, is highly cost-effective. Using this integrated approach to delivery, the interventions produce 8.7 times greater benefits than costs. The three integrated packages have an annual incremental cost of $6.2 billion in low-income countries and $12.4 billion in LMICs, at the per capita cost of $6.7 in LICs and $4.7 in LMICs, which reduce over time after the initial process has been set up. The package includes cost-effective nutrition services, including community management of severe acute malnutrition, several interventions for diarrhea, vitamin A and zinc supplementation, infant and young child feeding and education interventions, and nutrition interventions in pregnancy. Nutrition interventions such as treatment of severe acute malnutrition were found to be among the most cost-effective services.

However, malnutrition is a complex problem that the health sector cannot entirely solve. There are many ways in which policies and interventions outside the health sector can complement the work of the RMNCH CoC.

2 Social Protection Programs and Nutrition Action Through Non-health Sectors

While the RMNCH CoC is a cost-effective strategy for delivering high-impact nutrition interventions, a comprehensive and sustainable approach to end malnutrition must go beyond healthcare services. The health sector alone cannot address the causes that produce malnutrition in the first place.

While a broad set of factors outside the health system are associated with under- and overnutrition, the risk is higher for those who are socially and economically marginalized. Moreover, lower economic status is also associated with many other determinants of undernutrition, such as low maternal education, poor nutritional status of the mother, lower household income, large family size, child's age and birth order, and low birth weight [10]. Various socioeconomic factors also determine undernutrition among women. Similarly, among pregnant women in Africa, low socioeconomic status and its various associated issues, such as low education of the partner, are associated with undernutrition, whereas higher economic status is protective [11]. While addressing these determinants is beyond the preventive and curative remit of the health sector, policies to address these factors must be developed in the social sector to complement and reinforce the effects of services delivered through the RMNCH CoC.

2.1 What Are Social Protection Programs?

Social protection is an age-old idea implying how people in a society help those in times of distress. It spans several ideas that focus on risk reduction, humanitarian assistance, and promoting social justice. According to the World Bank, social protection systems "help individuals and families, especially the poor and vulnerable, cope with crises and shocks, find jobs, improve productivity, invest in the health and education of their children, and protect the aging population. They empower people to be healthy, pursue their education, and seek opportunity to lift themselves and their families out of poverty" [12]. Thus, social protection systems work under the objective of reducing the economic and social vulnerability of poor and marginalized groups in society (Fig. 1). Social protection has become necessary in the discourse on global health in the context of global financial crises, which has prompted the need for robust safety nets to make societies, particularly the most vulnerable, resilient to these shocks [13, 14].

On the other hand, proponents of a broader social protection agenda argue that it should be grounded in a more comprehensive program of long-term and sustainable poverty reduction [15]. In their link with nutrition, both conceptions of social protection have a role. While many social protection programs have a focus on particular sets of interventions for healthcare access and improving nutrition, the usefulness of the broader social development paradigm through economic development and sustainable poverty reduction, focused on the whole population rather than the most vulnerable, is an emerging paradigm among those who consider the traditional program-based approach to social protection reductionist [15]. While this is a reasonable focus for a broader agenda of social development, many social protection interventions have been tried in many LMICs, where governments have not been able to provide a comprehensive social protection across all sectors of society. Achieving this remains a long-term project. At the same time, it is precisely in these contexts that the most vulnerable are at the risk of social and economic vulnerability deeply tied to malnutrition.

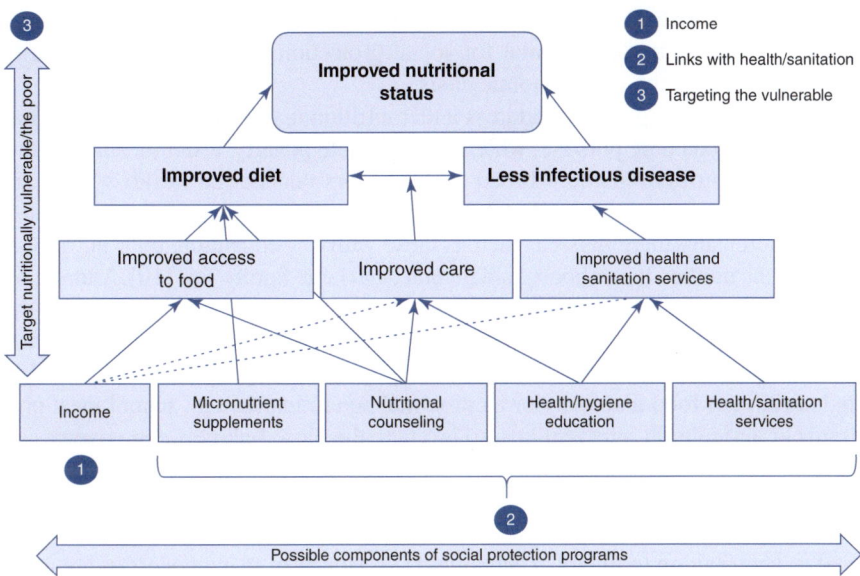

Fig. 1 Pathways of impacts of social protection programs on health and nutrition of nutritionally vulnerable populations. (Reproduced from: Laar et al. [37]. *[with permissions from Cambridge University Press]*)

2.2 Social Protection Programs and Malnutrition

Social protection interventions are vital in addressing nutritional challenges, particularly among vulnerable populations. The nexus between social protection and nutrition is intricate, as access to adequate food, healthcare, and education significantly influences the nutritional status of individuals, particularly women and children who are especially vulnerable. In this context, social protection encompasses a spectrum of policies, programs, and initiatives to safeguard individuals and communities from various risks that may affect their health and nutrition.

Malnutrition is a multidimensional issue with intractable underlying factors such as poverty and marginalization. It is unlikely to be solved by isolated interventions. However, social protection programs are increasingly recognized as an important part of the response because of their ability to address structural issues like poverty and exclusion [16]. Poor nutrition in the context of poverty and marginalization is closely related to issues of food insecurity. Food security is a multidimensional concept involving the availability of food in adequate quantity in the area; the ability of households to access food that is safe, healthy, and appropriate to its needs; utilization of food within the household and the body's uptake of nutrients; and stability of these factors across time [17]. Food insecurity due to inadequacy in one or more of these dimensions can be either chronic, related to long-term structural issues of poverty and lack of social safety nets, or acute, due to natural disasters or conflict [17]. Various social protection mechanisms can be deployed to relieve food insecurity and malnutrition in both contexts. The COVID-19 pandemic brought renewed attention to the potential for social protection to relieve food insecurity during an acute health and economic crisis.

Social protection programs address undernutrition in two key ways: first, by fulfilling their broad core purpose, which is to alleviate poverty, a significant determinant of malnutrition. While a broad set of factors outside the health system are associated with under- and overnutrition, the risk is higher for those who are socially and economically marginalized, such as those with low education, poor nutritional status of the mother, lower household income, and large family size [10]. Addressing poverty through social protection programs has the potential to allow families the means to have better access to many things, such as food, education, and healthcare, which impacts nutrition. Second, many social protection programs directly target malnutrition or food insecurity or its proximal determinants, e.g., school meal programs or agricultural interventions, to leverage the close link between poverty and poor nutrition to find common solutions to both.

Most social protection programs focused on nutrition in LMICs have historically provided food assistance as in-kind food focused on issues of food assistance as well as contribution to the local economy [18]. However, many countries are moving from in-kind food provision to food vouchers and cash transfers to meet nutritional needs [18].

2.3   Nutrition-Focused Social Protection Interventions and Their Impact

In-kind food transfers, such as distributions of various staple foods, have been commonly used as part of many social safety net systems. Although other mechanisms, such as cash transfers, have been shown to have broad effects on nutrition, e.g., increasing dietary diversity, in-kind programs remain a common strategy in LMICs. The reasons in-kind transfers remain common include ensuring the consumption of a minimum amount of food and political motivations. They remain common in many countries, even those that use cash and subsidy measures.

2.3.1   In-Kind Food Transfers

One of the most common food support programs implemented around the world is school meal programs. They are an instructive example of joint benefits offered by addressing nutrition as part of broader social protection interventions. While school feeding programs have positive effects, of different nature and degree, on both health and educational outcomes, Jomaa et al. (2011) argue that they are more appropriately characterized as transfer programs meant to provide a social safety net to vulnerable groups [19]. They assert that the current evidence suggests that the most substantial social protection impact of such programs is the transfer of income to low-income groups, and along with improvements in education outcomes and some nutritional benefits for families, they constitute an investment in human social capital. This indicates that there are positive complementarities between these components that promote human capital development and provide positive anti-poverty effects. The impact of school nutrition programs as effective social safety nets gained particularly strong recognition during the food and fuel crisis of 2007 and 2008 [20].

From a nutrition perspective, school feeding programs complement and consolidate the health gains made through the RMNCH CoC by supporting nutrition and health as children grow older. These programs positively affect children's nutrition knowledge and health behaviors [21], which could translate to lifelong healthy eating habits, thus preventing overweight and the development of nutrition-related noncommunicable diseases later in life. This prevention could be linked to both informational and behavioral impacts. Children in these programs tend to show higher knowledge about healthy nutrition and a preference for healthy foods, and with the availability of healthy foods through the programs, children are less likely to eat non-nutritious food, further strengthening healthy eating habits [22–24]. Despite such positive evidence on nutrition-related knowledge and behaviors, evidence about the actual health effects of these programs is mixed. While there is significant evidence that they conclusively improve micronutrient deficiencies and increase calorie intake, there is less certainty about the impact on physical growth or cognitive abilities [25]. However, there is strong evidence that school enrollment and attendance improve due to these programs, which could have generational effects on good nutrition and health.

2.3.2 Food Subsidies and Vouchers

Social protection programs that use food subsidies and vouchers include interventions that address food prices or increase purchasing power in the target population [17]. Vouchers, or food stamps, allow households to access food of a particular value or quantity from predefined outlets, often calibrated to allow access to a basket of goods such as staples and grains [18]. Food subsidies have often been used to achieve the twin objectives of improving the population's access to food and supporting local agriculture or the food manufacturing industry [18]. Food subsidies and voucher programs can provide support, in addition to interventions through the RMNCH system, in redressing nutritional inequities among mothers and young children by improving children's diets and health [26]. Food vouchers seem to have some effect on improving stunting, but the effect on wasting and dietary diversity seems to be minimal based on weak evidence. Food and nutrition subsidies, on the other hand, may improve dietary diversity among school children, but the evidence for this is also weak [17].

In many LMICs, food vouchers and subsidies have been in transitional stages of the evolution of food-related social protection between in-kind food support and cash transfers (CTs). There are two main kinds of cash transfer programs—conditional cash transfers (CCTs) and unconditional cash transfers (UCTs). In UCTs, the cash is given to families, and it is left to them to decide how to spend it. On the other hand, in CCTs, cash assistance is tied to specific behaviors such as school enrollment, utilization of health services, or health information meetings [27]. The choice of whether a country uses conditional or unconditional transfers is determined not just by the potential for effectiveness but also by social and institutional factors and the feasibility of implementation. Many countries in Latin America use CTs, whereas in sub-Saharan Africa, the use of UTs is more common [27]. The presumption is that the use of unconditional transfer in sub-Saharan Africa is because the supply side in health or other relevant sectors may not be able to fulfill the demand for services generated by CTs, accompanied by a lack of capacity for effectively implementing CTs [28]. Moreover, because of persistent and deep poverty, the programs in sub-Saharan Africa aim at immediate survival and food security and improving chronic poverty with the secondary aim of improving health [29–31].

De Groot. et al. (2017) hypothesize there are three potential pathways through which cash transfers improve child nutrition: (i) by reducing food insecurity; (ii) by improving health through direct utilization of health services or through better access to clean water and sanitation; (iii) by improved care via increasing the caregivers' knowledge, resources and autonomy, and reducing their stress and altering their practices [27]. Cash transfer programs have been shown to positively affect food security by increasing access to food, increasing dietary diversity, and promoting the consumption of healthier food [32]. UCTs have been shown to improve food security and may increase dietary diversity and reduce stunting, but they do not seem to improve cognitive function or development in children [17]. On the other hand, evidence for CCTs shows that they can produce a slight improvement in cognitive functions, may have some effect on improving dietary diversity, but not household expenditure on food, and may not have any impact on stunting or wasting among children [17]. However, these effects are moderated by how the transfers are used, and intra-household dynamics can have strong effects, such as food consumption patterns within households, which can differ by age and gender, or whether UCTs are used for other nutrition-related improvements, such as improved sanitation systems in the household [27].

One potentially harmful effect of interventions that increase access to food is the risk of overweight or obesity. This could be because calorie-dense and nutrient-poor food, such as ultra-processed products or sugar-sweetened beverages, might be used because of constrained resources, e.g., if calorie-dense foods are cheaper than healthier food, or because of a lack of information about good nutrition [16, 33]. This is why it has been argued that it may be additionally valuable for such programs to be accompanied by information and education about healthy nutrition.

In addition, a large number of agricultural interventions have been undertaken to address food insecurity and malnutrition. Reporting their systematic review, Bizikova et al. (2020) report various agricultural interventions to reduce food insecurity, from input subsidies to value chain improvements [34]. Their findings suggest that instead of the specific kind of intervention, effectiveness is more dependent on the design features of the intervention. They find that food security outcomes are better achieved when interventions have pro-poor features, respond to local context-specific food security issues, incorporate community engagement, and actively collaborate with local institutions.

In conclusion, effectively designed and implemented social protection programs can not only provide support in maintaining the gains made in the nutritional health of mothers and children but also be sources of sustaining them through longer-term measures and broader impact on the social and economic circumstances of households. Particularly for those households dealing with poverty and other socio-economic disadvantages, as well as those struggling with acute food crises, social protection programs can provide an invaluable source of resilience.

> **Box 1 The Role of Social Safety Nets in Sustaining and Improving Nutrition in Humanitarian Emergencies—Lessons from COVID-19**
>
> The importance of social safety nets has been widely recognized in humanitarian crises and emergencies, but it has gained particular significance during the COVID-19 pandemic. Various social safety net mechanisms, such as cash transfers, vouchers, and direct food distribution, were effective in protecting against malnutrition [35]. However, the choice of mechanism depends on the context. If food is available in the market, all of these mechanisms can potentially be effective. But if there are challenges with the supply of food, direct food distribution is more effective, although it tends to be more expensive due to higher administrative costs. In terms of overall benefit to the community, cash transfers and vouchers provide benefits that are twice and 1.5 times the amount provided to recipients, respectively, assuming food availability is not a barrier [35]. Direct food distribution does not provide this additional benefit. Cash transfers are also associated with a higher quality and diversity of food, as well as higher household savings than other mechanisms [35]. Furthermore, targeting women with conditional cash transfer programs has proven particularly effective in improving investment in the health and well-being of children in the household [35].
>
> Recent evidence based on COVID-19 era data suggests that nutrition-sensitive social safety measures have proven effective in preventing the expected worsening of nutrition indicators, particularly for the most vulnerable women and children. Abay et al. (2020) [36] report that household food insecurity increased by 11.7% during the pandemic in Ethiopia. However, this adverse effect was significantly reduced among households participating in Ethiopia's Productive Safety Net Program (PSNP). This program provides cash transfers and in-kind support, which is particularly useful for households with limited access to markets, especially during the pandemic, when supply chain disruptions may limit food availability in markets. The likelihood of being food insecure increased by only 2.4% among those who participated in the program, compared to the expected increase. This protective effect was more substantial for households that were poorer or living in remote areas. The PSNP households were 7.7% less likely than non-participating households to reduce expenditure on health and education. In PSNP households, mothers and children's diets changed little, except for a decline in the intake of animal-source foods.
>
> Therefore, if properly structured and delivered, nutrition-sensitive social safety measures such as cash transfers, food vouchers, and direct food supply can effectively mitigate the adverse nutritional consequences of emergencies and humanitarian crises.

References

1. Victora CG, Christian P, Vidaletti LP, Gatica-Domínguez G, Menon P, Black RE. Revisiting maternal and child undernutrition in low-income and middle-income countries: variable progress towards an unfinished agenda. Lancet. 2021;397(10282):1388–99.
2. NCD Risk Factor Collaboration. Trends in adult body-mass index in 200 countries from 1975 to 2014: a pooled analysis of 1698 population-based measurement studies with 19.2 million participants. Lancet. 2016;387(10026):1377–96.
3. World Health Organization. Levels and trends in child malnutrition: UNICEF/WHO/The World Bank Group joint child malnutrition estimates: key findings of the 2020 edition. Levels and trends in child malnutrition: UNICEF/WHO/The World Bank Group joint child malnutrition estimates: key findings of the 2020 edition. 2020.
4. Stenberg K, Sweeny K, Axelson H, Temmerman M, Sheehan P. Returns on investment in the continuum of care for reproductive, maternal, newborn, and child health. In: Black RE, Laxminarayan R, Temmerman M, Walker N, editors. Reproductive, Maternal, Newborn, and Child Health: Disease Control Priorities, Third Edition (Volume 2). Washington, DC: The International Bank for Reconstruction and Development / The World Bank; 2016.
5. Kerber KJ, de Graft-Johnson JE, Bhutta ZA, Okong P, Starrs A, Lawn JE. Continuum of care for maternal, newborn, and child health: from slogan to service delivery. Lancet. 2007;370(9595):1358–69.
6. Chou VB, Walker N, Kanyangarara M. Estimating the global impact of poor quality of care on maternal and neonatal outcomes in 81 low-and middle-income countries: a modeling study. PLoS Med. 2019;16(12):e1002990.
7. Nguyen PH, Khương LQ, Pramanik P, Billah SM, Menon P, Piwoz E, Leslie HH. Effective coverage of nutrition interventions across the continuum of care in Bangladesh: insights from nationwide cross-sectional household and health facility surveys. BMJ Open. 2021;11(1):e040109.
8. Bhutta ZA, Das JK, Rizvi A, Gaffey MF, Walker N, Horton S, et al. Evidence-based interventions for improvement of maternal and child nutrition: what can be done and at what cost? Lancet. 2013;382(9890):452–77.
9. Black RE, Levin C, Walker N, Chou D, Liu L, Temmerman M. Reproductive, maternal, newborn, and child health: key messages from disease control priorities 3rd edition. Lancet. 2016;388(10061):2811–24.
10. Katoch OR. Determinants of malnutrition among children: a systematic review. Nutrition. 2022;96:111565.
11. Desyibelew HD, Dadi AF. Burden and determinants of malnutrition among pregnant women in Africa: a systematic review and meta-analysis. PLoS One. 2019;14(9):e0221712.
12. The World Bank. The World Bank in Social Protection. Available at: https://www.worldbank.org/en/topic/socialprotection. Accessed: 10 Dec 2023.
13. Milazzo A, Grosh M. Social safety nets in World Bank lending and analytical work: FY2002-2007. World Bank SP Discussion Paper. 2008:810.
14. Development DfI. Social transfers and chronic poverty: emerging evidence and the challenge ahead. DFID London; 2005.
15. Devereux S, Sabates-Wheeler R. IDS working paper 232 transformative social protection. Development. 2004;36:36.
16. Ruel MT, Alderman H. Nutrition-sensitive interventions and programmes: how can they help to accelerate progress in improving maternal and child nutrition? Lancet. 2013;382(9891):536–51.
17. Durao S, Visser ME, Ramokolo V, Oliveira JM, Schmidt B-M, Balakrishna Y, et al. Community-level interventions for improving access to food in low-and middle-income countries. Cochrane Database Syst Rev. 2020;7
18. Alderman H, Gentilini U, Yemtsov R. The 1.5 billion people question: food, vouchers, or cash transfers? World Bank Publications; 2017.

19. Jomaa LH, McDonnell E, Probart C. School feeding programs in developing countries: impacts on children's health and educational outcomes. Nutr Rev. 2011;69(2):83–98.
20. Drake L, Fernandes M, Aurino E, Kiamba J, Giyose B, Burbano C, et al. School feeding programs in middle childhood and adolescence. Disease control priorities, Vol 8: Child and adolescent health and development; 2017. p. 147–64.
21. Colley P, Myer B, Seabrook J, Gilliland J. The impact of Canadian school food programs on children's nutrition and health: a systematic review. Can J Diet Pract Res. 2018;80(2):79–86.
22. Fung C, Kuhle S, Lu C, Purcell M, Schwartz M, Storey K, Veugelers PJ. From "best practice" to "next practice": the effectiveness of school-based health promotion in improving healthy eating and physical activity and preventing childhood obesity. Int J Behav Nutr Phys Act. 2012;9(1):1–9.
23. He M, Beynon C, Bouck MS, St Onge R, Stewart S, Khoshaba L, et al. Impact evaluation of the northern fruit and vegetable pilot programme—a cluster-randomised controlled trial. Public Health Nutr. 2009;12(11):2199–208.
24. Drapeau V, Savard M, Gallant A, Nadeau L, Gagnon J. The effectiveness of a school-based nutrition intervention on children's fruit, vegetables, and dairy product intake. J Sch Health. 2016;86(5):353–62.
25. Lawson TM. Impact of school feeding programs on educational, nutritional, and agricultural development goals: a systematic review of literature [Master's thesis]. St. Paul, MN: University of Minnesota; 2012. Accessed 27 Feb 2024. Available from: https://ageconsearch.umn.edu/record/142466/?v=pdf.
26. Hattersley L. Promoting equity in early childhood development for health equity through the life course: an evidence summary. Melbourne, Australia: Victorian Health Promotion Foundation (VicHealth); 2015 Accessed 26 February 2024. Available from: https://www.vichealth.vic.gov.au/sites/default/files/Health-Equity_Summary-Report_EarlyChildhoodDev.pdf.
27. De Groot R, Palermo T, Handa S, Ragno LP, Peterman A. Cash transfers and child nutrition: pathways and impacts. Dev Policy Rev. 2017;35(5):621–43.
28. Schubert B, Slater R. Social cash transfers in low-income African countries: conditional or unconditional? Dev Policy Rev. 2006;24(5):571–8.
29. Davis B, Gaarder M, Handa S, Yablonski J. Evaluating the impact of cash transfer programmes in sub-Saharan Africa: an introduction to the special issue. J Dev Eff. 2012;4(1):1–8.
30. Attanasio O, Battistin E, Fitzsimons E, Vera-Hernandez M. How effective are conditional cash transfers? Evidence from Colombia (IFS Briefing Notes BN54). 2005. London, UK: Institute for Fiscal Studies. Accessed 20 February 2024. Available from: https://discovery.ucl.ac.uk/id/eprint/14766/1/14766.pdf.
31. Paxson C, Schady N. Does money matter? The effects of cash transfers on child development in rural Ecuador. Econ Dev Cult Chang. 2010;59(1):187–229.
32. Merttens F, Jones E. Evaluation of the Uganda Social Assistance Grants for Empowerment (SAGE) Programme. Oxford Policy Management; 2014.
33. de Bem LJ, Sichieri R, Burlandy L, Salles-Costa R. Changes in food consumption among the Programa Bolsa Família participant families in Brazil. Public Health Nutr. 2011;14(5):785–92.
34. Bizikova L, Jungcurt S, McDougal K, Tyler S. How can agricultural interventions enhance contribution to food security and SDG 2.1? Glob Food Secur. 2020;26:100450.
35. International Initiative for Impact Evaluation. 2020. How effective are safety net programs at protecting people from the socio-economic effects of COVID-19? Accessed 26 Feb 2024. Available from: https://www.3ieimpact.org/evidence-hub/publications/other-briefs/how-effective-are-safety-net-programmes-protecting-people.
36. Abay KA, Berhane G, Hoddinott J, Tafere K. COVID-19 and food security in Ethiopia: do social protection programs protect? Econ Dev Cult Chang. 2023;71(2):373.
37. Laar AK, et al. Improving nutrition-sensitivity of social protection programmes in Ghana. Proc Nutr Soc. 2017;76(4):516–23.

Food Security and Agriculture

Narjis Fatima Hussain, Hamna Amir Naseem, and Jai K. Das

1 Background

The term "food security" first appeared in a policy context in the 1970s. Food security is a complex and pressing global issue affecting developing and developed countries. Ending hunger and achieving food security by 2030 is one of the United Nations' Sustainable Development Goals (SDG 2). However, several impeding factors, including climate change, economic inflation, conflicts, and resource restraints, have limited the progress.

According to the World Food Program (WFP), 45% of the population is food insecure [1]. The United Nations reports that 828 million people were affected by hunger in 2021—46 million more people than a year earlier and 150 million more from 2019 [2]. This increase is also reflected in the gender gap in food insecurity which has continued to rise in 2021—31.9% of women in the world were moderately or severely food insecure, compared to 27.6% of men—a gap of more than 4 percentage points, compared with 3 percentage points in 2020 [2].

In addition, supply chain disruptions due to COVID-19, increased consumer demand, and subsequent high prices across the globe have increased the severity of food insecurity for 811 million people around the world [3]. It may also push an additional 9.3 million children to the existing 13.6 million children into acute malnutrition [3]. Around 2.3 billion people in the world (29.3%) were moderately or

---

N. F. Hussain
Institute for Global Health and Development, Aga Khan University, Karachi, Pakistan

SickKids Centre for Global Child Health, The Hospital for Sick Children, Toronto, Canada
e-mail: narjisfatima.hussain@sickkids.ca; narjisfatima.hussain@mail.utoronto.ca

H. Amir Naseem · J. K. Das (✉)
Institute for Global Health and Development, Aga Khan University, Karachi, Pakistan
e-mail: hamna.amir@aku.edu; jai.das@aku.edu

© The Author(s), under exclusive license to Springer Nature
Switzerland AG 2025
Z. S. Lassi, R. A. Salam (eds.), *Nutrition Across Reproductive, Maternal, Neonatal, Child, and Adolescent Health Care*,
https://doi.org/10.1007/978-3-031-95721-5_14

severely food insecure in 2021—350 million more compared to before the outbreak of the COVID-19 pandemic [2]. Nearly 924 million people (11.7% of the global population) faced food insecurity at severe levels, an increase of 207 million in two years [2].

Furthermore, climate change also acts as a hunger risk multiplier exacerbating current vulnerabilities, with projections suggesting that the number of people at risk of hunger will increase by 10–20% by 2050, with 65% of this population in Sub-Saharan Africa, while the number of malnourished children could increase by up to 21% (24 million children) owing to food insecurity and the impact of climate change on the agricultural sector [4, 5].

Agriculture is a key driver of food security, playing a pivotal role in ensuring people have access to sufficient, safe, and nutritious food. It influences food availability, quality, diversity, and safety. Sustainable and efficient agricultural practices are essential for maintaining a stable food environment. According to the Food and Agriculture Organisation (FAO) of the United Nations, almost half the world's population lives in households engaged in agrifood systems [6]. Their research estimates that 3.83 billion people globally rely on agrifood systems, with the highest agrifood system-dependent population in Asia estimated at 2.359 billion [6]. Developing countries are home to roughly 80% of the world's population, 98% of humanity's hungry people, and 78% of harvested croplands [7]. Their farming systems have an essential role to play in addressing global food needs, as the relationship between food security and agriculture underscores the importance of addressing agricultural challenges to address global food security issues.

Farmers cultivate either food crops, cash crops, or both. Food crops are grown for human consumption and provide nutrition and sustenance, e.g., rice, wheat, and maize. These crops play a major role in addressing food security and ensuring a stable food supply. Conversely, cash crops are primarily grown for profit rather than consumption, e.g., cotton, coffee, and tobacco. Especially in developing countries, cash crops are grown on a large scale and sometimes compete with the land use and resource requirements of the local community [8]. As major cash crops are influenced by global market prices, farmers' revenues are impacted by the fluctuations, affecting the next cycle of production with latent effects on global food security.

The relationship between agriculture and global food security is complex and can be impacted by multiple issues such as climate change, economic inflation, the COVID-19 pandemic, and regional conflicts. Such factors can affect crop production and labor availability, disrupt supply chains and market dynamics, or introduce vulnerabilities that lead to widespread food insecurity as communities grapple with multiple simultaneous challenges.

This chapter will elaborate on the concepts and dimensions of food security, its trends over time, and its significance. It will then delve into the intricate relationship between food security and agriculture, explore the challenges and links between the concepts, and shed light on the innovations and strategies that shape our ability to feed a growing world population and our pathway to achieving SDG 2. In that, we will also examine the critical components of food security, the role of agriculture, and the implications of climate change, technology, and policy on the future of food security.

2 Defining Food Security

The FAO defines food security as a state where "all people, at all times, have physical and economic access to sufficient, safe, and nutritious food to meet their dietary needs and food preferences for an active and healthy life." [9] This definition includes not only the quantity of food available but also its quality, safety, and the ability of individuals and communities to obtain it.

Food security encompasses four key dimensions [10]:

1. Availability: The consistent and adequate supply of food within a specific region or community, and often related to food production and distribution.
2. Access: The ability of individuals and communities to obtain food, which is influenced by factors such as income, food prices, transportation, and physical proximity to food sources.
3. Utilization: The appropriate utilization of food, which refers to the quality, nutritional value, and safety of the food consumed.
4. Stability: The consistent and reliable state of access to food. Food security must be stable over time and should not be a temporary condition.

The four dimensions of food security (availability, access, utilization, and stability) are widely recognized and were established as a framework by the FAO. However, a growing recognition of the need to expand beyond the physical aspects of food to include social, economic, and cultural factors led to the development of an expanded framework that incorporates two additional dimensions. These are part of a broader and evolving discourse on food security, often advocated by researchers, nongovernmental organizations, and agencies to provide a more comprehensive understanding of food security. The fifth and sixth dimensions of food security [11] include:

5. Agency and Empowerment: The ability of individuals and communities to make informed choices and decisions regarding their food and nutrition, ensuring food that is culturally acceptable and respectful of people's traditions, preferences, and values. It addresses issues of self-determination, empowerment, and participation in shaping food systems that respect cultural diversity and identities.
6. Sustainability: The long-term ability of food systems to provide food security and nutrition in such a way that does not compromise the economic, social, and environmental bases that generate food security and nutrition for future generations.

Figure 1 illustrates the six dimensions of food security. While agency and sustainability have each been widely recognized in the scholarly literature as

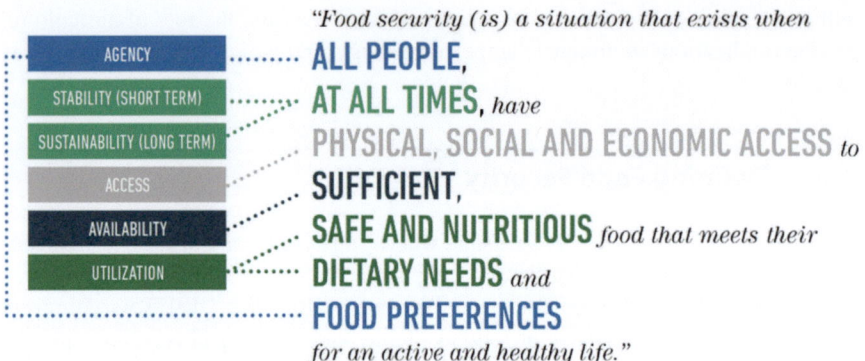

Fig. 1 Six dimensions of food security. (Source: HLP 15, 2020 [12])

being relevant to food security for several decades, Clapp et al. first proposed the six-dimensional framework for food security in the 15th report of the High-Level Panel of Experts on Food Security and Nutrition (HLPE), Food Security and Nutrition: Building a Global Narrative Towards 2030 (HLPE, 2020) [11]. Clapp et al. argue the need to formally embrace the expansion as it impacts the conceptualization of food security and has important implications for the design of policies and programs.

Including these additional dimensions in the concept of food security broadens the perspective to consider not only the physical aspects of food but also the social, economic, and cultural aspects. This more comprehensive view reflects a deeper understanding of food security and the factors that influence an individual's or community's well-being and quality of life.

Hence, these six dimensions offer a more holistic view of food security and reflect a deeper understanding of food security and its complexity, considering the broader context in which people gain access to safe, nutritious, and culturally acceptable food consistently and sustainably. It is a multidimensional concept that considers not only the quantity of food but also its quality, accessibility, and sustainability, to ensure "Zero Hunger."

3   Trends in Food Security

In 1990, it is estimated that a population ranging from 15 to 35 million individuals faced the threat of famine, with 786 million being susceptible to persistent malnutrition [13]. Additionally, hundreds of millions experienced deficiencies in micronutrients, as well as issues such as diarrhea, measles, malaria, parasites, and other nutritional deficiencies [13]. As of the World Bank's October 2023 World Food Security Outlook, preliminary estimates indicate that global food insecurity may have peaked at 11.9% during 2020–2022, with a slight improvement to 11.8%

expected for 2021–2023 and 11.6% for 2022/2023, although the long-term outlook remains uncertain [1].

Over the past three decades, the trajectory of food security research has exhibited a discernible upward trend, with a surge in activity from 2013 to 2019, particularly in developed regions such as Europe and America [1]. Advancements in agriculture and technology have contributed to increased food production, leading to improved food security in many regions. There has also been an increase in the awareness of the need to improve agricultural practices to ensure sustainability.

4 Significance of Food Security

Food security has paramount significance at all socioecological levels, from the individual to the society, and extends into public policy with large global implications. Apart from being one of the basic human needs for survival, food security is important for its role in nutrition to ensure proper growth, cognitive development, and overall mental and physical well-being.

Food security is essential for economic and social stability, contributing to livelihoods and a national Gross Domestic Product (GDP) [14]. In that, it empowers individuals and communities by ensuring that they have the resources and capacity to feed themselves, thereby reducing dependency and increasing self-sufficiency and resilience to shocks.

At a global level, food security is a key component in poverty reduction efforts and is significantly associated with global and political stability, leading to better international relations and lowered migration rates [15]. It also impacts global public health, leading to better health outcomes, especially for children who are most vulnerable to food insecurity, as this can lead to increased susceptibility to diseases as well as stunting, wasting, and delayed and impaired growth. It is estimated that 840 million people in developing countries are undernourished, 167 million children in developing countries are malnourished, and over 50% of deaths in children are linked to malnourishment [16]. One of the major causes of food insecurity in developing countries is the lack of access to food due to poverty. Achieving food security within a household may often compete with other expenditures that are necessities, such as healthcare, education, and housing [16]. Food security is also closely linked with nutrition security, which refers to having access to an adequate nutritional diet to maintain growth, recover from disease or illness, and ensure a healthy pregnancy, adequate lactation, and physical work capacity [16].

Socially, food security also contributes to better educational outcomes, as well-nourished and cognitively developed students are more likely to attend school regularly, concentrate better, and perform well academically [17]. Malnutrition can lead to decreased academic performance and hinder educational activities. Conversely, improved food security enhances students' health and cognitive abilities, fostering an environment conducive to effective learning. Integrating food security measures in educational settings not only addresses immediate nutritional needs but also contributes to breaking the cycle of poverty and facilitating better educational outcomes. Food security is also closely related to women's empowerment and agency, as such initiatives often empower women, who play a central role in food production and distribution [18].

Food security is essential not only for individuals' survival and well-being but also for broader economic, social, and global stability. It is a critical component of achieving a sustainable and prosperous future for the world's population. Efforts to address food security challenges are interconnected with many other aspects of human development and global stability, especially agriculture and associated practices.

5 Relationship Between Agriculture and Food Security

Agriculture plays a central role in safeguarding the global food supply and achieving the SDG 2 target of Zero Hunger by 2030. It involves the cultivation of crops, the raising of animals, and the production of food products. In addition, the agricultural sector is central to achieving food security and plays a strategic role in improving the availability of food, promoting sustainable agricultural practices, and ensuring the livelihoods of the poorest.

Agriculture affects all dimensions of food security: It influences the availability of food through production, access to food through income and market dynamics, utilization through the quality and safety of food, stability through resilient agricultural systems, agency and empowerment through rural livelihoods and preservation of cultural food traditions, and sustainability through the promotion of sustainable agriculture practices.

The relationship between agriculture and food security is impacted owing to various factors, especially population growth, coupled with the increased intensity of environmental events such as floods, droughts, and extreme variability in temperature or rainfall, which often pose a threat to food security [14]. Furthermore, due to greater food demand and reduced crop productivity, higher food prices along with income inequalities may negatively affect food access and availability for poor households. It is important to note that poverty, war and conflict, natural disasters, and climate change, as well as population growth, are the main causes of hunger and malnutrition [14].

According to the most recent FAO data, around 13% of the population living in developing countries suffer from undernourishment [19], reflecting that the challenge of feeding the world's population is likely to become even more serious in the future [20]. The global population exceeded 7.6 billion people in 2018 [21] and is predicted to reach 9.2 billion by 2050 [22], with a projected increased food demand of 59–102% [23, 24]. Consequently, it seems necessary to increase agricultural production by about 60–70% to provide food for the global population in 2050 and meet the needs of the human population [22].

According to Maslow's classification of needs by urgency and intensity, the need to alleviate hunger and thirst is foremost [25]. In "An Essay on the Principle of Population, As It Affects the Future Improvement of Society," published in

1798, Malthus claimed that the population size grows geometrically, beyond control, while the production of food grows only arithmetically [26]. As such, Malthus asserted that if the population grows while the supply of natural resources (especially land) remains constant, productivity in agriculture tends to decline, leading to a reduction in supply, followed by famine. The primary failure of the Malthusian approach was its inability to account for technological progress that enabled food production growth without the need to acquire new land resources. This was addressed by Boserup in the Boserupian model, which states that innovations and technology allow for faster food production when compared to population size [27].

Hence, the agricultural sector and its advancement play a strategic role in improving the availability of food and achieving food security. It also has a much greater impact on reducing poverty and improving food security than the other sectors of the economy. Therefore, the relationship between agriculture and food security underscores the importance of addressing agricultural challenges to address global food security issues.

6   Challenges to Agriculture and Food Security

The Malthusian population theory, formulated at the end of the eighteenth century, has been demonstrated to be largely wrong about the relationship between agriculture and food security [28, 29]. Furthermore, from the eighteenth century onward, the food supply has almost always increased faster than population growth [30]. Despite that, the undernourished population is still more than 800 million [21], and food insecurity is at a rise: Therefore, a question arises concerning the underlying causes and challenges.

6.1   Population Growth

While agriculture is integral to food security, several challenges threaten the stability and accessibility of the world's food supply. According to Poleman [31], food production has been growing much faster than the world's population, but only in developed countries. For developing countries, the food production rates are close to population growth rates, thus having minimal impact. Poleman further sees the main cause of food insecurity as insufficient incomes, and numerous studies assessing the relationship between income and food consumption reveal the existence of a positive association [31].

6.2   Social and Political Factors

Agricultural systems are situated within social and political environments that have tremendous influence on how they operate. A wide range of social and political factors affect agricultural systems. The factors can be divided into three categories: internal social factors, external social factors, and political factors [32]. Internal social factors have a direct influence as they are part of a farmer's environment and can include factors such as land tenancy, system of ownership, size of holdings, availability of labor and capital, religion, level of technological development, accessibility to the market, and irrigation facilities [32]. External social factors do not directly impact agriculture or food security but can influence it through internal factors, including social norms (gender inequality and cultural preferences), through market trends for agricultural products, and political processes [32]. Political factors can impact agriculture directly or indirectly through government plans, international policies, conflict and displacement, and global trade policies [32]. As such, social and political environments can have a close impact on agricultural activities and subsequent food security.

6.3 Urban Development

Urban development, particularly with the creation of alternate employment opportunities and generations moving to new fields, has significantly impacted agriculture and food security [33]. As more individuals shift from rural areas to urban centers in pursuit of diverse job opportunities, there is a reduction in the labor force available for agriculture, thus reducing productivity. This shift can lead to a decline in traditional farming practices, affecting both crop production and rural livelihoods [33]. Moreover, the conversion of agricultural land for urban development can limit the available arable land, exacerbating food production challenges.

6.4 Food Crops Versus Cash Crops

Food security among rural agriculturists involved in food crops and cash crops depends on many factors such as region, type of crop, and the conditions of the local economy. Rural agriculturists who are working in food crops have a direct impact on food security in their households, as staple food crops contribute to a consistent source of food for families [34]. Cultivating cash crops that are grown for sale rather than personal consumption provides farmers with income. However, depending on cash crops alone can lead to some risks and challenges. There may be external factors, such as market price fluctuations, leading to decreased affordability of food, while expanded cash crop production can affect the availability of food due to reduced diversity of food products [34].

6.5 Land Degradation

Land degradation owing to soil erosion, deforestation, overgrazing, and intensive agricultural practices has diminished agricultural productivity. The Global

Assessment of Soil Degradation (GLASOD) estimates that during the last 40 years, about one-third of global total arable land was permanently damaged in some way by soil erosion, with continued rates of erosion at ten million hectares per year [37, 38]. Since the dawn of agriculture, GLASOD establishes that 1.97 billion hectares of land (23% of global land) have been degraded [38]. This is compounded by water scarcity in many regions since agriculture is a water-intensive industry and requires efficient irrigation and water management.

6.6 Water

In the last 100 years, the demand for water worldwide has grown twice as fast as the human population [39]. Water scarcity is already an issue on every continent with agriculture, presenting a major threat to food security. Furthermore, agricultural water scarcity is expected to increase in more than 80% of the world's croplands by 2050 [40]. Agricultural water use is the world's largest water user and is significantly affected by climate change, socioeconomic development, and population [41, 42]. Intensification of agricultural water scarcity can affect food production, threatening food security, particularly for the poor and disadvantaged groups [40]. Conversely, increased water use in economic sectors can deleteriously affect freshwater ecosystems, which might further aggregate agricultural water scarcity and impair the sustainability of food production in the future [40]. Water scarcity has become an increasing threat to food security, and the situation is expected to aggravate under future climate change [43]. Hence, understanding agricultural water scarcity under climate change is, therefore, important given the increasing food demands and consequently intensified irrigation and expansion of cropland in the future.

6.7 Climate Change

Climate change not only impacts water availability but is a major challenge for agriculture and subsequent food security through various pathways (Fig. 2). Direct pathways include changes in temperature levels and rainfall distribution [44]. Indirect factors that affect production include changes in pollinators, pests, disease vectors, and invasive species [44].

Climate change threatens to reverse the progress made so far in the fight against hunger and to achieve SDG 2. The Intergovernmental Panel on Climate Change (IPCC) states that climate change augments and intensifies risks to food security for the most vulnerable countries and populations [45]. Four out of the eight key risks induced by climate change identified by IPCC AR5 have direct consequences for food security: loss of rural livelihoods and income; loss of marine and coastal ecosystems and livelihoods; loss of terrestrial and inland water ecosystems and livelihoods; and food insecurity and breakdown of food systems [45].

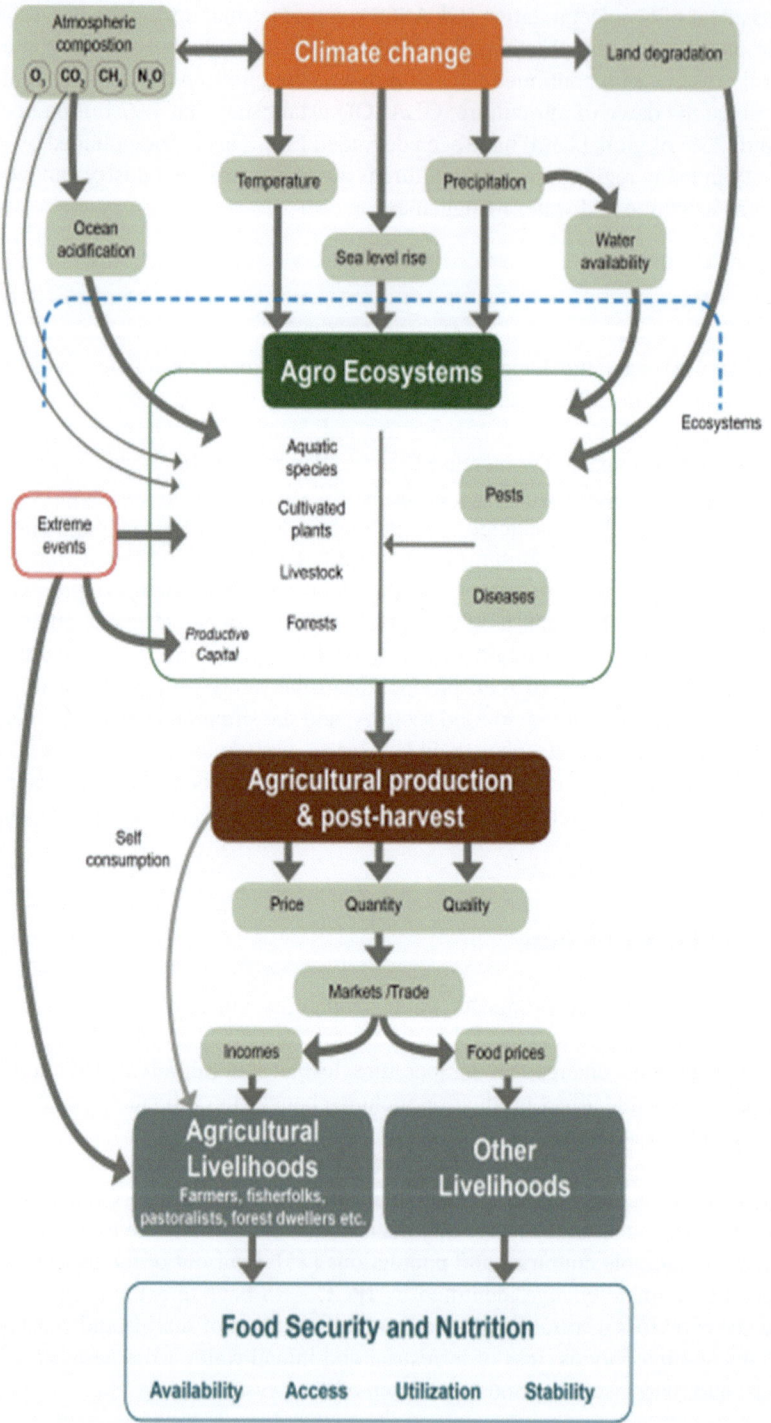

Fig. 2 Schematic representation of the cascading effects of climate change impacts on food security and nutrition. (Source: FAO, 2015 [44])

Climate change has already negatively affected wheat and maize yields globally. Modeling estimates have predicted that a mean effect on yields of four crop groups (coarse grains, oil seeds, wheat, and rice, accounting for about 70% of global crop harvested area) will decrease by 17% globally by 2050 [44–46]. It also affects livestock production; in various countries in Sub-Saharan Africa, 20–60% losses in animal numbers were recorded during serious drought events in the past decades [44]. In South Africa, dairy yields may decrease by 10–25% because of climate change [44]. Climate change and climate variability also impact forests, fisheries, and the development of aquaculture in marine and freshwater environments [44].

Climate change affects food security in many dimensions: access, availability, utilization, stability, agency, and sustainability. It impacts food production, livelihoods, and incomes of small-scale producers, leading to higher food prices and volatility, limiting access and agency. Effects of climate change on nutrition include potential changes in the nutritional quality of some foods (e.g., reduced concentration of proteins and in some vitamins and minerals). Increased climate variability, increased frequency, and intensity of extreme events, as well as slow ongoing changes, will also affect the stability and sustainability of food supply, access, and utilization.

6.8 COVID-19 and Other Potential Pandemics

The COVID-19 pandemic also had a major impact on the global agricultural sector and food security. To prevent the spread of the disease, strict restrictions were placed on labor mobility, which significantly impeded the normal functioning of agricultural activities. This disruption in the supply chain, coupled with issues in the transportation of agricultural products, resulted in decreased productivity [35]. As a result, the COVID-19 pandemic had a significant impact on global food security, causing many regions to experience disruptions in the availability and affordability of food items.

6.9 Conflicts

Regional conflict can also have profound effects on agriculture and food security. In areas that are affected by conflict, agricultural activities can be disrupted due to the displacement of communities, damaged infrastructure, and abandoned land. This, coupled with the unstable economic structure, can lead to farmers facing challenges in producing crops, resulting in food shortages and price inflation, which can be of significant concern to food security in the region [36].

7 Innovations in Agriculture and Food Security

Innovations in agriculture and food production are critical in addressing the challenges to food security. These innovations come in various forms, including technological advancements, sustainable farming, including community practices, and social and political changes.

7.1 Technological Advancements in Agriculture

Technological advancements can boost production and yield through improved crop varieties based on genetic modification to increase crop resistance to pests, diseases, and environmental stress [47, 48]. This also contributes to food safety as such crops reduce the need for chemical pesticides and enhance nutritional content. Furthermore, climate-resilient crops are varieties that are specially engineered to withstand the challenges posed by rapidly changing climate conditions. These crops have been bred to thrive and grow in extreme conditions and stresses such as increased temperatures, altered precipitation patterns, and other climate-related stressors, including droughts, through genetic modification. This can ensure more stable yields in the event of unpredictable environmental conditions, lending resiliency to food systems and subsequent food security [49–52].

Further advancements also promote crop diversification by reducing risks associated with mono-cropping to ensure soil health, enhance dietary diversity, and contribute to sustainable and resilient agriculture. Crop diversification also provides smallholder farmers with an improved income and nutrition security, leading to a decrease in cases of malnutrition [53]. Crop diversification is a dynamic tool to ensure food security sustainably and can also mitigate the adverse effects of climate change [54].

Apart from crop modifications, technology in agricultural techniques allows for efficient resource use, promoting sustainable practices. Methods like precision agriculture leverage technology like the Global Positioning System, sensors, and drones to optimize farming practices such as irrigation. This approach helps farmers make data-driven decisions, reducing resource wastage and increasing efficiency [55]. It also allows for optimal use of resources like water, fertilizers, and pesticides. This efficiency not only reduces costs but also minimizes the environmental footprint of agriculture [55].

Similar to precision agriculture, the drip irrigation method directs water straight to plant roots, reducing waste and optimizing resource utilization. This technique enhances crop yields across different farming systems by ensuring effective water distribution and promoting water conservation [56]. A global meta-analysis concluded that in the case of water shortage, drip irrigation can save water and ensure a crop yield comparable to other forms of irrigation [56]. Furthermore, increasing amounts of drip irrigation can significantly increase crop yields by 2.32–28.92% when compared to other irrigation approaches [56]. Moreover, the drip irrigation approach can also reduce fertilizer leaching and soil salinity, leading to improved soil health [56].

In addition to innovations that enhance food production, advanced methods of storage and transportation also help in reducing post-harvest losses to ensure greater food availability and accessibility. Such methods can include cold storage facilities [57], modified atmosphere packaging [58], vacuum sealing [59], solar-powered storage [57], smart solution using Internet of Things [60], and blockchain technology [61].

7.2 Sustainable Agriculture

While technological advancements work to increase agricultural productivity, ensuring availability and access to safe and nutritious food, it is also crucial to consider stability and sustainability through effective agricultural practices. As such, sustainable agriculture is an approach to farming that aims to produce food while preserving the environment, supports the well-being of farmers and their communities, and ensures food security for future generations.

Apart from approaches that optimize resource use, other techniques, such as agroecology, focus on sustainable farming practices that work in harmony with local ecosystems. It promotes biodiversity, soil health, and resilience in agricultural systems [62]. Moreover, identifying synergies between ecosystem services like pest control and pollination, and the agronomic and economic advantages, could heighten farmer engagement [62]. This presents an opportunity to expand sustainable agroecological practices, particularly if they align with current agricultural methods. In addition, urban agriculture methods like vertical farming and hydroponics allow food production in densely populated areas, reducing the need for long-distance transportation of food, increasing access, and ensuring food security while promoting sustainability [63].

Other sustainable farming practices include crop rotation, as alternating the types of crops grown in a specific field from season to season can help prevent soil degradation and nutrient depletion while reducing the buildup of pests and diseases [64]. Moreover, planting cover crops, such as legumes or grasses, between main crops can protect the soil from erosion, add organic matter, and improve soil health. It can also promote biodiversity and boost productivity.

Additional sustainable approaches include no-till or reduced-till practices that minimize soil disturbance, retain more moisture, reduce erosion, and sequester carbon in the soil. This protects the nutritional content of food and preserves land resources for longer use [65]. Land resources are also conserved through sustainable livestock management, which promotes rotational grazing, providing access to open pastures, and reducing the use of antibiotics can make livestock farming more sustainable, while water conservation can be encouraged through efficient irrigation methods and rainwater harvesting.

Sustainable agriculture practices also support the cultivation of local and indigenous crop varieties to help preserve agricultural biodiversity and adapt to local environmental conditions. Such initiatives should be supported by policies that encourage farmers to shift toward sowing local crop varieties rather than those with higher profits.

7.3 Agency and Empowerment—Social and Political Factors

Increasing agency and empowerment in the domain of food security in agriculture is vital for ensuring that individuals and communities have the knowledge, resources, and decision-making capacity to shape their food systems. These strategies can vary by region and farming system, and they often work best when integrated into a comprehensive, holistic approach to sustainable agriculture. Approaches to agency and empowerment encompass social and political factors. It is crucial to provide education and training on sustainable farming practices, modern technologies, and market knowledge to empower farmers with the skills and information they need to make informed decisions.

Supporting such programs and communities is crucial in providing the necessary structure for implementation. In terms of policy advocacy, supporting farmers' organizations in advocating for policies that benefit small-scale farmers and promote sustainable agriculture can empower them to shape the agricultural landscape. Such policies should acknowledge and incorporate traditional and indigenous knowledge in agricultural practices that respect local cultures and traditions, empowering communities to preserve their heritage.

Apart from this, policy changes are also crucial in creating conducive environments that encourage sustainable and resilient agricultural practices. Such policies can include those policies that prioritize public and private investments in agriculture, land tenure policies to incentive investment in land especially for small-scale farmers, policies that facilitate access to credit and financial services for farmers, subsidies for sustainable agriculture, trade agreements, risk management such as crop insurance, social safety net programs, policies focusing on climate-smart agriculture, nutrition promotion, and resource allocation for agricultural research and innovation. Furthermore, effective policy formulation and implementation should be facilitated through collaborations between government agencies, civil society, and the private sector to ensure that policies address the complex and interconnected issues related to agriculture and food security.

7.4 Women Empowerment

Furthermore, it is important to consider gender equity when targeting empowerment. Women make up 43% of the global agricultural labor force [66], yet face significant discrimination when it comes to land and livestock ownership, equal pay, and decision-making. It should be noted that improvements in women's empowerment in agriculture are associated with higher levels of productivity and efficiency [67].

Furthermore, social aspects concerning agriculture and food security are an important consideration. Techniques such as home/kitchen gardening refer to the practice of growing plants, primarily vegetables, herbs, and fruits, at home. It allows for easy access to fresh and nutritious produce, increases dietary diversity, and reduces costs. In addition, communal spaces for agriculture involve the cultivation of crops on shared land or community-owned plots. They not only promote food security by providing a collective source of food for the community but also enhance resource efficiency and agency by empowering the community to make crucial choices for their well-being.

Case Study: Enhancing Food Security Through Sustainable Agriculture [68]
In the semi-arid region of Sub-Saharan Africa, where food security challenges are pronounced, a transformative initiative emerged to address the pressing issues. The project, "African Sustainable Agriculture Project" (ASAP), represents a holistic approach to food security and agriculture.

The ASAP project works to empower farmers and communities in Africa through creation of sustainable agriculture practices focused on entrepreneurship and education. The project is implemented in collaboration with local communities and international organizations and emphasizes sustainable agricultural practices to expand the status of farming in Africa beyond the current level of subsistence and sub-subsistence farming to a production system that creates sustainable commerce, thereby producing jobs and improving the health of communities for generations to come. By promoting entrepreneurship endeavors, such as quality seeds, enhanced feed to increase yields, and quality livelihood programs such as "Let's Raise Chickens for Profit!," the initiative has boosted local economy and access to quality food.

One striking success of the ASAP project is the empowerment of women farmers as well as genocide victims. With access to resources, training, and support, women have taken the lead in sustainable farming, contributing not only to increased food production but also to greater gender equality in the community.

Moreover, the project has integrated nutritional education, enhancing not only the quantity of food but also its quality. The diversity of crops cultivated, coupled with community-led nutrition programs, has led to improved dietary diversity and reduced malnutrition.

As of now, ASAP established the first commercial feed mill in Rwanda in 2014 and maintains a 10,000-hen operation to provide eggs to the community. Further, in partnership with international organizations, ASAP has initiated a small holder farmer broiler project, doubling household incomes and enabling farmers to send their children to school for better life outcomes.

The ASAP project underscores the intricate relationship between agriculture and food security, demonstrating that sustainable farming practices can not only address the immediate challenge of food availability but also promote long-term food security, social empowerment, and environmental resilience. This case study highlights the transformative potential of sustainable agriculture in achieving comprehensive food security in vulnerable regions.

7.5 Organic Farming/Biofortification

The integration of traditional and innovative knowledge is also integral in building capacity in local contexts to encourage organic farming practices for biofortification and sustainable food production. Organic farming refers to an agricultural approach that relies on natural and ecological processes to grow crops and raise livestock. It avoids the use of synthetic chemicals, such as synthetic fertilizers, pesticides, herbicides, and genetically modified organisms (GMOs). Instead, organic farmers utilize techniques like crop rotation, composting, biological pest control, and the use of organic fertilizers to maintain soil fertility, control pests and diseases, and promote sustainability.

These strategies are interrelated and should be implemented in a comprehensive and context-specific manner to effectively enhance agency and empowerment in agriculture, ultimately contributing to food security and sustainable development.

8 Way Forward

The intricate relationship between food security and agriculture is vital, resonating deeply with the well-being of individuals, communities, and nations. Agriculture is not merely a source of sustenance; it is a cornerstone of economic development, a guardian of environmental integrity, and a reflection of social equity.

The multidimensional nature of food security, as exemplified by its six dimensions, underscores the complexity of ensuring access to safe, nutritious, and sufficient food for all. Beyond the immediate dimensions of availability and access, the aspects of utilization, stability, sustainability, and agency broaden our understanding of the challenges and opportunities at hand.

Throughout this chapter, we have explored the importance of sustainable agriculture as a linchpin for addressing food security. Sustainable farming practices offer the promise of greater productivity, resilience to environmental changes, and the preservation of natural resources. They are the foundation upon which a more secure and equitable food future can be built.

In the ever-evolving landscape of agriculture and food security, innovation, policy changes, and community empowerment are essential tools. Whether it is the adoption of climate-resilient crops, the implementation of circular economy principles, or the formulation of inclusive and adaptive policies, we have seen that proactive measures can make a profound impact.

As we navigate the challenges and opportunities on the horizon, let us be guided by the belief that sustainable agriculture is not merely a technical endeavor; it is a testament to our shared responsibility to safeguard the future of our planet and to nourish the well-being of all its inhabitants. Through collective efforts, sustainable practices, and innovative solutions, we can cultivate a world where food security is not a dream but a steadfast reality for generations to come, paving the way to achieve SDG 2 by 2030 with its aim of "Zero Hunger."

References

1. World Bank Group. Food security update| the bank's response to rising food insecurity. World Bank Group; 2023.
2. UN Report. Global hunger numbers rose to as many as 828 million in 2021 [Internet]. Newsroom. FAO; 2022 [cited 2023 Dec 13]. Available from: https://www.fao.org/newsroom/detail/un-report-global-hunger-SOFI-2022-FAO/en.
3. COVID-19 brief: Impact on food security – [Internet]. USGLC. U.S. Global Leadership Coalition; 2020 [cited 2023 Dec 13]. Available from: https://www.usglc.org/coronavirus/global-hunger/.
4. Parry M, Evans A, Rosegrant MW, Wheeler T. Climate change and hunger: responding to the challenge. Intl Food Policy Res Inst. 2009;
5. Nelson GC, Rosegrant MW, Koo J, Robertson R, Sulser T, Zhu T, Ringler C, Msangi S, Palazzo A, Batka M, Magalhaes M. Climate change: impact on agriculture and costs of adaptation. Intl Food Policy Res Inst. 2009;
6. Estimating global and country-level employment in agrifood systems [Internet]. FAO; 2023. Available from: https://www.fao.org/3/cc4337en/cc4337en.pdf.
7. McArthur JW, Rasmussen K. Where does the world's food grow? [Internet]. Brookings. 2016 [cited 2023 Dec 13]. Available from: https://www.brookings.edu/articles/where-does-the-worlds-food-grow/.
8. Glossary: Cash crops [Internet]. Europa.eu. [cited 2023 Dec 13]. Available from: https://ec.europa.eu/eurostat/statistics-explained/index.php?title=Glossary:Cash_crops.
9. Definitions [Internet]. Fao.org. [cited 2023 Dec 13]. Available from: https://www.fao.org/3/w4979e/w4979e05.htm.
10. Gunaratne MS, Radin Firdaus RB, Rathnasooriya SI. Climate change and food security in Sri Lanka: towards food sovereignty. Humanit Soc Sci Commun [Internet]. 2021;8(1) Available from: https://doi.org/10.1057/s41599-021-00917-4.
11. Clapp J, Moseley WG, Burlingame B, Termine P. Viewpoint: the case for a six-dimensional food security framework. Food Policy [Internet]. 2022;106(102164):102164. Available from: https://www.sciencedirect.com/science/article/pii/S0306919221001445.
12. HLPE. Food security and nutrition: building a global narrative towards 2030. Report by the high level panel of experts on food security and nutrition of the committee on world food security, Rome. 2020.
13. Chen RS, Kates RW. World food security: prospects and trends. Food Policy [Internet]. 1994;19(2):192–208. Available from: https://www.sciencedirect.com/science/article/pii/0306919294900698.
14. Pawlak K, Kołodziejczak M. The role of agriculture in ensuring food security in developing countries: Considerations in the context of the problem of sustainable food production. Sustainability [Internet]. 2020 [cited 2023 Dec 13];12(13):5488. Available from: https://www.mdpi.com/2071-1050/12/13/5488.
15. Food security and political stability [Internet]. Dkiapcss.edu. [cited 2023 Dec 13]. Available from: https://dkiapcss.edu/Publications/Report_Food_Security_98.html.
16. Smith LC, El Obeid AE, Jensen HH. The geography and causes of food insecurity in developing countries. Agric Econ [Internet]. 2000;22(2):199–215. Available from: https://doi.org/10.1111/j.1574-0862.2000.tb00018.x.
17. The impact of education across sectors: Food security [Internet]. Epdc.org. [cited 2023 Dec 13]. Available from: https://www.epdc.org/sites/default/files/documents/Impact%20of%20Education%20Across%20Sectors%20-%20Food%20Security.pdf.
18. Ishfaq S, Anjum A, Kouser S, Nightingale G, Jepson R. The relationship between women's empowerment and household food and nutrition security in Pakistan. PLoS One [Internet]. 2022;17(10):e0275713. Available from: https://doi.org/10.1371/journal.pone.0275713.

19. Ritchie H, Rosado P, Roser M. Hunger and Undernourishment. Our World in Data [Internet]. 2023 [cited 2023 Dec 13]; Available from: https://ourworldindata.org/hunger-and-undernourishment.
20. Porkka M, Kummu M, Siebert S, Varis O. From food insufficiency towards trade dependency: a historical analysis of global food availability. PLoS One [Internet]. 2013;8(12):e82714. Available from: https://doi.org/10.1371/journal.pone.0082714.
21. FAOSTAT [Internet]. Fao.org. [cited 2023 Dec 13]. Available from: https://www.fao.org/faostat/en/#data/OA.
22. Feeding the world in 2050 and beyond – Part 1: productivity challenges [Internet]. Agriculture. 2018 [cited 2023 Dec 13]. Available from: https://www.canr.msu.edu/news/feeding-the-world-in-2050-and-beyond-part-1.
23. Elferink M, Schierhorn F. Global demand for food is rising. Can we meet it? Harvard business review [Internet]. 2016 Apr 7 [cited 2023 Dec 13]; Available from: https://hbr.org/2016/04/global-demand-for-food-is-rising-can-we-meet-it
24. Fukase E, Martin W. Economic growth, convergence, and world food demand and supply. World Dev [Internet]. 2020;132(104954):104954. Available from: https://www.sciencedirect.com/science/article/pii/S0305750X20300802.
25. Maslow AH, Frager R, Fadiman J, McReynolds C, Cox R. Motivation and personality. 3rd ed. New York; 1987.
26. Malthus TR. An essay on the principle of population.. 1826.
27. Boserup E. Population and technology. Oxford: Blackwell; 1981.
28. Smith K. The malthusian controversy. Routledge; 2013.
29. Foster P, Leathers HD. The world food problem: tackling the causes of undernutrition in the Third World. Lynne Rienner Publishers; 1999.
30. Dowd DF. Inequality and the Global economic crisis. Pluto Press; 2009.
31. Poleman TT. Quantifying the nutrition situation in developing countries. 1979.
32. Archer DW, Dawson J, Kreuter UP, Hendrickson M, Halloran JM. Social and political influences on agricultural systems. Renew Agric Food Syst [Internet]. 2008;23(4):272–84. Available from: http://www.jstor.org/stable/44490597.
33. Steenkamp J, Cilliers EJ, Cilliers SS, Lategan L. Food for thought: addressing urban food security risks through urban agriculture. Sustainability [Internet]. 2021 [cited 2023 Dec 13];13(3):1267. Available from: https://www.mdpi.com/2071-1050/13/3/1267
34. Longhurst R. Cash crops, household food security and nutrition. IDS Bull [Internet]. 1988;19(2):28–36. Available from: https://doi.org/10.1111/j.1759-5436.1988.mp19002005.x.
35. Okolie CC, Ogundeji AA. Effect of COVID-19 on agricultural production and food security: A scientometric analysis. Humanit Soc Sci Commun [Internet]. 2022 [cited 2023 Dec 13];9(1):1–13. Available from: https://www.nature.com/articles/s41599-022-01080-0.
36. Weldegiargis AW, Abebe HT, Abraha HE, Abrha MM, Tesfay TB, Belay RE, et al. Armed conflict and household food insecurity: evidence from war-torn Tigray, Ethiopia. Confl Health [Internet]. 2023;17(1):22. Available from: https://doi.org/10.1186/s13031-023-00520-1.
37. Pimentel D, Harvey C, Resosudarmo P, Sinclair K, Kurz D, McNair M, et al. Environmental and economic costs of soil erosion and conservation benefits. Science [Internet]. 1995 [cited 2023 Dec 13];267(5201):1117–23. Available from: https://pubmed.ncbi.nlm.nih.gov/17789193/.
38. Hossain A, Krupnik TJ, Timsina J, Mahboob MG, Chaki AK, Farooq M, et al. Agricultural land degradation: processes and problems undermining future food security. In: Environment C, editor. Plant and vegetation growth. Cham: Springer International Publishing; 2020. p. 17–61.
39. Water scarcity predicted to worsen in more than 80% of croplands globally this century [Internet]. Preventionweb.net. 2022 [cited 2023 Dec 13]. Available from: https://www.preventionweb.net/news/water-scarcity-predicted-worsen-more-80-croplands-globally-century.
40. Liu X, Liu W, Tang Q, Liu B, Wada Y, Yang H. Global agricultural water scarcity assessment incorporating blue and green water availability under future climate change. Earths Future [Internet]. 2022;10(4) Available from: https://doi.org/10.1029/2021ef002567.

41. Gerten D, Heck V, Jägermeyr J, Bodirsky BL, Fetzer I, Jalava M, et al. Feeding ten billion people is possible within four terrestrial planetary boundaries. Nat Sustain [Internet]. 2020 [cited 2023 Dec 13];3(3):200–8. Available from: https://www.nature.com/articles/s41893-019-0465-1.
42. Ward FA, Pulido-Velazquez M. Water conservation in irrigation can increase water use. Proc Natl Acad Sci U S A [Internet]. 2008;105(47):18215–20. Available from: https://doi.org/10.1073/pnas.0805554105.
43. Jägermeyr J, Pastor A, Biemans H, Gerten D. Reconciling irrigated food production with environmental flows for Sustainable Development Goals implementation. Nat Commun. 8, 15900.
44. Climate change and food security: risks and responses [Internet]. FAO. [cited 2023 Dec 14]. Available from: https://www.fao.org/3/i5188e/I5188E.pdf
45. Food Security [Internet]. IPCC. [cited 2023 Dec 14]. Available from: https://www.ipcc.ch/srccl/chapter/chapter-5/
46. Zhao C, Liu B, Piao S, Wang X, Lobell DB, Huang Y, et al. Temperature increase reduces global yields of major crops in four independent estimates. Proc Natl Acad Sci U S A [Internet]. 2017 [cited 2023 Dec 14];114(35):9326–31. Available from: https://doi.org/10.1073/pnas.1701762114.
47. Abdul Aziz M, Brini F, Rouached H, Masmoudi K. Genetically engineered crops for sustainably enhanced food production systems. Front Plant Sci [Internet]. 2022;13. Available from: https://doi.org/10.3389/fpls.2022.1027828.
48. Datta A. Genetic engineering for improving quality and productivity of crops. Agric & Food Secur [Internet]. 2013;2(1) Available from: https://doi.org/10.1186/2048-7010-2-15.
49. Gaba Y, Pareek A, Singla-Pareek SL. Raising climate-resilient crops: journey from the conventional breeding to new breeding approaches. Curr Genomics [Internet]. 2021 [cited 2023 Dec 14];22(6):450–67. Available from: https://doi.org/10.2174/1389202922666210928151247.
50. Benitez-Alfonso Y, Soanes BK, Zimba S, Sinanaj B, German L, Sharma V, et al. Enhancing climate change resilience in agricultural crops. Curr Biol [Internet]. 2023;33(23):R1246–61. Available from: https://www.sciencedirect.com/science/article/pii/S096098222301429X.
51. Cooper M, Messina CD. Breeding crops for drought-affected environments and improved climate resilience. Plant Cell [Internet]. 2023 [cited 2023 Dec 14];35(1):162–86. Available from: https://academic.oup.com/plcell/article/35/1/162/6825320.
52. Dhankher OP, Foyer CH. Climate resilient crops for improving global food security and safety. Plant Cell Environ [Internet]. 2018;41(5):877–84. Available from: https://doi.org/10.1111/pce.13207.
53. Mango N, Makate C, Mapemba L, Sopo M. The role of crop diversification in improving household food security in Central Malawi. Agric Food Secur [Internet]. 2018;7(1) Available from: https://doi.org/10.1186/s40066-018-0160-x.
54. Ijaz M, Nawaz A, Ul-Allah S, Rizwan MS, Ullah A, Hussain M, et al. Crop diversification and food security. In: Agronomic crops. Singapore: Springer Singapore; 2019. p. 607–21.
55. Tantalaki N, Souravlas S, Roumeliotis M. Data-driven decision making in precision agriculture: the rise of big data in agricultural systems. J Agric Food Inf [Internet]. 2019;20(4):344–80. Available from: https://doi.org/10.1080/10496505.2019.1638264.
56. Yang P, Wu L, Cheng M, Fan J, Li S, Wang H, et al. Review on drip irrigation: Impact on crop yield, quality, and water productivity in China. Water (Basel) [Internet]. 2023 [cited 2023 Dec 14];15(9):1733. Available from: https://www.mdpi.com/2073-4441/15/9/1733.
57. Adeyeye SAO. The role of food processing and appropriate storage technologies in ensuring food security and food availability in Africa. Nutr Food Sci [Internet]. 2017;47(1):122–39. Available from: https://doi.org/10.1108/nfs-03-2016-0037.
58. Opara UL, Caleb OJ, Belay ZA. Modified atmosphere packaging for food preservation. In: Food quality and shelf life. Elsevier; 2019. p. 235–59.
59. Mk M. Vacuum packaging technology: a novel approach for extending the storability and quality of agricultural produce. Adv Plants Agric Res [Internet]. 2017;7(1) Available from: https://doi.org/10.15406/apar.2017.07.00242.

60. Qureshi T, Saeed M, Ahsan K, Malik AA, Muhammad ES, Touheed N. Smart agriculture for sustainable food security using internet of things (IoT). Wirel Commun Mob Comput [Internet]. 2022;2022:1–10. Available from: https://doi.org/10.1155/2022/9608394.
61. Yadav VS, Singh AR, Raut RD, Cheikhrouhou N. Blockchain drivers to achieve sustainable food security in the Indian context. Ann Oper Res [Internet]. 2023;327(1):211–49. Available from: https://doi.org/10.1007/s10479-021-04308-5.
62. Knapp J, Sciarretta A. Agroecology: protecting, restoring, and promoting biodiversity. BMC Ecol Evol [Internet]. 2023;23(1):29. Available from: https://doi.org/10.1186/s12862-023-02140-y.
63. Yuan GN, Marquez GPB, Deng H, Iu A, Fabella M, Salonga RB, et al. A review on urban agriculture: technology, socio-economy, and policy. Heliyon [Internet]. 2022;8(11):e11583. Available from: https://www.sciencedirect.com/science/article/pii/S2405844022028717.
64. Fabiansson SU. Safety of food and beverages: safety of organic foods. In: Encyclopedia of food safety. Elsevier; 2014. p. 417–21.
65. Soares JC, Santos CS, Carvalho SMP, Pintado MM, Vasconcelos MW. Preserving the nutritional quality of crop plants under a changing climate: importance and strategies. Plant Soil [Internet]. 2019;443(1–2):1–26. Available from: https://doi.org/10.1007/s11104-019-04229-0.
66. Women in agriculture [Internet]. Fao.org. [cited 2023 Dec 14]. Available from: https://www.fao.org/reduce-rural-poverty/our-work/women-in-agriculture/en/.
67. Mobarok MH, Skevas T, Thompson W. Women's empowerment in agriculture and productivity change: the case of Bangladesh rice farms. PLoS One [Internet]. 2021 [cited 2023 Dec 14];16(8):e0255589. Available from: https://doi.org/10.1371/journal.pone.0255589
68. Projects—[Internet]. African Sustainable Agriculture Project. [cited 2023 Dec 14]. Available from: https://sustainableagafrica.org/projects-1.

Nutritional Empowerment Through Food Fortification and Biofortification

Maha Azhar, Rahima Yasin, and Jai K. Das

1   Background

Foods, well-balanced in micronutrients, play a critical role in human growth and development [1]. Yet, in most developing countries, the burden of undernutrition and micronutrient deficiencies remains a multifaceted challenge due to a multitude of factors such as poverty, economic instability, and limited agricultural resources. Population growth, coupled with the effects of global climate change and the COVID crisis [2], has resulted in aggravated existing malnutrition and hidden hunger in poverty-stricken regions where there is a lack of sufficient food and essential nutrients to sustain the entire population. Moreover, the transition from rural to urban areas has also led to abandoning traditional diets for processed foods that often contain high levels of salt, sugar, and saturated fat, while being deficient in essential nutrients and fiber.

Malnutrition is characterized by an imbalance of nutrients in the human body, resulting in adverse health effects [3]. *Hidden hunger*, otherwise known as micronutrient deficiency, is a form of undernutrition stemming from the consumption of calorie-rich foods that are deficient in essential minerals and vitamins [4, 5]. Together these contribute significantly to an unacceptably high rates of mortality and morbidity and are associated with conditions such as anemia, poor immunity, growth retardation, birth defects, and developmental delays [6–8]. These are

M. Azhar · R. Yasin
Institute for Global Health and Development, The Aga Khan University, Karachi, Pakistan
e-mail: maha.azhar2@aku.edu; rahima.yasin@aku.edu

J. K. Das (✉)
Institute for Global Health and Development, The Aga Khan University, Karachi, Pakistan

Division of Women and Child Health, The Aga Khan University, Karachi, Pakistan
e-mail: jai.das@aku.edu

© The Author(s), under exclusive license to Springer Nature Switzerland AG 2025
Z. S. Lassi, R. A. Salam (eds.), *Nutrition Across Reproductive, Maternal, Neonatal, Child, and Adolescent Health Care*,
https://doi.org/10.1007/978-3-031-95721-5_15

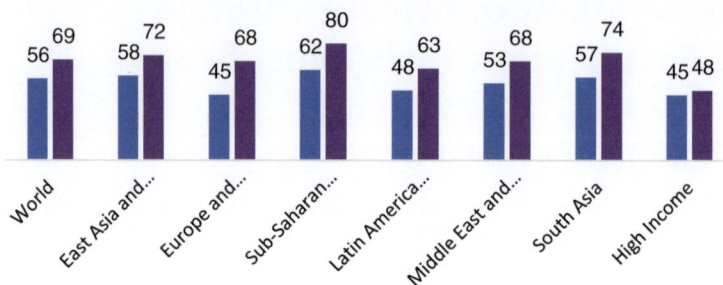

Fig. 1 Prevalence of any micronutrient deficiency. (Source: [1])

persistent global health problems, with an estimated two billion people affected worldwide by micronutrient deficiencies, while around one-third of the population is at risk of at least one micronutrient deficiency. Evidence depicts that approximately 200 million children in low- and middle-income countries (LMICs) are affected by stunting or wasting, and nearly twice as many suffer from deficiencies in essential vitamins and nutrients, notably folic acid, iron, iodine, zinc, and vitamin A [9]. According to the findings in *The Lancet Global Health 2022*, it is estimated that half of preschool-aged children and two-thirds of women of reproductive age globally experience at least one micronutrient deficiency [1]. The *State of Food Security and Nutrition in the World Report 2019* indicates a persistent increase in the number of undernourished individuals over several consecutive years [10]. Simultaneously, there is a concerning rise in the number of overweight and obese individuals worldwide [11]. Back in the mid-twentieth century, *the Green Revolution* commenced in the developing world to alleviate malnutrition and poverty, with the aim to increase agricultural productivity through the adoption of high-yielding varieties of crops with a particular emphasis on rice and wheat. While the Green Revolution had a significant impact on food security and economic growth, the focus on monoculture (rice and wheat) led to the loss of biodiversity while raising concerns about nutritional security [12]. Global prevalence of any micronutrient deficiency is shown in Fig. 1.

The causes of micronutrient deficiencies worldwide are intricate, with unhealthy diets standing out as one of the primary contributors to the global burden of disease. In 2016, unhealthy diets were recognized as the second-leading risk factor for deaths and disability-adjusted life-years (DALYs) on a global scale [13]. By 2017, these diets contributed to around 11 million deaths and 255 million DALYs [14]. The optimal solution for addressing hidden hunger and malnutrition involves the consumption of a diverse and varied diet, ensuring an adequate intake of micronutrients to fulfill an individual's physiological requirements at every stage of life. Sustainable healthy diets are accessible, affordable, safe, equitable, and culturally acceptable [15]. These dietary patterns not only promote health but also have a low environmental footprint, as defined by the Food and Agriculture Organization (FAO) and the World Health Organization (WHO) in 2019 [15]. Regrettably, such diverse diets are frequently unavailable or economically unattainable for numerous households, particularly in the LMICs. An estimated 3 billion people in these regions are unable to afford a nutritious diet. Food-based approaches, involving the enhancement of the micronutrient content in commonly consumed foods and condiments through industrial fortification or biofortification, have been demonstrated to be effective, cost-efficient, and scalable solutions for enhancing micronutrient intakes and improving associated health outcomes [12].

The United Nations (UN) established the second Sustainable Development Goal (SDG) to eradicate malnutrition and tackle hidden hunger [16, 17]. In light of this, governments globally, in collaboration with various stakeholders, have introduced initiatives to address these challenges. Notable programs include the Global Alliance for Improved Nutrition (GAIN), the New Alliance for Food Security and Nutrition, the Health Gain Initiative, the Scaling Up Nutrition Movement, and the Harvest Plus Challenge Program. The WHO and the FAO have outlined four key strategies to combat micronutrient malnutrition. These strategies encompass nutrition education to enhance diet diversity and quality, food fortification and biofortification, supplementation, and disease control measures. Each of these approaches plays a crucial role in alleviating the burden of micronutrient malnutrition [18]. In this chapter, we discuss food fortification and biofortification, highlighting their complementary roles as key food system interventions.

2   Defining Food Fortification

Fortification refers to the deliberate augmentation of the content of a micronutrient, such as a vitamin or mineral (inclusive of trace elements), in a food item [19]. This practice contributes to enhancing the nutritional quality of the food supply to help consumers reach the recommended dietary allowances (RDAs) for those nutrients, contributing to a public health benefit without causing any adverse effects. A *food vehicle* is a selected food item in which a nutrient or nutrients are intentionally added during its regular processing, essentially serving as a carrier of these nutrients. Typically, it is a commonly consumed staple food or condiment. Different types of food fortification include the following:

2.1   Mass or Large-Scale Fortification (LSFF)

To correct a demonstrated micronutrient deficiency in the general population by adding micronutrients to foods that are commonly or frequently consumed, including staple food items and/or condiments. LSFF programs can be categorized as either *mandatory*—meaning they are initiated and regulated by the government—or *voluntary*, where food processors add nutrients to their foods on their own volition but are still governed by regulatory limits.

2.2   Targeted Fortification

To correct a demonstrated micronutrient deficiency in specific population groups with unique nutritional requirements, such as infants, children, pregnant women, and beneficiaries of social protection programs. Examples are complementary foods for young children, special foods designed for expectant or lactating mothers, and emergency rations.

2.3   Point-of-Use Fortification

When vitamins and minerals are not incorporated into foods during the processing phase but are instead added just before consumption, either at home, in schools, or in childcare facilities.

Food fortification programs have a history dating back to the 1920s, marked by the initiation of salt iodization programs in Switzerland and Michigan, USA. Looking back, at the 1921 American Medical Association (AMA) convention, two physicians from Ohio presented their clinical trial findings, illustrating the efficacy of sodium iodide treatments in preventing goiter among schoolgirls in Akron. Drawing from the early achievements of reducing goiter incidence through salt iodization, the practice of food fortification saw expansion and scaling up. This broader initiative included fortifying milk (with vitamin D), flour and bread (with B vitamins and iron), and other staples and condiments. The enforcement of mandatory wheat flour fortification was initially implemented in 1942, and to date, 85 countries have made it a compulsory practice. In North and South America, the addition of folic acid to wheat flour is obligatory as a preventive measure against birth defects. Edible oils are increasingly utilized as a common vehicle for fortification, with 27 countries currently mandating the fortification of oil with vitamin A. Additionally, 14 countries have made milk fortification mandatory, where 11 countries fortify milk with both vitamin A and D. Notably, Costa Rica incorporates iron and folic acid in its milk fortification efforts, while China and Canada go a step further by adding calcium in addition to vitamins A and D [18]. The fortification of sugar with vitamin A commenced in the 1970s in Latin America, with Guatemala being the pioneer to implement this practice in 1975. Guatemala's successful implementation served as a model for other countries, leading to a nearly threefold increase in vitamin A intake and a reduction in vitamin A deficiency from 22% to 5% within just one year [20]. In Africa, mandatory sugar fortification programs are in place in Malawi, Mozambique, Nigeria, Rwanda, Zambia, and Zimbabwe. Presently, more than 140 countries worldwide have established guidance or regulations for fortification programs, with the majority being compulsory [21]. Additionally, nearly 140 countries have initiated national salt iodization programs, out of which 102 have made it mandatory [22]. Furthermore, 85 countries enforce the fortification of at least one type of cereal grain (maize, rice, or wheat) with iron and folic acid, while over 40 countries mandate the fortification of edible oils, margarine, and/or sugar with vitamin A and/or vitamin D [21]. Peru introduced a mandatory fortification law, passed in 2021, in efforts to scale up food fortification as presented in the box below.

> **Case Study: Rice Fortification in Peru**
> Although it is recognized as a national priority, anemia remains a persistent public health challenge in Peru, mirroring similar situations in numerous other countries. In 2021, 38.8% of children under 3 and 18.8% of women in their reproductive years were impacted. Regrettably, progress toward the anaemia target established at the World Health Assembly in 2014 has shown little advancement. Notably, Peru stands as a noteworthy rice producer, cultivating around two million tons annually. A significant 83% of the population includes rice in their daily diet. Given its widespread consumption and production, fortifying rice with various micronutrients emerged as a sensible approach. In 2017, the World Food Programme initiated efforts to incorporate fortified rice into the national social assistance programs that cater to millions of Peruvians, particularly those among the most economically disadvantaged and nutritionally vulnerable. Given that rice was already included in these programs, the transition from unfortified to fortified rice was viewed as an easily attainable goal. This approach presented an opportunity to enhance dietary quality by leveraging existing distribution networks and demanding only minimal behavioral adjustments from program participants. Efforts to enhance the capabilities of rice millers, establish consistent demand, and instill widespread belief in the advantages of fortified rice laid the foundation for the enactment of a law mandating rice fortification, officially passed in 2021 [24].

3 Defining Biofortification

Biofortification, alternatively referred to as nutrient enrichment, involves the use of traditional crop breeding methods to create varieties with higher levels of bioavailable vitamins and minerals. This strategy is designed not only to boost productivity but also to enhance resistance to both biotic and abiotic stresses, improve climate resilience, and enhance the palatability of staple crops [23].

The concept of biofortification was developed in the 1990s and evolved into a programmatic strategy with the establishment of the *HarvestPlus program* under the Consultative Group on International Agricultural Research in 2003 [24]. The goal was to take the initiative in combating micronutrient deficiencies in major food crops of common beans, maize, sweet potatoes, pearl millet, cassava, and rice in Asian and African countries. The target is to reach 1 billion people with a supply of biofortified crops by 2030. The delivery of biofortified planting material commenced through pilot projects in Uganda and Mozambique in 2006–2007 [25].

Table 1 Common nutrients added to food vehicles through fortification and biofortification

Food vehicle	Large-scale food fortification	Biofortification
Beans	–	Iron and zinc
Cassava	–	Vitamin A
Maize	Iron, calcium, zinc, folic acid, vitamin B12, vitamin A, thiamine, niacin, vitamin B6, and/or vitamin D	Vitamin A or zinc
Milk	Vitamin A and/or vitamin D	–
Oil	Vitamin A, vitamin D, and/or vitamin K	–
Pearl millet	–	Iron
Rice	Iron, folic acid, vitamin B12, vitamin A, zinc, thiamine, niacin, and/or vitamin B6	Zinc
Salt	Iodine, iron	–
Sweet potato	–	Vitamin A
Wheat	Iron, calcium, zinc, folic acid, vitamin B12, vitamin A, zinc, thiamine, niacin, vitamin B6, and/or vitamin D	Zinc

Source: [24]

Subsequently, programs were implemented in various countries, including Bangladesh, the Democratic Republic of the Congo, India, Nigeria, Pakistan, Rwanda, and Zambia. Worldwide, biofortified crops have been introduced in 40 countries, spanning across Africa, Asia, and Latin America. The proposition that it represents a cost-effective approach to combat malnutrition and its potential to seamlessly complement other strategies, such as food fortification and food supplementation (that involves the consumption of micronutrients through capsules, tablets, or syrup), is a key point of discussion. Table 1 shows common nutrients added to food vehicles through food fortification and biofortification.

4 Types of Biofortification

Biofortification can be achieved through various approaches, including conventional (involving traditional crop breeding), agronomic methods (such as soil or foliar application), and transgenic (utilizing biotechnology). Although the transgenic approach targets a broader range of crops, the most commonly adopted method for biofortification is through conventional breeding. Figure 2 shows the different methods employed for biofortification.

4.1 Plant Breeding

Traditional plant breeding is a method of improving the nutritional content of crops by selecting for desired traits through controlled crosses between different plant varieties. The process involves selecting plants with desirable traits, such as higher micronutrient content, and crossing them with other plants to create a hybrid with improved characteristics. Over time, this process is repeated, and the offspring are screened for desired traits. There are three main techniques employed for plant breeding.

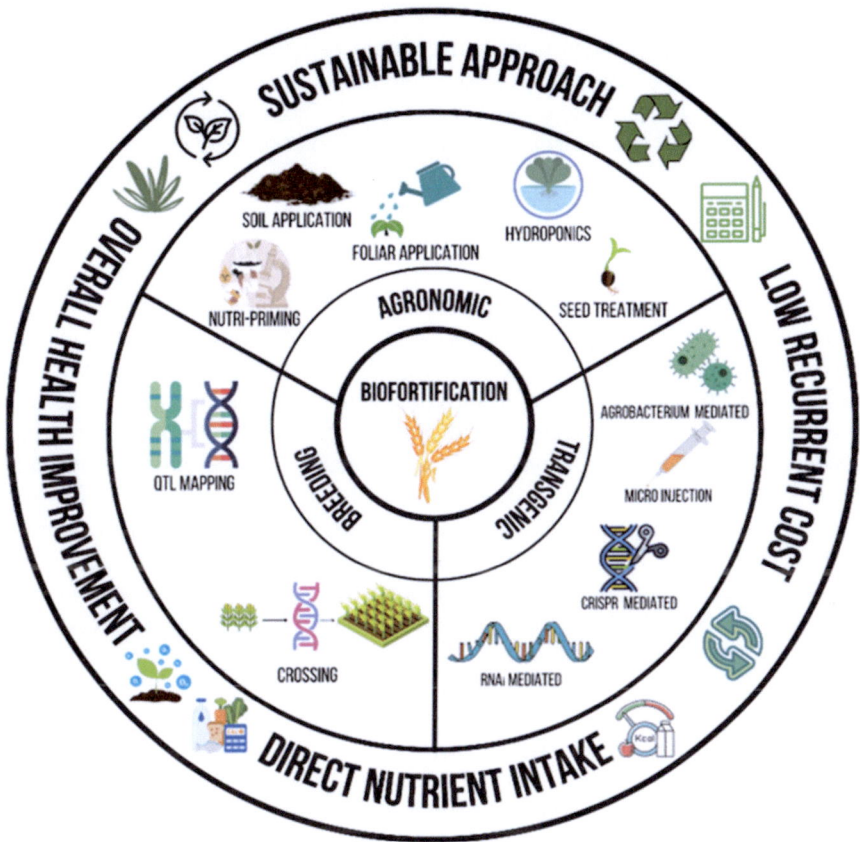

Fig. 2 Methods of biofortification. (Source: [12])

4.1.1 Conventional Breeding

Conventional breeding stands as the most prevalent and widely accepted method for plant breeding in the context of biofortification [26, 27]. The breeding entails crossing crops with genotypic features characterized by high nutrient density and other favorable agronomic traits [26]. As of now, more than 299 biofortified crop varieties have been introduced in over 30 countries through conventional breeding [28]. An illustrative example of a crop biofortified through conventional breeding is Orange Fleshed Sweet Potato (OFSP), which has been enhanced with provitamin A and increased yield traits [28]. Quality Protein Maize is another product of conventional breeding [29]. Recent instances of conventionally bred biofortified plant-based foods encompass varieties like "Zincol" and "Akbar-2019," released in 2015 and 2019, respectively, featuring enhanced iron (Fe) and zinc (Zn) contents.

4.1.2 Mutation Breeding

Mutation breeding diverges from conventional breeding in that distinctions in genetic traits among crops are induced by introducing mutations through chemical treatments or physical methods like irradiation [27, 30]. Recently, mutation breeding has been employed to enhance the biofortification of resilient chickpea mutants, such as Pusa-408 (Ajay), Pusa-413 (Atul), Pusa-417 (Girnar), and Pusa-547, developed at the Indian Agricultural Research Institute (I.A.R.I.), India [31].

4.1.3 Molecular Breeding

Biofortification through molecular breeding involves pinpointing the location of a gene responsible for enhancing nutritional quality and identifying closely linked markers associated with that specific gene. Using these markers, desirable traits can be introduced into the crop through conventional breeding methods [32]. Molecular breeding serves to swiftly determine the presence or absence of a desired trait in a specific crop during its developmental stages, making it a faster process compared to other forms of plant breeding. This approach, also known as molecular or *marker-assisted breeding*, has been instrumental in developing numerous maize varieties with enhanced provitamin A content. These varieties have the potential to fulfill 25–50% of the estimated average requirements for vitamin A in women and children [27, 33]. Such biofortified maize varieties have been introduced in countries like Zambia, Nigeria, and India.

4.2 Agronomic Biofortification

Agronomic biofortification refers to the process of enriching the nutritional value of crops through fertilization and soil management. It offers an efficient and timely solution that is the quickest and most affordable way to produce nutrient-dense food, albeit it only offers a short-term fix. The majority of crops can benefit from this very simple method of biofortifying with iron, zinc, iodine, and selenium. To boost the content of micronutrients in the plant's edible parts, micronutrient-containing organic/inorganic fertilizers or biofertilizers are applied to the plant by foliar or soil application. Micronutrient concentration depends on the source of fertilizer used, method and rate of fertilizer application, stage of application, and translocation of nutrients within plants. Due to variations in mineral mobility, mineral accumulation among plant species, and soil compositions in the particular geographic region of each crop, the success of agronomical biofortification is highly variable. The effectiveness of agronomic biofortification has increased with the development of high-specialized fertilizers with high nutrient uptake efficiency and greater nutrient translocation to the consumable sections of a crop plant, which include water-soluble fertilizers, chelated fertilizers, and nanofertilizers. However, in similarity with supplements and fortification, agronomic intervention is most effectively utilized in specific scenarios or in conjunction with other strategies. One limitation of agronomic intervention is the expense and consequences of fertilizers. The use of fertilizers is anticipated to raise the overall cost of food, potentially limiting its accessibility for the most economically disadvantaged individuals. Given that costly fertilizers need regular application, and with no immediate yield incentive for farmers in developing nations, there is a likelihood that the intervention may be neglected to cut costs, despite the fact that seeds produced in mineral-rich conditions exhibit more robust germination than those in impoverished soils.

4.3 Genetic Engineering/Transgenic Approach

Genetic engineering (GE) represents the newest tool in the arsenal against mineral deficiency, employing advanced biotechnological methods to directly introduce genes into breeding varieties. These genes can be sourced from various origins, including animals and microbes, and are strategically designed to achieve one or more of the following objectives:

(a) Enhance the efficiency of mineral mobilization in the soil
(b) Decrease the presence of anti-nutritional compounds
(c) Elevate the levels of nutritional enhancer compounds, like inulin

Genetic engineering, also known as rDNA (recombinant DNA), is a method that provides increased speed and expansiveness by transferring specific genes with desired traits from a source organism, without the necessity of being a related organism, directly into the living DNA of a target organism. This transgenic trait is introduced without relying on regular biological reproduction. However, once integrated into the plant, it becomes heritable through normal reproductive processes. Scientists initially developed this technique in the laboratory in 1973, and since the 1980s, they have been utilizing it to modify agricultural crop plants. Once a beneficial gene is identified, a process that often involves extensive research and numerous years, it is linked to marker and promoter genes and then introduced into a plant, typically utilizing a nonviable virus called *Agrobacterium* as a carrier. Genetic engineering (GE) results in the creation of plants known as transgenics or, more broadly, genetically modified organisms (GMOs). GE is highly impactful as it can introduce valuable traits not present in the seeds of individual plant species. The application of GE was crucial in the development of golden rice, incorporating the precursor to vitamin A from a daffodil plant. This trait was absent in rice plants and could not be introduced through conventional means, as daffodils cannot be conventionally crossbred with rice plants [34].

Plant breeding and genetic engineering are frequently juxtaposed because, unlike agronomic interventions, both entail altering the genotype of a specific crop. Despite having a shared objective, these two processes differ in their scope. Both endeavors aim to develop plant lines harboring genes conducive to the optimal accumulation of bioavailable minerals. Plant breeding achieves this by crossbreeding the most high-performing plants and selecting those with favorable traits over numerous generations. In contrast, genetic engineering accesses genes from any source and directly introduces them into the crop.

4.4 Others

4.4.1 Biofortification Using Microorganisms

The presence of beneficial soil microorganisms with symbiotic association in plant roots provides the production of plant growth hormones and enhances the availability of mineral nutrients. The soil microorganisms, like *Bacillus* and *Pseudomonas*, are applied to promote the phytoavailability of micronutrients and are mainly used as seed inoculants. These microorganisms promote plant growth through the production of antibiotics, chitinases, siderophores, and growth hormones. The use of plant growth-promoting microorganisms in iron fortification is very useful because they can chelate iron through the generation of siderophore compounds, solubilize phosphorus, and prevent the growth of plant pathogens.

4.4.2 The Role of Nanotechnology in Fortification

Nanotechnologies encompass technologies comprising particles, either natural or synthetic, constituting a minimum of 50% of the total, within the size range of 1–100 nanometers, equivalent to one billionth of a meter [35]. Nano-sized particles or *nanoliposomes* are utilized to improve the absorption and bioavailability of nutrients in fortified foods through encapsulating vitamins, minerals, or other bioactive chemicals. This encapsulation preserves nutrients from degradation through the process of food preparation, storage, and digestion, preserving their integrity and bioavailability, and improving agricultural productivity. Nanocarriers can be developed to release nutrients at specific sites in the body in a regulated or targeted manner, guaranteeing maximum absorption and utilization [36]. Nanofertilizers outperform traditional fertilizers because they can exponentially increase the nutrients' efficacy, minimize the need for chemical fertilizers, make crops drought and disease resistant, and are less harmful to the environment [37]. Nanopesticides are pesticide formulations that are nano-sized and use nanotechnology to increase the efficiency, effectiveness, and targeted delivery of active pesticide components. These formulations attempt to improve pest control while decreasing environmental impact and the amount of insecticides required for effective use [38]. There are some negative effects of nanomaterials on biological systems and the environment caused by nanoparticles, like chemical hazards on edible plants after treatment with high concentrations of nanosilver. Also, in some cases, nanomaterials generate free radicals in living tissue, leading to DNA damage. Therefore, nanotechnology should be carefully evaluated before use [37].

> **Case Study: Biofortification in Zimbabwe and Rwanda**
> In Zimbabwe, within the framework of a program promoting conservation agriculture to enhance climate resilience and agricultural productivity, participating farmers embraced biofortified varieties of various crops. The adoption of climate-resilient techniques not only led to increased productivity but also enhanced the availability of micronutrients in households involved in the program. Meanwhile, in Rwanda, farmers swiftly embraced iron-biofortified beans. By the close of 2018, an estimated 20% of the country's bean production comprised iron-biofortified varieties, with 15% of the population incorporating them into their diets. Regular consumption of these fortified beans was found to meet up to 80% of daily iron requirements. Furthermore, the iron-biofortified varieties demonstrated yields with iron levels 20% higher than other varieties, making them an appealing choice for farmers [10].

5 How Effective and Cost-Effective Are Fortification and Biofortification?

The efficacy of LSFF has been well-established [39, 40]. Consequently, there is widespread acknowledgment that fortifying foods with micronutrients holds the potential to notably elevate serum micronutrient concentrations and alleviate clinical and physiological signs of deficiencies [39, 41]. This improvement extends to various micronutrients, such as iron, folic acid, iodine, vitamin A, vitamin D, and zinc, and spans a range of food vehicles, including wheat flour, maize flour, rice, salt, oil, sugar, soy and fish sauces, bouillon, and milk. The effectiveness of LSFF has been similarly demonstrated in high-income countries and to a lesser extent in LMICs. In numerous high-income countries, LSFF has been acknowledged for its beneficial effects on various micronutrient deficiency disorders. These include the eradication of pellagra and beriberi through the fortification of flour with B vitamins (niacin and thiamine, respectively), a decrease in neural tube defects (NTDs) resulting from fortifying cereal grains with folic acid, the elimination of rickets through milk fortification with vitamin D, and a reduction in goiter prevalence through salt iodization. A systematic review of randomized controlled trials (RCTs) and quasi-trials indicated that fortifying foods with iron led to a significant increase in hemoglobin (0.42 g/dL, 95% confidence interval [CI]: 0.28–0.56) and serum ferritin (1.36 mg/L; 95% CI: 1.23–1.52). Additionally, there was a reduced risk of anemia (risk ratio [RR]: 0.59; 95% CI: 0.48–0.71) and iron deficiency (RR: 0.48; 95% CI: 0.38–0.62). However, no discernible effects were observed on the rates of infections, physical growth, or mental and motor development [42]. In LMICs, measurable improvements in micronutrient and health status have also been demonstrated, including reductions in anemia (from iron fortification), goiter (salt iodisation), NTDs (folic acid fortification), and vitamin A deficiency. A systematic review assessing the effect of LSFF with key micronutrients demonstrated that anemia was decreased by 34% (RR: 0.66; 95% CI: 0.59, 0.74), the likelihood of goiter was reduced by 74% (odds ratio (OR): 0.26; 95% CI: 0.16, 0.43), and the odds of neural tube defects decreased by 41% (OR: 0.59; 95% CI: 0.49, 0.70). Additionally, the findings indicated that the use of LSFF with vitamin A could prevent vitamin A deficiency in nearly three million children annually [43]. Another systematic review reported that fortification of iron, vitamin A, and iodine can increase the level of hemoglobin, serum ferritin, and serum retinol and median urine iodine excretion, especially in toddlers and schoolchildren [44]. A systematic review comprising RCTs showed that vitamin D fortification of foods such as milk, cereal, juice, bread, yogurt, and cheese led to an improvement in 25(OH)D concentration (mean difference (MD): 15.51 nmol/L (95% CI 6.28–24.74). Additionally, the prevalence of vitamin D deficiency decreased (RR 0.53 (95% CI 0.41, 0.69), and cognitive function showed improvement (MD 1.22 (IQ) points (95% CI 0.65, 1.79) [45]. LSFF adds essential vitamins and minerals to widely consumed foods during processing. It is one of the most cost-effective interventions to reduce micronutrient deficiencies with an average cost/benefit ratio of 1:27, meaning every $1 invested generates $27 on average in economic return from averted disease, improved earnings, and enhanced work productivity [46, 47].

Intake of vitamin A-biofortified OFSP led to elevated circulating beta-carotene levels and exerted a moderate impact on vitamin A status [48]. The efficacy of biofortified staple crops in reducing micronutrient deficiencies is well-demonstrated for several biofortified crops, including iron-biofortified beans [49, 50], iron-biofortified pearl millet [51], vitamin A-biofortified cassava [52, 53], vitamin A-biofortified maize [54–56], and vitamin A-biofortified sweet potato [57–59] among children under five, school children, adolescent/young women, and women of reproductive age in LMICs. The introduction of OFSP in rural Uganda led to heightened vitamin A intakes in children and women, contributing to an enhanced vitamin A status among children. Furthermore, women who obtained more vitamin A from the crop demonstrated a reduced likelihood of experiencing marginal vitamin A deficiency [59]. In Kenya, provitamin A cassava proved effective in enhancing the vitamin A status of schoolchildren [52]. Studies have also shown that consumption of biofortified crops resulted in significant improvements in functional, cognitive, and health outcomes, such as improved memory and ability to pay attention and improved reaction time [60]. For iron-biofortified crops, studies have found improved ability to do everyday physical tasks, also known as work efficiency [61]. For vitamin A-biofortified crops, research has identified reductions in prevalence and duration of diarrhea for children under 5 [62]; protection from age-related retinal degeneration [63]; improved ability to see in dim light [55]; and improved vitamin A content of breast milk [54]. Efficacy of zinc biofortification and LSFF for reducing zinc deficiency is difficult to establish due to the dearth of zinc biomarkers sensitive enough to detect the effect of food-based zinc interventions on zinc outcomes. In lieu of zinc deficiency biomarkers, several health outcomes related to zinc deficiency have been investigated. For example, zinc-biofortified wheat was found to result in significant reductions in morbidity outcomes, such as days spent sick with pneumonia, vomiting, and fever [64]. Studies comparing the

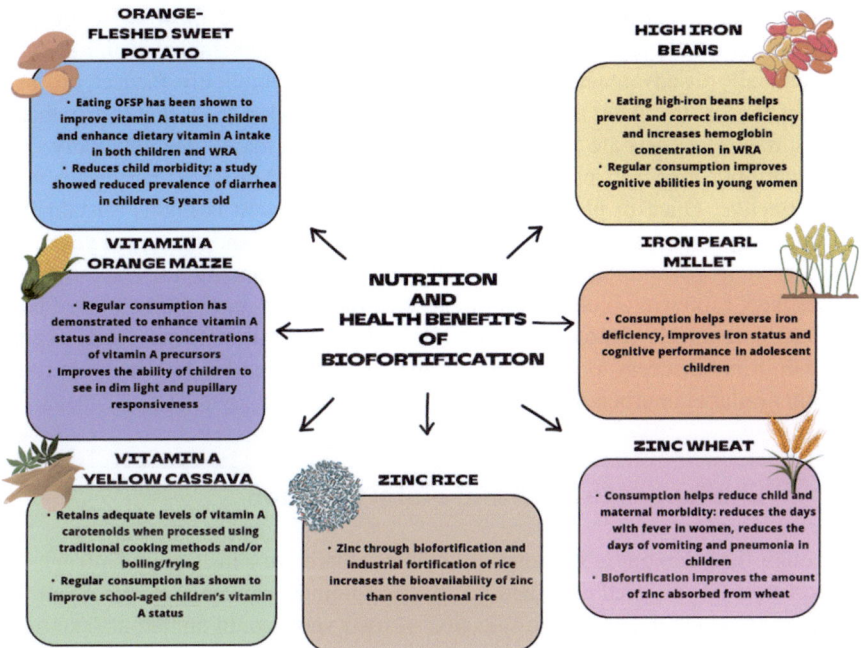

Fig. 3 Nutrition and health benefits of biofortification. (Source: [68])

absorption of zinc-biofortified rice and wheat to their zinc-fortified counterparts found zinc biofortification to be at least as good a source of bioavailable zinc as zinc fortification [65]. Since biofortification is a more recent intervention than LSFF, and given that effectiveness studies for agricultural-nutrition interventions such as biofortification require significant time and resource investments, the only completed effectiveness studies to date have been on vitamin A-biofortified sweet potato. These studies found delivery of this biofortified crop to result in significant adoption and consumption thereof; significant increases in vitamin A intakes among women and children; and significant improvement in vitamin A status for children in intervention households. Figure 3 shows the benefits of biofortification by nutrient and crop.

There is a significant body of ex-ante cost-effectiveness analyses of several biofortification interventions. These analyses found most biofortification interventions to be highly cost-effective according to the World Bank criteria of cost (in USD) per DALY saved. Based on such ex-ante analyses, the Copenhagen Consensus ranked interventions that reduce micronutrient deficiencies, including biofortification, among the highest value-for-money investments for economic development. As per their analysis, for every USD invested in biofortification, as much as 17 USD of benefits may be gained [66, 67]. Furthermore, the biofortification strategy aims to leverage the routine daily intake of substantial quantities of staple foods by every family member, particularly women and children who are most susceptible to micronutrient malnutrition. Due to the prevalence of food staples in the diets of economically disadvantaged individuals, this strategy implicitly focuses on low-income households. After a one-time investment to develop seeds that fortify themselves, recurrent costs are low, and germplasm may be shared internationally. It is this multiplier aspect of plant breeding across time and distance that makes it so cost-effective. Once in place, the biofortified crop system is highly sustainable. Nutritionally improved varieties will continue to be grown and consumed year after year, even if government attention and international funding for micronutrient issues fade. Moreover, biofortification has the potential to reach malnourished populations in relatively remote rural areas, delivering naturally fortified foods to people with limited access to commercially marketed fortified foods, which are more readily available in urban areas.

6 Challenges to Food and Biofortification

Although the potential advantages are evident, there are substantial challenges to biofortification that need to be addressed. The foremost challenge to effective food fortification is the inappropriate selection of food vehicles. In numerous countries, staple foods and condiments are required to be fortified due to their widespread consumption. However, the feasibility of fortifying the chosen food vehicle is often low, and governments face challenges in effectively enforcing compliance. This is especially problematic when the food vehicle is not produced by large formal industries or is not aggregated sufficiently to create opportunities for fortification. Additionally, numerous countries face a shortage of critical data and information, or they inadequately leverage existing data on industry structure, food supply chains, compliance, coverage, food intake, and nutrition status. These data-related challenges hinder program design, oversight, and evaluation. In several countries, prioritizing data quality, frequency, utility, and analysis is essential to establish efficient large-scale fortification programs. Laws and regulations concerning the monitoring, inspection, and enforcement of food fortification are frequently fragmented and inadequately integrated into legal frameworks, resulting in a deficiency of or weak enforcement. Considering the potential for excessive nutrient intake among groups not within the target population, continuous and vigilant monitoring of additional intakes and nutritional status linked to the consumption of fortified foods should be actively maintained as an essential component of any fortification program [18, 69]. For instance, in China, thorough monitoring has identified counties where a significant portion of the population is likely experiencing excessive iodine intake from the local water source, as indicated by urinary iodine levels. In response to this, efforts are being made to decrease the iodine content in the distributed iodized salt in these areas [70]. Commercially fortified products may be unaffordable for the most impoverished segments of societies, partially due to import duties and taxes on premixes or fortification equipment in some countries, leading to increased prices.

The inequality in access to fortified foods requires local research and contextual understanding, as the reasons for limited accessibility can vary within countries and households. Programs often lack this specific understanding and fail to assess intrahousehold food distribution practices, which frequently disadvantage women and young children within households. LSFF also depends on international supply chains, and any disruption to global trade can have a significant impact. For instance, fortification initiatives in Africa heavily depend on imported premix (the essential vitamins and minerals for fortification), and fortifiable staples such as grains and edible oil are usually brought in before processing and fortification within the country. In essence, the success of fortification programs in LMICs relies on favorable international trade conditions. Successful food fortification programs additionally hinge on robust quality control and surveillance systems at the country level, involving key contributions from major private sector enterprises, small- and medium-sized enterprises, government, and civil society. However, limited budgets are frequently recognized as a constraint on ensuring sufficient quality control and compliance.

An obstacle involves convincing farmers of the economic benefits and sustainability of cultivating biofortified crops. Additionally, the transgenic approach necessitates substantial investments in financial, temporal, and human resources during the research and developmental phases, and consumers may harbor concerns about the safety and long-term effects of GMOs [5, 30, 32]. The repeated use of mineral fertilizers through an agronomic approach can result in accumulation, potentially leading to toxicity [32, 71]. Moreover, the growing demand for mined minerals like selenium may contribute to depletion and have adverse environmental effects [71, 72]. Regulatory monitoring bodies and consumer protection organizations frequently fail to proactively safeguard consumers against underfortified or nonfortified foods and deceptive labeling practices. This situation can mislead consumers who rely on accurate information about vitamin and mineral content as stated on product packaging.

7 Way Forward

Foremost, there is a need for education about the benefits of cultivating biofortified crops and how they can enhance their livelihoods. This involves imparting knowledge about the potential increase in yield, improved pest resistance, and reduced dependency on chemical fertilizers and pesticides. Moreover, farmers require access to essential infrastructure, including reliable irrigation systems and storage facilities, to effectively cultivate and market biofortified crops, which may require extra funding. Overcoming these challenges is crucial for the successful adoption and acceptance of biofortified crops since the effectiveness of biofortification initiatives relies on the approval and adoption of biofortified crops by both farmers and consumers [73]. Since there is a potential for toxicity and adverse environmental effects with agronomic biofortification, mitigating these concerns necessitates thorough research and transparency. Therefore, scientists and regulatory bodies play a crucial role in conducting rigorous safety assessments to ensure that biofortified crops are safe for consumption and do not pose risks to the environment. This involves comprehensive evaluations of potential allergenicity and toxicity associated with GMOs. Offering precise and comprehensible information about the biofortified attributes of a product empowers consumers to make well-informed choices. Transparent labeling not only facilitates trust but also instills confidence in biofortified crops. This transparency allows consumers to comprehend the potential benefits, enabling them to make decisions that align with their preferences and values. Furthermore, to effectively reach populations in greatest need, opportunities to collaborate with social protection programs, for example, should be explored and better utilized.

8 Conclusion

Despite the undeniable potential benefits of genetically modified crops, it is imperative to carefully weigh the ethical implications linked to altering the genetic makeup of organisms. This necessitates continuous dialogue with stakeholders, including farmers, consumers, and environmental organizations, to guarantee that fortification and biofortification initiatives are carried out responsibly and with transparency. Political and regulatory obstacles, including apprehensions related to intellectual property rights, biosafety, and trade matters, may impede the development and dissemination of biofortified crops.

References

1. Stevens GA, Beal T, Mbuya MNN, Luo H, Neufeld LM, Addo OY, et al. Micronutrient deficiencies among preschool-aged children and women of reproductive age worldwide: a pooled analysis of individual-level data from population-representative surveys. Lancet Glob Health. 2022;10(11):e1590–9.
2. Global Alliance for Improved Nutrition (GAIN). COVID-19 is making it harder for vulnerable people to access healthy food [Internet]. 2020. Available from: https://www.gainhealth.org/sites/default/files/publications/documents/covid-19-is-making-it-harder-for-vulnerable-people-to-access-healthy-food.pdf
3. World Health Organization. Malnutrition [Internet]. Available from: https://www.who.int/health-topics/malnutrition#tab=tab_1
4. Gani GB, Bashir O, Bhat TA, Naseer B, Qadri T, et al. Hidden hunger and its prevention by food processing: a review. Int J Unani Integr Med. 2018;2(3):01–10.
5. Wakeel A, Farooq M, Bashir K, Ozturk L. Micronutrient malnutrition and biofortification: recent advances and future perspectives. In: Plant micronutrient use efficiency [internet]. Elsevier; 2018 [cited 2024 Jan 3]. p. 225–43. https://linkinghub.elsevier.com/retrieve/pii/B9780128121047000174.
6. Kiprop Choge J. Malnutrition: Current Challenges and Future Perspectives. In: Imran M, Imran A, editors. Malnutrition [Internet]. IntechOpen; 2020 [cited 2024 Jan 4]. Available from: https://www.intechopen.com/books/malnutrition/malnutrition-current-challenges-and-future-perspectives

7. World Food Programme. The Economic Consequences of Undernutrition in Pakistan [Internet]. 2017. Available from: https://docs.wfp.org/api/documents/WFP-0000112744/ download/#:~:text=The%20lost%20future%20workforce%20is,US%24%202.24%20 billion%20per%20year.&text=Cognitive%20deficits%20derived%20from%20 childhood,US%24%203.7%20billion%20per%20year
8. Castrogiovanni P, Imbesi R. The role of malnutrition during pregnancy and its effects on brain and skeletal muscle postnatal development. J Funct Morphol Kinesiol. 2017;2(3):30.
9. UNICEF. Advancing Large Scale Food Fortification UNICEF's Vision and Approach [Internet]. Available from: https://www.unicef.org/documents/LSFF-Vision
10. Food and Agriculture Organization of the United Nations. The State of Food Security and Nutrition in the World (SOFI): Safeguarding against economic slowdowns and downturns [Internet]. 2019. Available from: https://www.wfp.org/publications/2019-state-food-security-and-nutrition-world-sofi-safeguarding-against-economic
11. World Health Organization. Obesity and overweight [Internet] 2021. Available from: https://www.who.int/news-room/fact-sheets/detail/obesity-and-overweight#:~:text=Worldwide%20 obesity%20has%20nearly%20tripled,%2C%20and%2013%25%20were%20obese
12. Avnee, Sood S, Chaudhary DR, Jhorar P, Rana RS. Biofortification: an approach to eradicate micronutrient deficiency. Front Nutr. 2023;10:1233070.
13. Gakidou E, Afshin A, Abajobir AA, Abate KH, Abbafati C, Abbas KM, et al. Global, regional, and national comparative risk assessment of 84 behavioural, environmental and occupational, and metabolic risks or clusters of risks, 1990–2016: a systematic analysis for the Global Burden of Disease Study 2016. Lancet. 2017;390(10100):1345–422.
14. Afshin A, Sur PJ, Fay KA, Cornaby L, Ferrara G, Salama JS, et al. Health effects of dietary risks in 195 countries, 1990–2017: a systematic analysis for the global burden of disease study 2017. Lancet. 2019;393(10184):1958–72.
15. WHO TEAM, Nutrition and Food Safety (NFS). Sustainable healthy diets: guiding principles [Internet]. ISBN: 9789241516648, 2019. Available from: https://www.who.int/publications/i/item/9789241516648
16. Gil JDB, Reidsma P, Giller K, Todman L, Whitmore A, Van Ittersum M. Sustainable development goal 2: improved targets and indicators for agriculture and food security. Ambio. 2019;48(7):685–98.
17. Saint Ville A, Po JYT, Sen A, Bui A, Melgar-Quiñonez H. Food security and the Food Insecurity Experience Scale (FIES): ensuring progress by 2030. Food Secur. 2019;11(3):483–91.
18. Osendarp SJM, Martinez H, Garrett GS, Neufeld LM, De-Regil LM, Vossenaar M, et al. Large-scale food fortification and biofortification in low- and middle-income countries: a review of programs, trends, challenges, and evidence gaps. Food Nutr Bull. 2018;39(2):315–31.
19. Fortification assessment coverage toolkit (FACT) [Internet]. Global Alliance for Improved Nutrition (GAIN), Oxford Policy Management; 2019. Available from: https://www.gainhealth.org/resources/reports-and-publications/fortification-assessment-coverage-toolkit-fact
20. Mejia LA, Bower AM. The global regulatory landscape regarding micronutrient fortification of condiments and seasonings. Ann N Y Acad Sci. 2015;1357(1):1–7.
21. Global Fortification Data Exchange [Internet]. Available from: https://fortificationdata.org/
22. Mkambula P, Mbuya MNN, Rowe LA, Sablah M, Friesen VM, Chadha M, et al. The unfinished agenda for food fortification in low- and middle-income countries: quantifying progress, gaps and potential opportunities. Nutrients. 2020;12(2):354.
23. Pfeiffer WH, McClafferty B. HarvestPlus: breeding crops for better nutrition. Crop Sci [Internet] 2007 Dec [cited 2024 Jan 3];47(S3). Available from: https://acsess.onlinelibrary.wiley.com/doi/10.2135/cropsci2007.09.0020IPBS
24. Global Alliance for Improved Nutrition (GAIN). Transforming food systems to deliver nutritious foods the vital roles of fortification and biofortification [Internet]. 2022. Available from: https://www.gainhealth.org/sites/default/files/publications/documents/GAIN-Discussion-Paper-Series-10-Transforming-food-systems-to-deliver-nutritious-foods-the-vital-roles-of-fortification-and-biofortification.pdf

25. Reaching and Engaging End Users (REU) Orange Fleshed Sweet Potato (OFSP) in East and Southern Africa [Internet]. HarvestPlus. Available from: https://www.researchgate.net/profile/Ricardo-Labarta/publication/290433361_Reaching_and_Engaging_End_Users_REU_Orange_Fleshed_Sweet_Potato_OFSP_in_East_and_Southern_Africa/links/5697b14e08aea2d74375b61e/Reaching-and-Engaging-End-Users-REU-Orange-Fleshed-Sweet-Potato-OFSP-in-East-and-Southern-Africa.pdf
26. Garg M, Sharma N, Sharma S, Kapoor P, Kumar A, Chunduri V, et al. Biofortified crops generated by breeding, agronomy, and transgenic approaches are improving lives of millions of people around the world. Front Nutr. 2018;5:12.
27. Sheoran S, Kumar S, Ramtekey V, Kar P, Meena RS, Jangir CK. Current status and potential of biofortification to enhance crop nutritional quality: an overview. Sustain For. 2022;14(6):3301.
28. Dhaliwal SS, Sharma V, Shukla AK, Verma V, Kaur M, Shivay YS, et al. Biofortification—a frontier novel approach to enrich micronutrients in field crops to encounter the nutritional security. Molecules. 2022;27(4):1340.
29. Teklewold A, Wegary D, Tadesse A, Tadesse B, Bantte K, Friesen D, et al. Quality protein maize (QPM): a guide to the technology and its promotion in Ethiopia [internet]. 2015. Available from: https://nume.cimmyt.org/wp-content/uploads/sites/15/2015/12/QPM-Ethiopia-2015-manual-web.pdf
30. Singh U, Praharaj CS, Singh SS, Singh NP. Biofortification of food crops [Internet]. New Delhi: Springer India; 2016 [cited 2024 Jan 3]. Available from: http://link.springer.com/10.1007/978-81-322-2716-8
31. Ofori KF, Antoniello S, English MM, Aryee ANA. Improving nutrition through biofortification—a systematic review. Front Nutr. 2022;9:1043655.
32. Jha AB, Warkentin TD. Biofortification of pulse crops: status and future perspectives. Plan Theory. 2020;9(1):73.
33. Saltzman A, Birol E, Bouis HE, Boy E, De Moura FF, Islam Y, et al. Biofortification: Progress toward a more nourishing future. Glob Food Secur. 2013;2(1):9–17.
34. Singh U, Praharaj CS, Chaturvedi SK, Bohra A. Biofortification: introduction, approaches, limitations, and challenges. In: Singh U, Praharaj CS, Singh SS, Singh NP, editors. Biofortification of food crops [internet]. New Delhi: Springer India; 2016 [cited 2024 Jan 4]. p. 3–18. http://link.springer.com/10.1007/978-81-322-2716-8_1.
35. United Nations. Nanotechnology in agricultural production [Internet]. Available from: https://sustainabledevelopment.un.org/content/documents/12872Policybrief_Agri.pdf
36. Manjunatha SB, Biradar DP, Aladakatti YR. Nanotechnology and its applications in agriculture: a review. 2016. https://www.phytojournal.com/archives/2019/vol8issue3/PartT/8-2-109-768.pdf
37. Elemike E, Uzoh I, Onwudiwe D, Babalola O. The role of nanotechnology in the fortification of plant nutrients and improvement of crop production. Appl Sci. 2019;9(3):499.
38. Prasad R, Bhattacharyya A, Nguyen QD. Nanotechnology in sustainable agriculture: recent developments, challenges, and perspectives. Front Microbiol. 2017;8:1014.
39. Das JK, Salam RA, Kumar R, Bhutta ZA. Micronutrient fortification of food and its impact on woman and child health: a systematic review. Syst Rev. 2013;2(1):67.
40. Bhutta ZA, Das JK, Rizvi A, Gaffey MF, Walker N, Horton S, et al. Evidence-based interventions for improvement of maternal and child nutrition: what can be done and at what cost? Lancet. 2013;382(9890):452–77.
41. Hennessy Á, Walton J, Flynn A. The impact of voluntary food fortification on micronutrient intakes and status in European countries: a review. Proc Nutr Soc. 2013;72(4):433–40.
42. Gera T, Sachdev HS, Boy E. Effect of iron-fortified foods on hematologic and biological outcomes: systematic review of randomized controlled trials. Am J Clin Nutr. 2012;96(2):309–24.
43. Keats EC, Neufeld LM, Garrett GS, Mbuya MNN, Bhutta ZA. Improved micronutrient status and health outcomes in low- and middle-income countries following large-scale fortification: evidence from a systematic review and meta-analysis. Am J Clin Nutr. 2019;109(6):1696–708.
44. Dewi NU, Mahmudiono T. Effectiveness of food fortification in improving nutritional status of mothers and children in Indonesia. Int J Environ Res Public Health. 2021;18(4):2133.

45. Al Khalifah R, Alsheikh R, Alnasser Y, Alsheikh R, Alhelali N, Naji A, et al. The impact of vitamin D food fortification and health outcomes in children: a systematic review and meta-regression. Syst Rev. 2020;9(1):144.
46. Semba RD, Askari S, Gibson S, Bloem MW, Kraemer K. The potential impact of climate change on the micronutrient-rich food supply. Adv Nutr. 2022;13(1):80–100.
47. Garrett G, Matthias D, Keats E, Mbuya M, Wouabe E. Doubling down on food fortification to fortify the future [Internet]. Bill & Melinda Gates Foundation. Available from: https://www.gatesfoundation.org/Ideas/Articles/food-fortification-to-fortify-the-future
48. Bouis HE, Saltzman A. Improving nutrition through biofortification: a review of evidence from HarvestPlus, 2003 through 2016. Glob Food Secur. 2017;12:49–58.
49. Finkelstein J, Mehta S, Villalpando S, Mundo-Rosas V, Luna S, Rahn M, et al. A randomized feeding trial of iron-biofortified beans on school children in Mexico. Nutrients. 2019;11(2):381.
50. Haas JD, Luna SV, Lung'aho MG, Wenger MJ, Murray-Kolb LE, Beebe S, et al. Consuming iron biofortified beans increases iron status in Rwandan women after 128 days in a randomized controlled feeding trial. J Nutr. 2016;146(8):1586–92.
51. Finkelstein JL, Fothergill A, Hackl LS, Haas JD, Mehta S. Iron biofortification interventions to improve iron status and functional outcomes. Proc Nutr Soc. 2019;78(02):197–207.
52. Talsma EF, Melse-Boonstra A, De Kok BPH, Mbera GNK, Mwangi AM, Brouwer ID. Biofortified cassava with pro-vitamin a is sensory and culturally acceptable for consumption by primary school children in Kenya. Vermund SH. PLoS ONE. 2013;8(8):e73433.
53. Afolami I, Mwangi MN, Samuel F, Boy E, Ilona P, Talsma EF, et al. Daily consumption of provitamin A biofortified (yellow) cassava improves serum retinol concentrations in preschool children in Nigeria: a randomized controlled trial. Am J Clin Nutr. 2021;113(1):221–31.
54. Palmer AC, Craft NE, Schulze KJ, Barffour M, Chileshe J, Siamusantu W, et al. Impact of biofortified maize consumption on serum carotenoid concentrations in Zambian children. Eur J Clin Nutr. 2018;72(2):301–3.
55. Gannon B, Kaliwile C, Arscott SA, Schmaelzle S, Chileshe J, Kalungwana N, et al. Biofortified orange maize is as efficacious as a vitamin A supplement in Zambian children even in the presence of high liver reserves of vitamin A: a community-based, randomized placebo-controlled trial. Am J Clin Nutr. 2014;100(6):1541–50.
56. Palmer AC, Siamusantu W, Chileshe J, Schulze KJ, Barffour M, Craft NE, et al. Provitamin A–biofortified maize increases serum β-carotene, but not retinol, in marginally nourished children: a cluster-randomized trial in rural Zambia. Am J Clin Nutr. 2016 Jul;104(1):181–90.
57. Van Jaarsveld PJ, Faber M, Tanumihardjo SA, Nestel P, Lombard CJ, Benadé AJS. β-Carotene–rich orange-fleshed sweet potato improves the vitamin A status of primary school children assessed with the modified-relative-dose-response test1–3. Am J Clin Nutr. 2005;81(5):1080–7.
58. Low JW, Arimond M, Osman N, Cunguara B, Zano F, Tschirley D. A food-based approach introducing orange-fleshed sweet potatoes increased vitamin A intake and serum retinol concentrations in young children in rural Mozambique,3. J Nutr. 2007;137(5):1320–7.
59. Hotz C, Loechl C, De Brauw A, Eozenou P, Gilligan D, Moursi M, et al. A large-scale intervention to introduce orange sweet potato in rural Mozambique increases vitamin A intakes among children and women. Br J Nutr. 2012;108(1):163–76.
60. Vaiknoras K, Larochelle C. The impact of iron-biofortified bean adoption on bean productivity, consumption, purchases and sales. World Dev. 2021;139:105260.
61. Luna SV, Pompano LM, Lung'aho M, Gahutu JB, Haas JD. Increased iron status during a feeding trial of iron-biofortified beans increases physical work efficiency in Rwandan women. J Nutr. 2020;150(5):1093–9.
62. Jones KM, De Brauw A. Using agriculture to improve child health: promoting Orange sweet potatoes reduces diarrhea. World Dev. 2015;74:15–24.
63. Giuliano G. Provitamin A biofortification of crop plants: a gold rush with many miners. Curr Opin Biotechnol. 2017;44:169–80.
64. Mitra-Ganguli T, Boyd K, Uchitelle-Pierce B, Walton J. Proceedings of the workshop 'Biofortified food—Working together to get more nutritious food to the table in India'. J Nutr Intermed Metab. 2019;18:100100.

65. Rehman A, Farooq M, Ullah A, Nadeem F, Im SY, Park SK, et al. Agronomic biofortification of zinc in Pakistan: status, benefits, and constraints. Front Sustain Food Syst. 2020;4:591722.
66. Meenakshi JV. Best Practice Paper Cost-Effectiveness of Biofortification [Internet]. Available from: https://copenhagenconsensus.com/sites/default/files/biofortification.pdf
67. Horton S, Alderman H.A. Rivera J. The challenge of hunger and malnutrition [Internet]. Copenhagen Consensus 2008 Challenge Paper; 2008. Available from: https://copenhagenconsensus.com/sites/default/files/imported/cp_hungerandmalnutritioncc08vol2.pdf
68. Harvestplus and Food and Agricultural Organization of the United Nations (FAO). Biofortification: a food-systems solution to help end hidden hunger [Internet]. 2019. Available from: https://www.ifpri.org/publication/biofortification-food-systems-solution-help-end-hidden-hunger
69. Dwyer JT, Wiemer KL, Dary O, Keen CL, King JC, Miller KB, et al. Fortification and health: challenges and opportunities. Adv Nutr. 2015;6(1):124–31.
70. Codling K, Yan Y. China: Improving USI to ensure optimal iodine nutrition for all. 2015; Available from: @inproceedings{Codling2015ChinaIU, title={China: Improving USI to ensure optimal iodine nutrition for all}, author={Karen Codling and Yan Y. https://www.api.semanticscholar.org/CorpusID:130600753
71. De Valença AW, Bake A, Brouwer ID, Giller KE. Agronomic biofortification of crops to fight hidden hunger in sub-Saharan Africa. Glob Food Secur. 2017;12:8–14.
72. Umar M, Nawaz R, Sher A, Ali A, Hussain R, Khalid MW. Current status and future perspectives of biofortification in wheat. Asian J Res Crop Sci. 2019;6:1–14.
73. Sharma TR, Deshmukh R, Sonah H, editors. Advances in Agri-food biotechnology [internet]. Singapore: Springer Singapore; 2020 [cited 2024 Jan 3]. Available from: https://link.springer.com/10.1007/978-981-15-2874-3

Anthelminthics and WASH Interventions: Evidence and Gaps

Rehana A. Salam and Zohra S. Lassi

1 Epidemiology and Burden

Helminths are parasitic worms. Common helminths found in humans are broadly classified as nematodes (also known as roundworms), cestodes (also known as tapeworms), and trematodes (also known as flukes). Most common nematodes include major intestinal worms (also known as soil-transmitted helminths (STHs)) and the filarial worms that cause lymphatic filariasis and onchocerciasis, whereas cestodes include tapeworms, and trematodes include the schistosomes. Helminths are transmitted to humans through food, water, or soil, as well as by arthropod and molluscan vectors. These can infect every organ and organ system, including the intestines, liver, lungs, blood, and occasionally the brain and other organs.

The 2023 Global Report on Neglected Tropcial Diseases (NTDs) indicates that NTDs combined account for almost 14.5 million disability-adjusted life years (DALYs) [1]. In 2021, 1.65 billion people were reported to require mass or individual treatment and care for NTDs, which is a 25% decline from 2.19 billion in 2010. In 2019, the estimated burden of disease for STH was 1.97 million disability-adjusted life years (DALYs), for schistosomiasis was 1.64 million, for lymphatic filariasis was 1.63 million, for onchocerciasis was 1.23 million, and for

R. A. Salam (✉)
The Daffodil Centre, The University of Sydney, a joint venture with Cancer Council NSW, Sydney, NSW, Australia
e-mail: rehana.abdussalam@sydney.edu.au

Z. S. Lassi
School of Public Health, University of Adelaide, Adelaide, SA, Australia

Robinson Research Institute, Adelaide Medical School, The University of Adelaide, Adelaide, SA, Australia
e-mail: zohra.lassi@adelaide.edu.au

© The Author(s), under exclusive license to Springer Nature Switzerland AG 2025
Z. S. Lassi, R. A. Salam (eds.), *Nutrition Across Reproductive, Maternal, Neonatal, Child, and Adolescent Health Care*,
https://doi.org/10.1007/978-3-031-95721-5_16

leishmaniasis was 697,000 DALYs. The majority of this burden lies in the low- and middle-income countries (LMICs) of sub-Saharan Africa and South Asia [2]. Southeast Asia had the largest number of people requiring interventions for NTDs (51.8% of the global total), followed by the African Region (35.3%) at the end of 2021, while the remaining four regions account for 12.9% of the global total requiring interventions. Additionally, endemic geographies not only harbour multiple helminthic infections but are also burdened with high prevalence of other infectious diseases, including intestinal protozoan infections, malaria, tuberculosis (TB), and human immunodeficiency virus (HIV) [3].

2   Health Impact of Helminthic Infections

Helminthic infections are a major public health concern since these parasites feed on blood and hence contribute to anaemia [4, 5]. STH may also lead to haemorrhage by releasing anticoagulant compounds, thereby leading to iron-deficiency anaemia. It is the leading cause of pathological blood loss in tropical and subtropical regions [6]. The worms increase malabsorption of nutrients, and roundworms, in particular, may possibly compete for vitamin A in the intestine. Some STH also cause loss of appetite and, therefore, can lead to a reduction of nutritional intake and physical fitness. Additionally, STH and schistosomiasis often occur with co-infections in areas where malnutrition is already prevalent [7]. In particular, *Trichuris trichiura* can cause diarrhoea and dysentery. Heavier infections can also lead to a range of symptoms including intestinal manifestations (diarrhoea and abdominal pain), malnutrition, general malaise and weakness, and impaired growth and physical development. Infections of very high intensity can cause intestinal obstruction that should be treated surgically. *Strongyloides stercoralis* may cause dermatological and gastrointestinal morbidity and is also known to be associated with chronic malnutrition in children. In case of reduced host immunity, the parasite can cause hyperinfection/dissemination syndrome that is invariably fatal if not promptly and properly cured and is often fatal despite the treatment. Moreover, with the existing polyparasitism and co-infection with major diseases, individuals infected with multiple infections potentially experience worse health consequences [3].

Children, adolescents, and women of reproductive age (WRA) are much more prone to adverse health consequences. Infection during pregnancy leads to an added demand for nutrients that are critical for fetal growth and development [8, 9]. Hookworms, in particular, along with other STH and *schistosomes*, have been associated with reductions in haemoglobin and iron deficiency during pregnancy [10–14]. Schistosomiasis can also lead to hepatic fibrosis and an associated increased risk of oesophageal varices among pregnant women, occurring at approximately the same rates as in non-pregnant individuals. Women in LMICs are especially prone to these infections since they may be pregnant or lactating for as much as half of their reproductive lives [15]. Estimates indicate that over 50% of pregnant women residing in LMICs have iron-deficiency anaemia [16, 17]. There is a direct association between the intensity of STH infection, blood loss, and consequent anaemia, especially for hookworm infections [11, 18, 19]. The association between anaemia during pregnancy and adverse pregnancy outcomes, including low birth weight (LBW), preterm birth, perinatal mortality, and infant survival, has already been documented [20, 21]. Furthermore, the chances of favourable pregnancy outcomes are reduced by 30% to 45% in anaemic mothers, with their infants having less than half of normal iron reserves [20]. A meta-analysis assessing the association between helminths and childhood stunting reported some association with wasting; however, there was no significant overall evidence that helminths lead to stunting in children, mainly owing to heterogeneous data and shorter duration of follow-ups to detect their impact on stunting [22].

3 Evidence-Based Interventions

Mass deworming (also called preventive chemotherapy) is the process of treating large numbers of people in areas with a high prevalence of these conditions. Along with the water, sanitation, and hygiene (WASH) interventions, it is considered to be an effective measure to prevent and treat helminthic infections in high-burden geographies. Preventive chemotherapy (either alone or in combination) has been used as a public health tool for preventing morbidity due to infection, usually with more than one helminth at a time, since many of the anthelminthic drugs are broad-spectrum. The recent World Health Organisation (WHO) guidelines recommend mass deworming as a public health intervention for all children, non-pregnant adolescent girls, and non-pregnant women of reproductive age (WRA) living in endemic areas [23]. For pregnant women, mass deworming is recommended after the first trimester in areas with a high prevalence (more than 20%) of hookworm and/or *T. trichiura* infection and a high prevalence (over 40%) of anaemia [23]. Deworming during pregnancy is often accompanied by iron supplementation to reduce anaemia.

3.1 Evidence on Mass Deworming

A Cochrane review [24] assessing the effect of mass deworming programmes suggested that the public health programmes to regularly treat all children with deworming drugs did not appear to improve height, haemoglobin, cognition, school performance, or mortality. However, studies conducted in two settings over 20 years ago showed large effects on weight gain, but this is not a finding in more recent, larger studies. An individual participant data (IPD) network meta-analysis [25] to explore the effects of different types and frequencies of deworming drugs on childhood anaemia, cognition, and growth across potential effect modifiers suggested that there were no statistically significant subgroup effects across any of the potential effect modifiers. However, analyses showed that there may be greater effects on weight for moderate to heavily infected children. A Cochrane review assessing the impact of mass deworming among pregnant women after the first trimester of pregnancy concluded that the existing evidence is insufficient to recommend the use of anthelminthic drugs for pregnant women [26]. An IPD analysis looking at the impact of mass deworming after the first trimester of pregnancy suggested that it might be associated with reducing anaemia, with no evidence of impact on any other maternal or pregnancy outcome [27]. A Cochrane review evaluating the impact of drugs to treat schistosomiasis in general population (including 52 trials) suggested that praziquantel 40 mg/kg is effective as the standard treatment for *Schistosoma mansoni* infection while oxamniquine, a largely discarded alternative (due to a lack of current consensus on the optimal dosing regimen) also appeared to be effective [28]. Another Cochrane review evaluating the effectiveness of drugs (including 30 trials) for urinary schistosomiasis in the general population suggested that praziquantel 40 mg/kg was the most studied drug for treating urinary schistosomiasis and had the strongest evidence base [29].

3.2 Mass Deworming: Mixed Findings and Interpretations

There has been a lot of discussion around routine mass deworming programmes, and their effectiveness has been questioned since the recent evidence synthesis suggested that these programmes have very little or no benefit for children and pregnant women [26, 30–32]. The key area for debate around mass deworming is not whether deworming medicine works but whether the benefits of mass deworming exceed the costs or whether it would be more prudent to invest in other interventions including education, sustainability of WASH programmes, communication to encourage high treatment uptake and better integration of helminthic control with other relevant programmes with existing wide-spread coverage. Additionally, a fundamental limitation of mass deworming programmes is that it does not kill immature worms and consequently cannot prevent reinfection. Deworming drugs such as levamisole, mebendazole, albendazole, praziquantel, and pyrantel have been reported to be efficacious with minimal side-effects, but a critical issue in evaluating current STH policies concerns who to treat, how frequently to treat, and how long to treat.

With regard to mass deworming during pregnancy, the data about the deworming drug use in pregnancy are scarce [23, 26]. Adverse events associated with deworming in girls and women themselves have rarely been published and usually only within the context of specific research studies. Although mass deworming is regarded as the most effective means of controlling morbidity and mortality with STH, the long-term safety when administered during pregnancy, particularly in terms of birth outcomes, has not been rigorously evaluated [33, 34]. However, existing evidence have not reported any serious adverse events [35]. A review investigating the scope of available evidence for benefits of deworming treatments in order to inform a decision about possible inclusion of deworming as an intervention in the Lives Saved Tool (LiST) found that deworming did not show consistent benefits for indicators of mortality, anaemia, or growth in children younger than 5 or WRA and hence did not recommend including deworming in the LiST model [36]. These concerns are further complicated by the lack of evidence supporting the health benefits of treating helminths during pregnancy on maternal and birth outcomes [26, 27]. Consequently, there is the question of undue exposure to deworming drugs as a result of routine mass deworming and the potential adverse effects on the foetus. Another barrier in considering WRA in mass deworming programmes is inadvertently administering deworming drugs to women who may not be aware that they are in their first trimester of pregnancy (at which time deworming is contraindicated) since a comprehensive approach for targeting WRA is currently lacking [37]. More recently, issues related to limited efficacy profiles of albendazole, mebendazole, levamisole, and pyrantel pamoate have also been raised with some evidence supporting co-administration of some deworming drugs [38, 39]. Furthermore, there are issues related to drug resistance associated with the scale-up of periodic mass deworming campaigns [38, 39].

3.3 Evidence on WASH Interventions

Existing literature highlights the lack of high-quality evidence on the impact of WASH measures on helminthic infections [40, 41]. Recent large-scale community-level programmes assessing the impact of community and school-based WASH interventions also report mixed findings. The Geshiyaro project from Ethiopia [42] suggested that the lack of access to WASH, such as improved drinking water and shared toilet and hand-washing facilities, was linked to an increased risk of infection with STH and schistosome parasites. These associations, however, were reported to be difficult to establish at an individual household level because of wide variability in access between houses but are detectable when coverage is aggregated at the community level. WinS project [43] found no impact of the intervention on any primary (pupil absence) or secondary (enrolment, dropout, grade progression, diarrhoea, respiratory infection, conjunctivitis, STH infection) outcomes. Even among schools with the highest levels of fidelity and adherence, the impact of the intervention on absence and health was minimal. WASG for WORMS [44] also found no evidence that the WASH interventions led to any additional reductions in STH infections beyond those achieved with deworming alone over the 2-year trial period. The role of WASH on STH infections over a longer period of time and in the absence of deworming remains to be determined.

Evidence from a Cochrane review [45] suggested that the WASH interventions may slightly protect against STH infection. WASH also serves as a broad preventive measure for many other diseases that have a faecal-oral transmission route of transmission. The review further states that despite the biological plausibility for WASH to interrupt transmission of STH, WASH interventions as currently delivered have shown lower than expected impacts. There is a need for more rigorous and targeted implementation research and process evaluations, along with consistent and standardized reporting of the intensity of infection to enable pooled analyses and comparisons. One systematic review evaluated the impact of community-based packaged delivery of interventions, including health education to promote general hygiene and sanitation along with drug administration, iron and β-carotene supplementation, snail control, constructing latrines, eliminating cattle from the residential areas, staff training, and community mobilization [46]. The findings from this review were based on 32 studies and suggested that community-based interventions reduced the prevalence of STH and schistosomiasis and also improved mean haemoglobin and reduced anaemia prevalence. However, there was no clear impact on ferritin, height, weight, LBW, or stillbirths. A feasibility modelling study suggested that the most important determining factors in the control of STH were underlying intensity of STH transmission, implementation of the NTD control programmes and whether countries receive large-scale external funding and strong health systems [47].

3.4 WASH Interventions: Mixed Findings and Interpretations

There are some potential explanations for the mixed impact of WASH interventions on helminthic infections [48]. Firstly, uptake and adherence to WASH interventions is a complex behavioural issue and is influenced by various personal, cognitive, economic, social, cultural, and structural factors that are often resistant to change [49]. Behaviour change interventions ought to involve engagement with the target population, understanding their motivation to change, and adapting context-specific interventions that facilitate change in behaviours for sustainable improvements in uptake and consequent long-term health outcomes [50, 51]. The trials to date are too complex and not context-specific, resulting in limited uptake and unsustainable use owing to inadequate behaviour change methods to consistently achieve desired WASH practices. Secondly, since all trial settings have some access to WASH measures, it is challenging to know what level of WASH intervention coverage is required to interrupt a sufficient number of exposure pathways and, in doing so, prevent reinfection. It is possible that there is a minimal required level of coverage and use of WASH interventions to have an impact, but this threshold will undoubtedly vary by intervention type, background reinfection rates, ongoing deworming, or other factors not yet well defined. Thirdly, it is also difficult to manage contamination between arms in trials evaluating WASH interventions where control communities might have some uptake of improved WASH practices, diluting the estimated effect of the intervention. Fourthly, there might be differences in transmission in various helminths, and hence some might show an impact while others might not. Alternatively, the species-specific effects may reflect underlying differences in epidemiology of infection, including age patterns, within the respective study populations. And finally, the impact of WASH interventions might vary according to the underlying prevalence of helminthic infections and the frequency of ongoing mass deworming programmes. At high levels of infection and environmental contamination, WASH interventions might require a longer follow-up period to see effects, and most of the evidence has shorter follow-up periods.

4 Evidence Gaps and Future Implications

The field of helminths in general lags in terms of model development and parameter estimation, and much of the existing treatment mechanisms are largely based on discussion and consensus, without detailed calculations [52]. The existing evidence hardly considers the dynamic nature of the transmission cycle, and the fact that not all intestinal worms are the same or respond to the same deworming drugs. Although existing studies have shown that treatment of some individuals leads to a reduction in transmission in the community as a whole, these studies do not adequately address the population dynamics of helminthic infection [53]. The majority of the studies on deworming have followed standard practice in clinical trials and considered untreated people as a control group. Since the current studies have been conducted in areas where most people have low-to-moderate intensity infection rather than high intensity infection, there is a potential for considerable and unknown variance in the intensity of individual infection. Consequently, the intensity is unknown in any individual, as is the likelihood of morbidity and the potential scale of benefit from treatment. Such studies tend to average out the effectiveness when population as a whole is studied rather than studying population subgroups with varying intensity of infections [54]. Another critical issue concerns the reach of these drugs to infected geographical pockets and the lack of focus on concomitant transmission control strategies like WASH interventions. At present, many endemic countries are not availing themselves of the freely donated drugs to treat children, partly due to the logistical challenges in getting the drugs to these populations. With this existing situation, the expansion of these programmes to target WRA would also require an increase in drug donations as well as effective targeting platforms to achieve high programme coverage for WRA. Even if the mass deworming coverage targets are reached, it might not be enough to eliminate transmission and the focus should be concomitant morbidity control, and ideally, the eventual elimination of transmission. Consequently, it is highly desirable to modify the existing guidelines with a concomitant emphasis on education and sustainability of current WASH programmes along with mass deworming to reduce transmission intensity and thereby enhance the impact of mass deworming programmes.

5 Way Forward

The WHO emphasizes coordinated implementation of five WHO-recommended strategic interventions: innovative and intensified disease management, preventive chemotherapy, vector control, veterinary public health, and WASH to control, eliminate, or eradicate NTDs [1]. Periodic mass deworming remains the mainstay of helminthic control; however, mass deworming in isolation might not be a long-term solution due to potential anthelmintic resistance and poor sanitation coverage leading to reinfections. Therefore, effective and sustainable control could potentially be achieved through simultaneous environmental and WASH interventions. There is a stronger need for evidence and guidance on the complementary role that WASH has for deworming programmes (especially in preventing reinfection), the specific WASH interventions that have the greatest impact, the WASH coverage levels that are required to have an impact, and the points in a control programme cycle at which they should be emphasized. The existing WASH indicators appear to be dismal, where three out ten people lack a facility with water and soap available to wash their hands at home, and 462 million children attend schools with no hygiene facilities [55, 56]. Implementing WASH interventions will require cross-sectoral collaboration, political will, and investment in WASH in developing countries.

References

1. World Health Organization. Global report on neglected tropical diseases. Global Report on Neglected Tropical Diseases; 2023. p. 20232023.
2. Vos T, Lim SS, Abbafati C, Abbas KM, Abbasi M, Abbasifard M, et al. Global burden of 369 diseases and injuries in 204 countries and territories, 1990–2019: a systematic analysis for the Global Burden of Disease Study 2019. Lancet. 2020;396(10258):1204–22.
3. Donohue RE, Cross ZK, Michael E. The extent, nature, and pathogenic consequences of helminth polyparasitism in humans: a meta-analysis. PLoS Negl Trop Dis. 2019;13(6):e0007455.
4. Hotez P, Cerami A. Secretion of a proteolytic anticoagulant by Ancylostoma hookworms. J Exp Med. 1983;157(5):1594–603.
5. Torlesse H, Hodges M. Anthelminthic treatment and haemoglobin concentrations during pregnancy. Lancet. 2000;356(9235):1083.
6. Pawlowski ZS, Schad G, Stott G. Hookworm infection and anaemia: approaches to prevention and controlcontinued. World Health Organization; 1991.
7. Martin M, Blackwell AD, Gurven M, Kaplan H. Make new friends and keep the old? Parasite coinfection and comorbidity in Homo sapiens. Primates, Pathogens, and Evolution: Springer; 2013. p. 363–87.
8. Abrams ET, Miller EM. The roles of the immune system in women's reproduction: evolutionary constraints and life history trade-offs. Am J Phys Anthropol. 2011;146(S53):134–54.
9. Blackwell AD, Snodgrass JJ, Madimenos FC, Sugiyama LS. Life history, immune function, and intestinal helminths: trade-offs among immunoglobulin E, C-reactive protein, and growth in an Amazonian population. Am J Hum Biol. 2010;22(6):836–48.
10. Gyorkos TW, Gilbert NL, Larocque R, Casapía M. Trichuris and hookworm infections associated with anaemia during pregnancy. Trop Med Int Health. 2011;16(4):531–7.
11. Larocque R, Casapia M, Gotuzzo E, Gyorkos TW. Relationship between intensity of soil-transmitted helminth infections and anemia during pregnancy. Am J Tropic Med Hygiene. 2005;73(4):783–9.
12. Muhangi L, Woodburn P, Omara M, Omoding N, Kizito D, Mpairwe H, et al. Associations between mild-to-moderate anaemia in pregnancy and helminth, malaria and HIV infection in Entebbe, Uganda. Trans R Soc Trop Med Hyg. 2007;101(9):899–907.
13. Ndyomugyenyi R, Kabatereine N, Olsen A, Magnussen P. Malaria and hookworm infections in relation to haemoglobin and serum ferritin levels in pregnancy in Masindi district, western Uganda. Trans R Soc Trop Med Hyg. 2008;102(2):130–6.
14. Nurdia D, Sumarni S, Hakim M, Winkvist A. Impact of intestinal helminth infection on anemia and iron status during pregnancy: a community based study in Indonesia. 2001.
15. Report of the WHO informal consultation on hookworm infection and anaemia in girls and women. Geneva: World Health Organization: Schistosomiasis, WHO Unit, Intestinal Parasites; 1994.

16. Mason JB. United Nations-administrative committee on coordination-subcommittee on nutrition. Geneva: WHO; 2000.
17. World Health Organization. Conquering suffering, enriching humanity: report of the director-general. World Health Organization; 1997.
18. Bundy D, Chan M, Savioli L. Hookworm infection in pregnancy. Trans R Soc Trop Med Hyg. 1995;89(5):521–2.
19. Chan M, Medley G, Jamison D, Bundy D. The evaluation of potential global morbidity attributable to intestinal nematode infections. Parasitology. 1994;109(03):373–87.
20. Rahman MM, Abe SK, Rahman MS, Kanda M, Narita S, Bilano V, et al. Maternal anemia and risk of adverse birth and health outcomes in low-and middle-income countries: systematic review and meta-analysis. Am J Clin Nutr. 2016;103:ajcn107896.
21. Sifakis S, Pharmakides G. Anemia in pregnancy. Ann N Y Acad Sci. 2000;900(1):125–36.
22. Raj E, Calvo-Urbano B, Heffernan C, Halder J, Webster J. Systematic review to evaluate a potential association between helminth infection and physical stunting in children. Parasit Vectors. 2022;15(1):135.
23. Organization WH. Guideline: preventive chemotherapy to control soil-transmitted helminth infections in at-risk population groups. World Health Organization; 2017.
24. Taylor-Robinson DC, Maayan N, Donegan S, Chaplin M, Garner P. Public health deworming programmes for soil-transmitted helminths in children living in endemic areas. Cochrane Database Syst Rev. 2019;9
25. Welch VA, Ghogomu E, Hossain A, Riddle A, Gaffey M, Arora P, et al. Mass deworming for improving health and cognition of children in endemic helminth areas: a systematic review and individual participant data network meta-analysis. Campbell Syst Rev. 2019;15(4):e1058.
26. Salam RA, Das JK, Bhutta ZA. Effect of mass deworming with antihelminthics for soil-transmitted helminths during pregnancy. Cochrane Database Syst Rev. 2021;5
27. Salam R, Cousens S, Welch V, Gaffey M, Middleton P, Makrides M, et al. Mass deworming for soil-transmitted helminths and schistosomiasis among pregnant women: a systematic review and individual participant data meta-analysis. Campbell Syst Rev. 2019;15(3):e1052.
28. Danso-Appiah A, Olliaro PL, Donegan S, Sinclair D, Utzinger J. Drugs for treating Schistosoma mansoni infection. Cochrane Database Syst Rev. 2013;2
29. Kramer CV, Zhang F, Sinclair D, Olliaro PL. Drugs for treating urinary schistosomiasis. Cochrane Database Syst Rev. 2014;8
30. Bundy DA, Appleby LJ, Bradley M, Croke K, Hollingsworth TD, Pullan R, et al. 100 years of mass deworming programmes: a policy perspective from the World Bank's disease control priorities analyses. Adv Parasitol. 2018;100:127–54.
31. Turner HC, Truscott JE, Hollingsworth TD, Bettis AA, Brooker SJ, Anderson RM. Cost and cost-effectiveness of soil-transmitted helminth treatment programmes: systematic review and research needs. Parasit Vectors. 2015;8(1):1–23.
32. Welch VA, Ghogomu E, Hossain A, Awasthi S, Bhutta Z, Cumberbatch C, et al. Deworming and adjuvant interventions for improving the developmental health and well-being of children in low-and middle-income countries: a systematic review and network meta-analysis. Campbell Syst Rev. 2016;12(1):1–383.
33. WHO. WHO report of the informal consultation on hookworm infection and Anaemia in girls and women. (WHO/CTD/SIP/96.1). Geneva: World Health Organization; 1994.
34. World Health Organization. Reaching girls and women of reproductive age with deworming: report of the Advisory Group on deworming in girls and women of reproductive age: Rockefeller Foundation Bellagio Center, Bellagio, Italy 28–30 June 2017. Rockefeller Foundation Bellagio Center, Bellagio, Italy: World Health Organization; 2018 28–30 June 2017.
35. Ndyomugyenyi R, Kabatereine N, Olsen A, Magnussen P. Efficacy of ivermectin and albendazole alone and in combination for treatment of soil-transmitted helminths in pregnancy and adverse events: a randomized open label controlled intervention trial in Masindi district, western Uganda. Am J Tropic Med Hygiene. 2008;79(6):856–63.

36. Thayer WM, Clermont A, Walker N. Effects of deworming on child and maternal health: a literature review and meta-analysis. BMC Public Health. 2017;17(4):830.
37. Mofid LS, Gyorkos TW. The case for maternal postpartum deworming. PLoS Negl Trop Dis. 2017;11(1):e0005203.
38. Moser W, Schindler C, Keiser J. Efficacy of recommended drugs against soil transmitted helminths: systematic review and network meta-analysis. BMJ. 2017;358:j4307.
39. Palmeirim MS, Hürlimann E, Knopp S, Speich B, Belizario V Jr, Joseph SA, et al. Efficacy and safety of co-administered ivermectin plus albendazole for treating soil-transmitted helminths: a systematic review meta-analysis and individual patient data analysis. PLoS Negl Trop Dis. 2018;12(4):e0006458.
40. Grimes JE, Croll D, Harrison WE, Utzinger J, Freeman MC, Templeton MR. The relationship between water, sanitation and schistosomiasis: a systematic review and meta-analysis. PLoS Negl Trop Dis. 2014;8(12):e3296.
41. Strunz EC, Addiss DG, Stocks ME, Ogden S, Utzinger J, Freeman MC. Water, sanitation, hygiene, and soil-transmitted helminth infection: a systematic review and meta-analysis. PLoS Med. 2014;11(3):e1001620.
42. Phillips AE, Ower AK, Mekete K, Liyew EF, Maddren R, Belay H, et al. Association between water, sanitation, and hygiene access and the prevalence of soil-transmitted helminth and schistosome infections in Wolayita, Ethiopia. Parasites Vectors. 2022;15(1):1–16.
43. Chard AN, Garn JV, Chang HH, Clasen T, Freeman MC. Impact of a school-based water, sanitation, and hygiene intervention on school absence, diarrhea, respiratory infection, and soil-transmitted helminths: results from the WASH HELPS cluster-randomized trial. J Glob Health. 2019;9(2)
44. Nery SV, Traub RJ, McCarthy JS, Clarke NE, Amaral S, Llewellyn S, et al. WASH for WORMS: a cluster-randomized controlled trial of the impact of a community integrated water, sanitation, and hygiene and deworming intervention on soil-transmitted helminth infections. Am J Tropic Med Hygiene. 2019;100(3):750.
45. Garn JV, Wilkers JL, Meehan AA, Pfadenhauer LM, Burns J, Imtiaz R, et al. Interventions to improve water, sanitation, and hygiene for preventing soil-transmitted helminth infection. Cochrane Database Syst Rev. 2022;6
46. Salam RA, Maredia H, Das JK, Lassi ZS, Bhutta ZA. Community-based interventions for the prevention and control of helmintic neglected tropical diseases. Infect Dis Poverty. 2014;3(1):23.
47. Brooker SJ, Nikolay B, Balabanova D, Pullan RL. Global feasibility assessment of interrupting the transmission of soil-transmitted helminths: a statistical modelling study. Lancet Infect Dis. 2015;15:941.
48. Vaz Nery S, Pickering AJ, Abate E, Asmare A, Barrett L, Benjamin-Chung J, et al. The role of water, sanitation and hygiene interventions in reducing soil-transmitted helminths: interpreting the evidence and identifying next steps. Parasit Vectors. 2019;12:1–8.
49. Becker MH, Haefner DP, Kasl SV, Kirscht JP, Maiman LA, Rosenstock IM. Selected psychosocial models and correlates of individual health-related behaviors. Med Care. 1977;15(5):27–46.
50. Barker M, Dombrowski SU, Colbourn T, Fall CH, Kriznik NM, Lawrence WT, et al. Intervention strategies to improve nutrition and health behaviours before conception. Lancet. 2018;391(10132):1853–64.
51. Watson D, Mushamiri P, Beeri P, Rouamba T, Jenner S, Proebstl S, et al. Behaviour change interventions improve maternal and child nutrition in sub-Saharan Africa: a systematic review. PLOS Global Public Health. 2023;3(3):e0000401.
52. Anderson RM, Turner HC, Truscott JE, Hollingsworth TD, Brooker SJ. Should the goal for the treatment of soil transmitted helminth (STH) infections be changed from morbidity control in children to community-wide transmission elimination? PLoS Negl Trop Dis. 2015;9(8):e0003897.
53. Bundy DA, Kremer M, Bleakley H, Jukes MC, Miguel E. Deworming and development: asking the right questions, asking the questions right. PLoS Negl Trop Dis. 2009;3(1):e362.

54. Bundy DA, Appleby LJ, Bradley M, Croke K, Hollingsworth TD, Pullan R, et al. 100 years of mass deworming programmes: a policy perspective from the World Bank's Disease Control Priorities Analyses. Adv Parasitol: Elsevier. 2018;100:127–54.
55. Prüss-Ustün A, Wolf J, Bartram J, Clasen T, Cumming O, Freeman MC, et al. Burden of disease from inadequate water, sanitation and hygiene for selected adverse health outcomes: an updated analysis with a focus on low-and middle-income countries. Int J Hyg Environ Health. 2019;222(5):765–77.
56. World Health Organization. State of the World's Hand Hygiene: A global call to action to make hand hygiene a priority in policy and practice. 2021. Report No.: 924003644X.

Women's Empowerment and Nutritional Status

Salima Meherali, Mariam Ahmad, Sobia Idrees, and Amyna Ismail Rehmani

1 Introduction

Women's empowerment signifies the "ability to make strategic life choices where that ability had been previously denied them" [1]. Empowerment, as a change process, affects the elevation and amplification of women's voices, choices, and control over their lives. Empowerment can also affect change in a multitude of ways, from individual women gaining autonomy to entire communities mobilizing change to help women reach their potential [2].

The importance of women's empowerment is significant, not only on an individual level but also on a broader social, economic, and community health level. Studies have shown that when women are empowered, they not only experience improved well-being but also contribute positively to the well-being of their families and communities [3, 4]. For low- and middle-income countries (LMICs) in particular, women's empowerment has been recognized as an important policy goal for improving not just the well-being of women themselves but also the positive impact it has on the nutritional status of households and communities [2, 5]. It is also one of the Sustainable Development Goals set by the United Nations, highlighting its global significance [5].

Research has shown a strong link between women's empowerment and nutritional status [6, 7]. Studies have consistently demonstrated that women's empowerment leads to significant improvements in the nutritional status of women and their families [3, 8]. This link can be attributed to several factors, such as decision-making

S. Meherali (✉) · M. Ahmad · S. Idrees · A. I. Rehmani
Faculty of Nursing, College of Health Sciences, University of Alberta, Edmonton, AB, Canada
e-mail: meherali@ualberta.ca; mariam2@ualberta.ca; sidrees@ualberta.ca; amynaism@ualberta.ca

power, economic empowerment, and education. Nutrition is not just about food. It is about access to resources, knowledge, decision-making power, and the means to make choices that affect health and well-being. Firstly, empowered women have greater decision-making power within the household, including deciding on food choices and allocation of resources [9]. When women are empowered, they often have a voice when it comes to household decisions. This includes decisions regarding health care, household resource allocation, and food choices [9–12]. Economic empowerment, by way of meaningful employment, land ownership, and microcredit programs, has a positive socioeconomic impact on women, allowing them to contribute to household finances [13, 14]. With these financial resources, women can ensure that funds are allocated toward nutritionally dense foods, healthcare, and educational resources related to health and nutrition [15, 16]. Finally, a woman who is educated is more likely to understand the intricacies of nutrition, nutrient-dense food, and the significance of early childhood nutrition [17]. Research has consistently shown the ripple effect of a woman's education on her family's health and nutrition [18]. Her ability to discern nutritional information, prioritize nutrient-dense foods, and emphasize early childhood nutrition can significantly reduce the risk of malnutrition and related diseases in the family. This underscores the broader need for societal investments in female education—not just for the sake of gender equality but also as a strategy for improved public health outcomes [16, 17].

The objectives of this chapter are to explore the historical context of women's role in relation to food and nutrition in LMICs, examine the theoretical framework that explores the relationship between women's empowerment and nutritional outcomes, discuss the factors that influence nutritional status through women's empowerment, identify the challenges to women's empowerment in achieving nutritional outcomes, and finally, propose strategies to enhance women's empowerment for better nutritional outcomes in LMICs.

2   Context of Women and Nutrition in LMICs

Historically, in many societies, women have been the pillars of food production, preparation, and distribution, and their roles are deeply intertwined with the sustenance of their families and communities. They have been integral to the farming process, engaging in cultivating and harvesting crops, as well as processing and preserving food [19, 20]. These responsibilities have endowed women with an intimate knowledge of local food resources and traditional food preparation methods, contributing to the diversity and nutritional quality of diets [21]. Their command over seasonal crops shaped planting cycles and food consumption patterns, while their skill in combining ingredients created a rich tapestry of culinary traditions, often maximized for nutrient retention. Women often supplemented their food sources through engagements in livestock rearing and small-scale fishing, further expanding the availability of nutritious food for their households [22]. However, despite their pivotal roles, women in traditional agricultural societies faced constraints that limited their empowerment. Particularly in the aftermath of colonization, power dynamics shifted, marginalizing women's roles in society and reducing their influence in food and nutrition decisions [23].

2.1 Shift in Power Dynamics and Its Impact on Nutrition

After colonization and the movement to industrialization, there was a noticeable shift in societal power dynamics. This shift marginalized women's roles in food production and nutrition [24]. Consequently, their control over resources and decision-making ability faced a significant decline. The allure of better opportunities and jobs in urban areas led to a massive migration of men from rural to urban regions, often leaving women with increased responsibilities in rural areas [25]. Yet, these women found themselves without enough resources or rights to make vital decisions. The shift affected the type and quality of food produced, pointing to potential nutritional deficiencies [26]. The industrial age also marked the introduction of processed foods. With men predominantly controlling finances in many societies and the diminishing influence of women on food choices, a gradual shift toward these cheaper, longer-lasting, but less nutritious food options ensued [26]. In many agrarian societies, women's roles were critical in ensuring the nutritional needs of the family were met. After colonization, their societal roles were marginalized [23]. Alongside these changes, a disruption in the transfer of knowledge linked to food and nutrition occurred. This disruption of knowledge transfer led to increased reliance on commercially available yet less nutritious food sources, negatively affecting individual and community health levels [26, 27]. The consequences of this shift had a far-reaching impact on women's ability to ensure sufficient access to nutritious food for themselves and their families [28]. Despite these transitions and the resulting disparities, the importance of women's empowerment has become evident and recognized, leading to efforts to address these inequalities [28]. Women's empowerment is now regarded as a crucial ingredient in improving their and their children's nutritional outcomes [29].

2.1.1 Theoretical Framework

The theoretical framework for understanding the relationship between women's empowerment and nutritional outcomes is multifaceted. Using a feminist framework, it is important to acknowledge the structural and systemic factors that contribute to women's disempowerment and their impact on nutritional outcomes [30]. Patriarchal norms and gender inequalities often limit women's access to education, employment opportunities, and resources, thereby affecting their ability to make informed decisions regarding nutrition and health [9, 22]. Furthermore, the capability approach, as proposed by Amartya Sen, provides insight into how women's empowerment can enhance nutritional outcomes [31]. Women's empowerment involves expanding their capabilities and freedoms, which can lead to improved choices and outcomes regarding nutrition [8]. Moreover, the intersectionality of race, class, and other social identities further exacerbates the challenges faced by marginalized women in achieving nutritional well-being [32]. Women from marginalized communities often face the burden of multiple barriers due to the intersection of gender-based discrimination with other forms of oppression [33, 34].

2.2 The Role of Gender Equity and Decision-Making Power in Nutrition

One of the key aspects of women's empowerment that has a direct impact on nutritional outcomes is decision-making power. Women's decision-making power within the household can influence food choices and health practices [9, 42]. For example, when women have the autonomy to decide what foods to purchase and prepare, they are more likely to prioritize nutritious options for themselves and their families [10, 11, 43]. The power of decision-making also extends beyond food. Women who are empowered are more likely to have access to resources, such as education and employment opportunities, which can contribute to improved household well-being and, subsequently, better nutrition [11].

Gender equity, or equal treatment and opportunities for people of all genders, is another crucial factor that can influence nutritional outcomes [44]. When women are given equitable access to resources, opportunities, and decision-making power, they are more likely to prioritize their own nutrition and the nutrition of their children.

Moreover, a feminist perspective highlights the importance of challenging social norms and institutions that perpetuate gender inequalities [24]. By challenging patriarchal systems, societies can create an environment that promotes women's empowerment and improves nutritional outcomes [44]. This includes addressing structural barriers such as limited access to education, healthcare services, and economic opportunities for women.

3 Factors Influencing Nutritional Status Through Women's Empowerment

There are several factors that influence nutritional status through women's empowerment. These factors include age, decision-making power, gender equality, education, economic independence, and social and political participation. Effective interventions require acknowledging and challenging entrenched gender and social norms, with community and male support being pivotal.

Age Women's nutritional status is deeply entwined with a myriad of socioeconomic and cultural determinants that can either hinder or progress women's empowerment. Among these determinants, age is especially pronounced in its influence. As women progress through life's phases, their societal roles, access to resources, and decision-making capabilities often transform [49]. Younger women, notably those in their early adulthood, grapple with challenges associated with premature marriages and childbearing, potentially exacerbating nutritional deficiencies and curtailing empowerment avenues [50]. This empowerment trajectory often peaks for women aged between 41 and 49, as compared to those in the 21–30 age bracket, with those having a marital duration between 13 and 18 years showing marked improvement in empowerment compared to those married for only 2–6 years [49]. As women age further, their roles, expectations, and societal perceptions shift, potentially granting increased agency in household and community matters, which can have ripple effects on their and their family's nutritional status. Additionally, women's decision-making prowess, intricately linked to factors such as literacy rates, number of offspring, and household socioeconomic standing, tends to amplify with age [49, 50]. This empowerment, especially in joint decision-making scenarios, can significantly mold economic and overall empowerment dimensions, directly impacting nutritional outcomes.

Gender Equality In LMICs, the intricate relationship between gender equality and women's nutritional status is underscored by the dynamics of women's empowerment. The pursuit of gender equality often centers around empowering women to have greater control over resources, decision-making processes, and access to opportunities [51–53]. When women are afforded equal rights and opportunities, they are better positioned to make informed choices about health, nutrition, and well-being, both for themselves and their families. Gender equality paves the way for enhanced education, awareness, and autonomy for women, which directly translates into better nutritional practices and outcomes [52]. For instance, an empowered woman is more likely to have the knowledge and means to access a balanced diet, seek healthcare services during pregnancy, or make decisions about family planning [52–54]. Conversely, in settings where gender disparities are pronounced, women's nutritional needs might be sidelined, and their ability to make decisions about food and health can be severely restricted [52, 54]. Thus, advancing gender equality can be a powerful lever to uplift the nutritional status of women, their families, and communities at large.

Decision-Making Power The connection between women's empowerment and nutritional status is profoundly shaped by their decision-making power, particularly in LMICs [42]. Women's autonomy to make decisions directly impacts their ability to access and allocate resources, which has immediate implications for nutrition. The spheres of influence range from choices about their own health, family planning, and household expenditure to broader decisions concerning agricultural practices, which determine food availability and quality [11]. While some women might possess the agency to prioritize nutritious food for themselves and their families, others may face systemic barriers rooted in traditional norms and values [10, 42]. Furthermore, empowerment is not uniform; a woman's decision-making power can be heightened or diminished by factors such as age, education, socioeconomic status, and marital dynamics [12]. For instance, older women, with accumulated life experiences, might possess enhanced authority in household matters, leading to improved nutritional outcomes. Conversely, younger women, especially those subjected to early marriages, might lack the requisite agency, potentially affecting their nutritional well-being [49]. In essence, the relationship between decision-making power and nutritional status is multifaceted, and interventions that seek to elevate women's empowerment can play a transformative role in bettering nutritional outcomes in these countries.

Education Education plays a crucial role in influencing the nutritional outcomes of individuals, especially women and children [55]. Numerous studies have demonstrated a substantial relationship between women's empowerment and maternal and child health outcomes, including dietary diversity and nutritional status [56]. This association highlights the significant ripple effect that education can have on improving nutrition. Neighbors and extended family members often seek her counsel, elevating the nutritional awareness of the broader community [57]. Thus, in these countries, investing in women's education is not just a matter of individual empowerment but a strategic intervention for community-wide nutritional betterment.

Economic Independence Economic independence stands as a cornerstone in women's empowerment, holding a substantial influence on nutritional outcomes. When women have financial autonomy, their decision-making capability is substantially amplified, enabling them to prioritize and invest in nutritionally rich food options for their families [58]. Research consistently shows that women's empowerment, particularly in terms of economic security, plays a vital role in shaping the nutritional status not only of themselves but also of their children [14, 30].

In LMICs, where resources can be scarce, the economic independence of women becomes a vital determinant of nutritional choices [14, 45, 50]. With enhanced purchasing power, women are not confined to a monotonous or staple-centric diet. Instead, they can afford a broader spectrum of foods, tapping into essential nutrients from diverse food groups, thereby directly enhancing the overall nutrition of their households [58]. This diversity is particularly crucial in regions where certain food groups might be seasonally available or scarce. Furthermore, financial autonomy allows women to prioritize food quality over mere quantity [59]. In contexts where marketplaces might be flooded with cheaper, calorie-dense but nutritionally poor foods, economically empowered women can make discerning choices, prioritizing nutrient-rich options over the more filling, yet nutritionally empty alternatives.

4 Challenges to Women's Empowerment in Achieving Nutritional Outcomes

There are several challenges that hinder women's empowerment in achieving better nutritional outcomes. Cultural and societal barriers pose significant challenges to women's empowerment [60]. For LMICs especially, limited access to resources is often a barrier to women's empowerment in achieving better nutritional outcomes [61]. Gender norms and biases also play a role in hindering women's empowerment and can impact food allocation within households, as well.

4.1 Cultural and Societal Barriers

Cultural and societal barriers, such as deeply ingrained gender norms and biases, can limit women's autonomy and participation in decision-making processes. These barriers may restrict women's access to education, economic opportunities, and political participation—all of which are essential for their empowerment [52, 53]. The impact of cultural and societal barriers on women's empowerment in the context of maternal and child health outcomes has been widely studied [62]. Multiple studies from the developing world have shown a strong association between women's empowerment and various aspects of nutrition, including nutritional status and dietary diversity [6, 59].

Traditionally, in many LMICs, patriarchal norms and gender biases have limited women's decision-making capacities, even though they are often at the forefront of food selection, procurement, preparation, and feeding practices [63]. Societal expectations and stringent gender roles can sometimes dictate that women prioritize the nutritional needs of male family members or even compromise on their own nutritional intake during times of scarcity [63].

Furthermore, these societal norms can create barriers for women, impeding their access to education and information about health and nutrition [6]. Without this knowledge, even the act of food selection can become a challenge, with women potentially opting for cheaper, calorie-dense but nutritionally poor food options. Cultural barriers further compound this issue. For instance, certain societies might have taboos against women eating specific nutrient-rich foods or discourage them from participating actively in community dialogues about health and nutrition [64].

4.2 Limited Access to Resources

Inadequate access to resources, such as land, financial capital, and productive assets, poses a significant impediment to women's empowerment in improving nutritional outcomes [19]. This challenge is particularly pronounced in low- and middle-income countries, where women encounter various barriers that restrict their ownership and control over land and property [65]. These obstacles encompass discriminatory inheritance laws, limited availability of credit and financial services tailored to women's needs, and prevailing social norms that prioritize male ownership rights [66]. Consequently, women experience constraints on their ability to engage in agricultural production and activities generating income [44].

Promoting gender equity within these contexts necessitates addressing the crucial issue of resource access among women [67]. By enhancing female control over agricultural practices along with economic decision-making power concerning food allocation strategies or investments devoted to nutrition-centered interventions, more favorable nutrition-related outcomes can feasibly be achieved [68]. However challenging it may be, though, since sociocultural factors play critical roles by shaping an individual's practices or behaviors leading directly toward improved nutritional statuses, through empowering initiatives, successful implementation could occur even amidst the complexities present within LMIC societies [67].

4.3 Gender Norms and Their Impact on Food Allocation

Gender norms and their impact on food allocation represent another significant challenge to women's empowerment in achieving better nutritional outcomes. In some LMICs, deeply rooted societal norms and cultural beliefs often dictate the division of food and resources within households, with women and girls frequently receiving an inequitable share [69]. These gender norms perpetuate unequal power dynamics, limiting women's ability to make decisions about what food to purchase, prepare, and consume [70]. Addressing these gender norms requires comprehensive strategies that challenge patriarchal structures and promote gender equality [55].

Women face various economic, social, and political barriers, resulting in lower access compared to men to productive resources like land or credit, due partly to traditional gender roles and cultural biases that tend to limit women's economic opportunities [68]. These barriers hinder women's ability to generate income and make independent decisions about purchasing nutritious food for themselves and their families. Therefore, it is crucial to implement strategies that enhance women's empowerment and address these barriers [67].

5 Strategies to Enhance Women's Empowerment for Better Nutritional Outcomes

Research indicates that empowering women plays a significant role in improving various aspects of public health, including maternal healthcare utilization, agricultural productivity, and child nutrition [71]. In fact, studies suggest that women's empowerment is even more important than household poverty when it comes to determining the nutritional status of children [53, 62, 72]. When given the freedom to make decisions about household income allocation or food choices, empowered women have shown the ability to positively affect their families' diets and improve overall nutritional status [64]. To enhance women's empowerment for better nutritional outcomes, several strategies can be implemented:

Educational programs tailored specifically for women and girls can play a pivotal role in empowering them to make informed decisions about nutrition, health, and overall well-being [73]. These programs should focus on providing comprehensive knowledge on topics such as health, hygiene, food groups, balanced diets, and proper food preparation techniques [74].

Women have key responsibilities for food acquisition and preparation as well as child feeding and care. Therefore, it is crucial to address the roles of women in ensuring adequate nutrition outcomes for children and households [70]. Numerous studies have shown that agricultural interventions like home gardening or livestock production may increase food production but do not necessarily significantly impact nutrition or health outcomes among participating households. However, research has suggested that projects with components enabling gender empowerment, along with providing relevant nutritional education, are more likely to positively influence dietary intake quality, growth, presence of micronutrients, and morbidity incidence among children [38, 68]. Thus, it emphasizes the importance of holistic approaches linking agriculture, nutrition, and healthcare.

Cultural practices, social context, and social norms also contribute significantly toward determining nutritional outcomes in general [2, 56, 75]. Furthermore, the role individuals fulfill within their partnerships, in this case, women who serve as spouses to household heads, can significantly determine their nutritional status. Women's utilization of time constitutes an influential factor driving both their social status/empowerment level and the overall nutritional status of themselves and their children [38, 56].

Economic initiatives that prioritize women's empowerment have the potential to greatly impact their nutritional choices and overall well-being. These initiatives include microfinance programs, entrepreneurial training focused on women's economic viability, and equal wage policies [13, 39]. By providing women with access to financial resources and opportunities, these interventions can enable them to make healthier food choices.

Microfinance is a powerful tool that allows women to gain control over their own finances and invest in income-generating activities such as small-scale agriculture or home food production [39]. This not only gives them more decision-making power regarding production choices but also enables them to allocate resources within their households for better nutrition outcomes [2, 13].

Entrepreneurial training programs targeted at empowering women economically can equip them with the necessary skills and knowledge needed for successful business ventures related to food production or distribution [76]. By improving their economic status, these programs enhance women's ability to provide nutritious meals for themselves and their families [2, 38].

Promoting gender equality in governance processes through policies can have a positive impact on women's influence over decision-making related to nutrition and health. By increasing the representation of women in political offices and implementing inclusive planning strategies for healthcare services, we can take crucial steps toward ensuring better nutritional outcomes for both individuals and households [58, 71, 77].

Equal wage policies are essential in ensuring fair compensation for female workers across various industries. Closing gender pay gaps helps address financial disparities faced by women, enabling them to afford higher-quality foods that support better health outcomes [51, 56, 63, 74].

In conclusion, implementing economic initiatives like microfinance opportunities, entrepreneurial training programs catered specifically toward promoting female economic viability, and enacting equal wage policies are crucial steps toward advancing both the nutritional choices of women and overall household well-being.

5.1 Case Studies of the Impact of Women's Empowerment on Improved Nutrition

Programs, interventions, and initiatives aimed at empowering women in LMICs have demonstrated the positive impact of empowering women on improving nutritional outcomes. A systematic review, conducted by Santoso, examined that women's empowerment interventions improve nutrition-related outcomes, with the largest effects on food security as well as food affordability and availability [35]. The review also pointed out that as a whole, women's empowerment interventions positively impact food security, affordability, availability, and diet quality [35].

Table 1 summarizes some of the programs and initiatives, their empowering strategies, and the impact on nutrition outcomes. Case studies from various countries further illustrate the positive impact of women's empowerment on nutritional improvement and household well-being [47]. A study in Pakistan has shown that women's decision-making power has a direct impact on investment in human development, particularly in the form of education and better nutrition within the

Table 1 Summaries of programs and initiatives, the foundational empowering strategy guiding the program or initiative and the impact on nutrition outcomes

Country/region	Program/initiative	Empowering strategy	Impact on health/nutrition outcomes
Kenya	Green Belt movement	Tree planting for environmental conservation, biodiversity conservation, and indigenous food production	Improved household nutrition through increased availability of indigenous foods
Bangladesh	Microcredit initiatives	Providing microcredit to women for income-generating activities, increasing purchasing power, and access to food	Enhanced household nutrition, food security, and dietary diversity
Mexico	PROGRESA program	Cash transfer program targeting mothers to improve child health and nutrition, empowering women with resource control	Improved child health and nutrition; shifts in women's freedom, confidence, and household influence
West Senegal	Vegetable production project	Increasing women's income and control over it through vegetable production	Increased women's income and social status; however, limited direct improvement in nutrition

household [45]. When women have the authority to make decisions about resource allocation, they are more likely to prioritize the nutritional needs of their children, leading to a reduction in childhood stunting [46]. In northern Ghana, a study by Tsiboe et al. found that women's empowerment in agriculture, encompassing three key dimensions—production, income control, and leadership—positively influences nutrient availability in the household [48].

In 1977, Kenyan female activist Wangari Maathai initiated the Green Belt Movement, emphasizing tree planting as a means of environmental conservation [36]. This movement had a far-reaching influence, resulting in women's empowerment to conserve biodiversity, produce indigenous foods, and improve household nutrition [37]. Numerous studies have found evidence linking women's empowerment with improved diet and nutritional status among women and young children [18, 38]. Moreover, impact assessments of nutrition- and gender-sensitive agricultural development programs suggest that these programs can both empower women and improve nutritional outcomes for both women and children [38].

In Bangladesh, the implementation of microcredit initiatives aimed at empowering women has led to enhanced household nutrition [13, 39]. These microcredit initiatives have resulted in improved food security and dietary diversity for households, leading to enhanced nutritional outcomes [38]. The provision of microcredit to women allowed them to start income-generating activities, which in turn increased their purchasing power and access to nutritious food for their families. These findings highlight the importance of holistic approaches that address gender dynamics within households as key factors in promoting better nutrition outcomes [38].

The PROGRESA program in Mexico further illuminates the interplay between women's empowerment and nutritional outcomes [38, 40]. PROGRESA, a nationwide anti-poverty initiative, implemented a cash transfer program that specifically targeted mothers to improve child health and nutrition. The program recognized the growing evidence that empowering women by giving them control over resources leads to significant advancements in these areas [38, 40]. By directly providing cash benefits to mothers, PROGRESA aimed to enhance their empowerment and influence within households. Through PROGRESA, many women experienced shifts in their freedom of movement, self-confidence, and broadened horizons, while also confronting new challenges such as increased tensions and time burdens [40].

A vegetable production project in Kumbija, West Senegal, initiated in 1969, was assessed for its nutritional impact on households [38, 41]. Despite significantly increasing women's income and their control over it, the project did not show a direct improvement in nutrition, primarily because a small portion of the produced vegetables were consumed by families, and the income from sales was rarely used for food purchases [41]. The increased income empowered women, freeing them from financial dependence on their husbands, but women did use their increased purchasing power for non-food items, potentially enhancing their social status [38, 41].

6   Conclusion

In conclusion, it is evident that families play a crucial role in effecting change and empowering girls and women. Through education, employment, and political participation, gender equality can be achieved. However, access to these resources is often determined by cultural norms within the family structure. Grassroots programs and policies have proven successful in promoting gender equality by providing education, training, and self-empowerment opportunities for girls and women.

Furthermore, studies have shown that gender equality and the empowerment of women contribute to poverty reduction and economic growth at both the individual/family level and the macro level. The ability of women to exercise their rights and make decisions within their households has been linked to decreased poverty rates while improving productivity.

Another critical aspect of empowered women is their influence on health outcomes for themselves as mothers and also for their children. Women tend to allocate more resources toward the well-being of their families; however, persistent gender inequalities often limit their autonomy when making key health-related decisions or implementing necessary measures due to a lack of household decision-making power or sufficient resources. Encouraging dialogue among women through group involvement has emerged as an effective strategy not only for empowering them but also for potentially improving maternal-child healthcare outcomes.

It is important that developing countries embrace interventions such as the promotion of education among females, eradicating harmful traditional practices, and gender biases that hinder women's empowerment and access to resources. Investment in education tailored specifically for women and girls is crucial to empower them and improve their nutritional knowledge. Additionally, economic initiatives such as microfinance, entrepreneurial training, and equal wage policies can enhance women's economic independence, allowing them to make healthier nutritional choices and improve overall household nutrition. Moreover, policies that promote women's participation in politics and governance are essential in ensuring their voices are heard and their needs are addressed. Addressing and challenging cultural and societal barriers that limit women's empowerment is also crucial. Overall, women's empowerment plays a critical role in improving nutritional status and achieving better health outcomes.

References

1. Malhotra A, Schulte J, Patel P. Innovation for women's empowerment and gender equality. International Center for Research on Women (ICRW); 2009.
2. Scaling Up Nutrition. Empowering women and girls to improve nutrition: building a sisterhood of success [Internet]. Scaling Up Nutrition; 2016 [cited 2023 Oct 13]. Available from: https://scalingupnutrition.org/wp-content/uploads/2016/05/IN-PRACTICE-BRIEF-6-EMPOWERING-WOMEN-AND-GIRLS-TO-IMPROVE-NUTITION-BUILDING-A-SISTERHOOD-OF-SUCCESS.pdf

3. Bayeh E. The role of empowering women and achieving gender equality to the sustainable development of Ethiopia. Pac Sci Rev B Humanit Soc Sci. 2016;2(1):37–42.
4. OECD. Gender and sustainable development: maximising the economic, social and environmental role of women [Internet]. Paris: Organisation for Economic Co-operation and Development; 2008 [cited 2023 Sep 23]. Available from: https://www.oecd-ilibrary.org/environment/gender-and-sustainable-development_9789264049901-en
5. United Nations: Gender equality and women's empowerment [Internet]. United Nations Sustain Dev [cited 2023 Sep 25]. Available from: https://www-un-org.login.ezproxy.library.ualberta.ca/sustainabledevelopment/gender-equality/
6. Cunningham K, Ruel M, Ferguson E, Uauy R. Women's empowerment and child nutritional status in South Asia: a synthesis of the literature. Matern Child Nutr 2015;11(1):1–19, 1.
7. Ishfaq S, Anjum A, Kouser S, Nightingale G, Jepson R. The relationship between women's empowerment and household food and nutrition security in Pakistan. PLoS One. 2022;17(10):e0275713.
8. Narayanan S, Fontana M, Lentz E, Kulkarni B. Rural women's empowerment in nutrition: a proposal for diagnostics linking food, health and institutions [internet]. Rochester, NY; 2017 [cited 2023 Sep 25]. Available from: https://papers.ssrn.com/abstract=3336461
9. Moore EV, Singh N, Serra R, Mc Kune SL. Household decision-making, women's empowerment, and increasing egg consumption in children under five in rural Burkina Faso: Observations from a cluster randomized controlled trial. Front Sustain Food Syst [Internet]. 2022 [cited 2023 Sep 25];6. Available from: https://www.frontiersin.org/articles/10.3389/fsufs.2022.1034618
10. Agaba M, Azupogo F, Brouwer ID. Maternal nutritional status, decision-making autonomy and the nutritional status of adolescent girls: a cross-sectional analysis in the Mion District of Ghana. J Nutr Sci. 2022;11:e97.
11. Mallick R, Chouhan P. Impact of decision-making autonomy of women on nutritional status of under-five children in India: a cross-sectional study based on the national family health survey. SN Soc Sci. 2023;3(1):19.
12. Yu S, Desai S, Chen F. Aligning household decision-making with work and education: a comparative analysis of women's empowerment. Demogr Res. 2023;48(19):513–48.
13. Afrin S, Islam N, Ahmed S. Micro credit and rural women entrepreneurship development in Bangladesh: a multivariate model [internet]. Rochester, NY; 2010 [cited 2023 Sep 25]. Available from: https://papers.ssrn.com/abstract=2856217
14. Fabiyi EF, Akande KE. Economic empowerment for rural women in Nigeria: Poverty Alleviation through Agriculture. 2015 [cited 2023 Sep 25]; Available from: http://repository.futminna.edu.ng:8080/jspui/handle/123456789/15876
15. Petrovici DA, Ritson C. Factors influencing consumer dietary health preventative behaviours. BMC Public Health. 2006;6(1):222.
16. Rustad C, Smith C. Nutrition knowledge and associated behavior changes in a holistic, short-term nutrition education intervention with low-income women. J Nutr Educ Behav. 2013;45(6):490–8.
17. Fallah F, Pourabbas A, Delpisheh A, Veisani Y, Shadnoush M. Effects of nutrition education on levels of nutritional awareness of pregnant women in Western Iran. Int J Endocrinol Metab. 2013;11(3):175–8.
18. Lufuke M, Bai Y, Fan S, Tian X. Women's empowerment, food security, and nutrition transition in Africa. Int J Environ Res Public Health. 2022;20(1):254.
19. Doss CR. Is risk fully pooled within the household? Evidence from Ghana. Econ Dev Cult Change. 2001;50(1):101–30.
20. Pena C, Webb P, Haddad L. Women's economic advancement through agricultural change: a review of donor experience [Internet]. [cited 2023 Sep 25]. Available from: https://lib.icimod.org/record/9994
21. Ogato GS, Boon EK, Subramani J. Gender roles in crop production and management practices: a case study of three rural communities in Ambo District, Ethiopia. J Hum Ecol. 2009;27(1):1–20.

22. Njuki J, Parkins J, Kaler A. Transforming gender and food security in the global south. New York: Routledge; 2016.
23. Toulmin EB Su Fei Tan, Camilla. Woman's role in economic development. London: Routledge; 2013. p. 306.
24. Agarwal B. "Bargaining" and Gender relations: within and beyond the household. Fem Econ. 1997;3(1):1–51.
25. Deshingkar P. Migration, remote rural areas and chronic poverty in India. Oxf Dev Stud. 2010;38(3):231–50.
26. Popkin BM. An overview on the nutrition transition and its health implications: the Bellagio meeting. 2002 Feb
27. Pingali P. Westernization of Asian diets and the transformation of food systems: implications for research and policy. Food Policy. 2007;32(3):281–98.
28. Smith LC, Ramakrishnan U, Ndiaye A, Haddad L, Martorell R. The importance of women's status for child nutrition in developing countries: international food policy research institute (Ifpri) research report abstract 131. Food Nutr Bull. 2003;24(3):287–8.
29. Malhotra A, Schuler SR, Boender C. Measuring women's empowerment. World Bank Wash DC; 2002.
30. O'Brien C, Leavens L, Ndiaye C, Traoré D. Women's empowerment, income, and nutrition in a food processing value chain development project in Touba, Senegal. Int J Environ Res Public Health. 2022;19(15):9526.
31. Sen A. Commodities and capabilities. Amsterdam: North-Holland; 1985.
32. Rao M. Gender, water, and nutrition in India: an intersectional. Perspective. 2019;12(3)
33. Laster Pirtle WN, Wright T. Structural gendered racism revealed in pandemic times: intersectional approaches to understanding race and gender health inequities in COVID-19. Gend Soc. 2021;35(2):168–79.
34. Seng JS, Lopez WD, Sperlich M, Hamama L, Meldrum CDR. Marginalized identities, discrimination burden, and mental health: empirical exploration of an interpersonal-level approach to modeling intersectionality. Soc Sci Med. 1982;75(12):2437–45.
35. Santoso MV, Kerr RB, Hoddinott J, Garigipati P, Olmos S, Young SL. Role of women's empowerment in child nutrition outcomes: a systematic review. Adv Nutr. 2019;10(6):1138–51.
36. Muthuki J. Challenging patriarchal structures: Wangari Maathai and the Green Belt Movement in Kenya: Agenda: Vol 20, No 69 [Internet]. 2011 [cited 2023 Sep 25]. Available from: https://www.tandfonline.com/doi/abs/10.1080/10130950.2006.9674752?src=recsys
37. Scott K. Peace profile: Wangari Maathai and the Green Belt movement. Peace Rev. 2013;25(2):299–306.
38. van den Bold M, Quisumbing AR, Gillespie S. Women's empowerment and nutrition: an evidence review [Internet]. Rochester; 2013 [cited 2023 Sep 26]. Available from: https://papers.ssrn.com/abstract=2343160
39. Khandker SR. Microfinance and poverty: evidence using panel data from Bangladesh. World Bank Econ Rev. 2005;19(2):263–86.
40. Adato M, De la Briere B, Mindek D, Quisumbing AR. The impact of progresa on women's status and intrahousehold relations; final. Report. 2000;
41. Brun T, Reynaud J, Chevassus-Agnes S. Food and nutritional impact of one home garden project in Senegal. Ecol Food Nutr. 1989;23(2):91–108.
42. Girma S, Alenko A. Women's involvement in household decision-making and nutrition related-knowledge as predictors of child global acute malnutrition in southwest Ethiopia: a case–control study. Nutr Diet Suppl 2020 12:87–95.
43. Sinclair K, Thompson-Colón T, Bastidas-Granja AM, Del Castillo Matamoros SE, Olaya E, Melgar-Quiñonez H. Women's autonomy and food security: connecting the dots from the perspective of indigenous women in rural Colombia. SSM—Qual Res Health. 2022;2:100078.
44. Harris-Fry H, Nur H, Shankar B, Zanello G, Srinivasan C, Kadiyala S. The impact of gender equity in agriculture on nutritional status, diets, and household food security: a mixed-methods systematic review. BMJ Glob Health. 2020;5(3):e002173.

45. Rehman A, Ping Q, Razzaq A. Pathways and associations between women's land ownership and child food and nutrition security in Pakistan. Int J Environ Res Public Health. 2019;16(18):3360.
46. Kamiya Y, Nomura M, Ogino H, Yoshikawa K, Siengsounthone L, Xangsayarath P. Mothers' autonomy and childhood stunting: evidence from semi-urban communities in Lao PDR. BMC Womens Health. 2018;18(1):70.
47. Singh SK, Srivastava S, Gudakesh VY, Gupta J. Whether recent upswing in women's empowerment has a potential to address malnutrition among women and children? Evidence from Fourth Round of Indian Demographic Health Survey. 2017;2:1–16.
48. Tsiboe F, Zereyesus YA, Popp JS, Osei E. The effect of women's empowerment in agriculture on household nutrition and food poverty in northern Ghana. Soc Indic Res. 2018;138(1):89–108.
49. Batool S, Jadoon A. Women's Empowerment and Associated Age-Related Factors. 2019 Apr 29;
50. Kabir A, Rashid MM, Hossain K, Khan A, Sikder SS, Gidding HF. Women's empowerment is associated with maternal nutrition and low birth weight: evidence from Bangladesh demographic health survey. BMC Womens Health. 2020;20(1):93.
51. Klasen S, Lamanna F. The impact of Gender inequality in education and employment on economic growth: new evidence for a panel of countries. Fem Econ. 2009;15(3):91–132.
52. Ma J, Grogan-Kaylor AC, Lee SJ, Ward KP, Pace GT. Gender inequality in low- and middle-income countries: associations with parental physical abuse and moderation by child Gender. Int J Environ Res Public Health. 2022;19(19):11928.
53. Njuki J, Eissler S, Malapit HJ, Meinzen-Dick R, Bryan E, Quisumbing AR. A review of evidence on gender equality, women's empowerment, and food systems. International Food Policy Research Institute; 2021.
54. Sey-Sawo J, Sarr F, Bah HT, Senghore T. Women's empowerment and nutritional status of children in The Gambia: further analysis of the 2020 Gambia demographic and health survey. BMC Public Health. 2023;23(1):583.
55. Carlson GJ, Kordas K, Murray-Kolb LE. Associations between women's autonomy and child nutritional status: a review of the literature. Matern Child Nutr. 2015;11(4):452–82.
56. Pratley P. Associations between quantitative measures of women's empowerment and access to care and health status for mothers and their children: a systematic review of evidence from the developing world. Soc Sci Med. 2016;169:119–31.
57. Shrimpton R, Plessis LM du, Delisle H, Blaney S, Atwood SJ, Sanders D, et al. Public health nutrition capacity: assuring the quality of workforce preparation for scaling up nutrition programmes. Public Health Nutr 2016;19(11):2090–2100.
58. Ahmed S, Creanga AA, Gillespie DG, Tsui AO. Economic status, education and empowerment: implications for maternal health service utilization in developing countries. PLoS One. 2010;5(6):e11190.
59. Paul P, Saha R. Is maternal autonomy associated with child nutritional status? Evidence from a cross-sectional study in India. PLoS One. 2022;17(5):e0268126.
60. Gonzalez Parrao C, Shisler S, Moratti M, Yavuz C, Acharya A, Eyers J, et al. Aquaculture for improving productivity, income, nutrition and women's empowerment in low- and middle-income countries: a systematic review and meta-analysis. Campbell Syst Rev. 2021;17(4):e1195.
61. Jacobs B, Ir P, Bigdeli M, Annear PL, Van Damme W. Addressing access barriers to health services: an analytical framework for selecting appropriate interventions in low-income Asian countries. Health Policy Plan. 2012;27(4):288–300.
62. Shroff M, Griffiths P, Adair L, Suchindran C, Bentley M. Maternal autonomy is inversely related to child stunting in Andhra Pradesh, India. Matern Child Nutr. 2009;5(1):64–74.
63. Akbar M, Asif AM, Hussain F. Does maternal empowerment improve dietary diversity of children? Evidence from Pakistan demographic and health survey 2017–18. Int J Health Plann Manag. 2022;37(6):3297–311.
64. Ali W, Fani MI, Afzal S, Yasin G. Cultural barriers in women empowerment: a sociological analysis of Multan, Pakistan. Eur J Soc Sci. 2010;18:147–55.

65. Peterman A, Behrman JA, Quisumbing AR. A review of empirical evidence on Gender differences in nonland agricultural inputs, technology, and services in developing countries. In: Quisumbing AR, Meinzen-Dick R, Raney TL, Croppenstedt A, Behrman JA, Peterman A, editors. Gender in agriculture: closing the knowledge gap [Internet]. Dordrecht: Springer [cited 2023 Sep 25]; 2014. p. 145–86. https://doi.org/10.1007/978-94-017-8616-4_7.
66. Peters H, Irvin-Erickson Y, Adelstein S, Malik A, Derrick-Mills T, Valido A, et al. Qualitative evidence on barriers to and facilitators of women's participation in higher or growing productivity and male-dominated labour market sectors in low- and middle-income countries. Lond EPPI Cent Soc Sci Res Unit UCL Inst Educ Univ Coll Lond; 2019.
67. Akter S, Rutsaert P, Luis J, Htwe NM, San SS, Raharjo B, et al. Women's empowerment and gender equity in agriculture: a different perspective from Southeast Asia. Food Policy. 2017;69:270–9.
68. Malapit HJL, Quisumbing AR. What dimensions of women's empowerment in agriculture matter for nutrition in Ghana? Food Policy. 2015;52:54–63.
69. Hadley C, Lindstrom D, Tessema F, Belachew T. Gender bias in the food insecurity experience of Ethiopian adolescents. Soc Sci Med. 1982;66(2):427–38.
70. Ruel MT, Quisumbing AR, Balagamwala M. Nutrition-sensitive agriculture: what have we learned so far? Glob Food Secur. 2018;17:128–53.
71. Yaya S, Odusina EK, Uthman OA, Bishwajit G. What does women's empowerment have to do with malnutrition in Sub-Saharan Africa? Evidence from demographic and health surveys from 30 countries. Glob Health Res Policy. 2020;5:1.
72. Bhagowalia P, Menon P, Quisumbing AR, Soundararajan V. What Dimensions of Women's Empowerment Matter Most for Child Nutrition? Evidence Using Nationally Representative Data from Bangladesh: IFPRI Discuss Pap [Internet]. 2012 [cited 2023 Sep 26]; Available from: https://ideas.repec.org//p/fpr/ifprid/1192.html
73. Jayachandran S. The roots of gender inequality in developing countries. Annu Rev Econ. 2015;7(1):63–88.
74. Prasetyo YB, Permatasari P, Susanti HD. The effect of mothers' nutritional education and knowledge on children's nutritional status: a systematic review. Int J Child Care Educ Policy. 2023;17(1):11.
75. Kerr RB, Berti PR, Chirwa M. Breastfeeding and mixed feeding practices in Malawi: timing, reasons, decision makers, and child health consequences. Food Nutr Bull. 2007;28(1):90–9.
76. Bandiera O, Buehren N, Burgess R, Goldstein M, Gulesci S, Rasul I, et al. Women's empowerment in action: evidence from a randomized control trial in Africa. Am Econ J Appl Econ. 2020;12(1):210–59.
77. McKenna CG, Bartels SA, Pablo LA, Walker M. Women's decision-making power and undernutrition in their children under age five in The Democratic Republic of the Congo: a cross-sectional study. PLoS One. 2019;14(12):e0226041.

The Political Economy of Multi-sectoral Programming of Adolescent Nutrition: Global Discourse and Emerging Lessons from Pakistan

Shehla Zaidi

1 Adolescent Health and Its Reliance on Collaborative Multi-sector Governance

Adolescent health is increasingly featured in global policy discourse on sustainable development. Adolescents are an increasing proportion of low- and middle-income country populations. Investments in adolescent health and well-being can break the cyclical log jam of health issues that take root in the adolescent period and transform the lives of youth around the world [1]. Experts prioritise mental health, nutrition, tobacco, sexual health, and HIV as key areas for adolescent health interventions [2]. Adolescent health interventions rely on collaborative governance across health care, schools, youth, and community support services for effective implementation [3]. Considerable efforts are underway in an increasing number of countries to test and iterate effective interventions for adolescent nutrition as well as other adolescent health issues; however, progress has often floundered because the political economy of adolescent health has not been placed at the centre stage of programming adolescent health interventions [4]. The political economy underlying planning and resourcing decisions must be openly discussed and navigated for any meaningful headway in addressing adolescent nutrition as well as adolescent health issues.

S. Zaidi (✉)
Global Business School for Health, University College London, London, UK

Aga Khan University, Karachi, Pakistan
e-mail: shehla.zaidi@ucl.ac.uk

© The Author(s), under exclusive license to Springer Nature Switzerland AG 2025
Z. S. Lassi, R. A. Salam (eds.), *Nutrition Across Reproductive, Maternal, Neonatal, Child, and Adolescent Health Care*, https://doi.org/10.1007/978-3-031-95721-5_18

2 Political Economy Lessons from Adolescent Health Interventions

Despite global calls for more joined-up working across relevant sectors, less is known about how to effectively co-opt other sectors for programming of globally recommended adolescent health measures in a collaborative governance model.

Who Leads? A closer look at adolescent health interventions shows that the health sector is centrally dependent on other sectors for shaping, delivering, and resourcing adolescent health interventions. This changes the power paradigm from health to other sectors that are often more important in delivering adolescent health. Yet policy, resourcing, and implementation of adolescent health interventions continue to be led by the health sector, assuming that other sectors will naturally join and play a subordinate role. Governance approaches are critical for brokering the relationships and interactions in multi-sectoral action for adolescent health [4]. There is no single model of collaborative leadership, varying from distributed leadership across relevant sectors to binary leadership models between the two most instrumental sectors [5]. Leadership building requires investment in building capacity across sectors, and levels of government and cultivating champions in different sectors who can agree on common objectives [6].

Can We Be More Inclusive in Framing? The framing of adolescent health interventions can play a substantial role in influencing who controls the resources and where resources will be spent. The role of framing of health issues has traditionally been overlooked in political analysis but is now getting increasing attention. The narratives of adolescents' health can be driven by moral, societal, and development world ideologies that need to be deconstructed, understood, and appropriately framed for the inclusion of relevant societal stakeholders and sectors [7]. In practice, adolescent health has traditionally been underwritten by development sector goals and ideologies, emphasising prescriptive clinical top-down framing around fertility control and teen pregnancies, tobacco cessation, or anaemia reduction that have encountered either cultural resistance or poor social uptake. A shift to more socially inclusive framing is necessary and tailored to country contexts. Beyond ideology, framing will need to be supported by a clear set of interventions defined inclusively with non-health sectors for multi-sector programming.

Overlooking Male Adolescents There are questionable silences regarding male adolescents within adolescent health discourse, resourcing, and programming. Jacobs et al. 2021 unpack adolescent health policy discourse in South Africa which has been traditionally 'problematised' with fertility and HIV lenses, featuring on issues of adolescent girls, with boys featuring as a late and tokenish inclusion [8]. Issues particularly salient to male adolescents such as mental health, violence, tobacco use, substance abuse, and nutrition have not been at the centre of resourcing decisions. There has been little power-sharing with stakeholders relevant to developing and implementing socially constructed strategies for adolescent health. A coalition of stakeholders driving adolescent health needs to be broadened as many stakeholders are those who were involved with population and reproductive health and have continued to be the decision-makers for adolescent health.

Youth Representation and Agency Marginalised discourses also extend to the relative participation of youth in the design and implementation of responsive solutions [9]. Youth are taken as intended categorical recipients of adolescent health interventions, but there has been little representation of youth groups and sectors interfacing with youth such as sports, culture, and media sectors, in the design, resourcing, and decision-making of adolescent health interventions. Better inclusivity of youth-centric actors would likely shift the discourse from medical and health lenses to social, societal, and communication lenses that are critical for the effective programming of interventions.

Understanding Dynamics of National and Sub-National Governance Architecture Probably one of the least understood areas within adolescent health interventions is catalysing change within national contexts. Content of adolescent health interventions and the approach to implementation continues to be spearhead from international networks; however, adolescent health issues given their social complexity and reliance on stakeholders beyond the health sector are inherently reliant on local collaborative governance arrangements. This involves not only time spent on deconstructing and framing the issue within the local context as discussed earlier, but also understanding adaptive capability, financing, and power-sharing within state bureaucracies [10]. Sub-national contexts and power-sharing arrangements are particularly important, but often the most overlooked in adolescent health programming. Important questions around where the interventions will be housed, how resourcing will be shared, whether there are joint accountability indicators, and who takes the lead for oversight and accountability must be squarely addressed in defining a governance architecture [6, 11]. Sub-national contexts may also be complicated by power-sharing arrangements with central governments [12]. Needless to say, sub-national arrangements can sustain or flounder adolescent health initiatives but have been given almost no recognition.

Health as a Lead Actor or Contributing Actor for Adolescent Health Interventions?

The importance of health as a key actor but not always the lead actor has been emphasised by experts. A multi-country study by George et al. [4] applied lead actor mapping for intervention areas for adolescent sexual-reproductive health, HIV, mental health, and violence prevention to sectors responsible for them using a framework that highlights settings, roles, and alignment. Out of 11 intervention areas, health is the lead actor for one and a possible lead actor for two other interventions depending on the implementation context. All other interventions take place outside of the health sector, with the health sector playing a range of bilateral, trilateral supporting roles or in several cases a minimal role [4].

Framing of Adolescent Health Is Underwritten by Shifting Development World Ideologies

The framing of an issue in terms of shared benefit across sectors or narrower concentration of benefits within one sector influences collaboration from other sectors [5]. Akwara and Idele [13] deconstructed narratives related to adolescent—young peoples' sexual-reproductive health (AYSRH) policies and programmes in Kenya. Pre-MDG period was dominated by issue-based policies of population growth and high fertility rates in the married population with strong cultural and religious barriers to AYSRH; early to mid-MDG was mainly influenced by the threat of HIV/AIDS, driven by medical narratives and religious-cultural opposition to AYSRH. Late-MDG saw more progressive policies leaning towards liberal social reforms with a refocus on sexual-reproductive health due to sustained early childbearing, culminating in the revised Adolescent Sexual and Reproductive Health Policy of 2015 [13].

Missing Constituencies

Mental health problems and suicide are the leading causes of ill-health in young people globally. Stress, anxiety, and depression were commonly identified as mental health concerns in India [14]. Diverse platforms such as community, family, school, digital, and health facilities were devised to deliver preventive interventions through peers and non-specialist providers supported with treatment interventions through speciality providers. There was very little engagement of young people in the development of these policies or in their implementation, hence despite well-defined interventions, underlying social determinants such as supportive schools were only occasionally addressed, whereas social norms remained unaddressed [14].

Catalysing Change Through National Contexts Is Less Understood and Often Taken for Granted

The right solution framing, pre-converted champions, and inclusive coalitions have come together during policy openings to spearhead adolescent health interventions into effective programming. For example, Mississippi and Nigeria two socially conservative places unlikely to prioritise sexuality education took forward sexuality education interventions in schools supported by similar drivers [15]. These included the presence of committed local individuals and organisations, the opening of a policy window requiring a solution to a pressing social problem of teen pregnancy in Mississippi and HIV/AIDS in Nigeria, and external resources to support implementation costs [15].

3 Programming Nutrition for Adolescent Health

Whereas undernutrition has been an ongoing recognised chronic issue within adolescents, obesity has become an epidemic requiring worldwide action [16]. Evidence on processes and pathways for nutrition interventions in adolescents has focused on supplementation-driven undernutrition programmes [17, 18] or school health obesity interventions [19]. Discussion of political drivers is rare, and where it occurs, it focuses on specific interventions rather than multipronged strategies that bring together obesity and undernutrition paradigms into single inclusive policy programming. Fragmented siloed narratives have been highlighted underscoring the need for transformational and more distributive leaderships [17], as the business-as-usual approach to adolescent nutrition is unlikely to make headway. The issues of institutional ownership and strengthening [20] are repeatedly cited as chronic blocks both for adult and adolescent nutrition. However, exploration of political economy has too often focused on policy discourses but not on institutional dynamics and governance arrangements that must be better understood to co-opt other sectors in the leadership and delivery of adolescent health interventions. We draw on Pakistan's attempts to realise adolescent nutrition, looking more closely at the underlying political drivers linked with the governance architecture for moving towards more expansive and sustainable programming of adolescent nutrition.

4 Discourse from Pakistan—Unpacking Governance of Adolescent Health Interventions

4.1 The Landscape of Adolescent Nutrition

Pakistan lends well to a political economy case analysis of adolescent health due to the high burden of adolescent health malnutrition in Pakistan as well as the governance complexities of multi-sector action in a devolved country setting. Pakistan is home to an estimated 40 million adolescents [21], approximately a quarter of the total country population. It has traditionally lagged behind other South Asian countries in access to health services [22] and school enrolment [23], hence limiting opportunities for access to health education, counselling, and referral services for adolescents. Fifty-six per cent of adolescent girls are anaemic, whereas one in eight adolescent girls and one in five adolescent boys are underweight [24]. Undernutrition and anaemia are exacerbated by marriages of adolescent girls, unmet needs for contraception, food insecurity, as well as water and sanitation issues. Obesity was for the first time highlighted in Pakistan in the National Nutrition Survey of 2017–2019, which showed a slight decrease in stunting but a rise in overweight persons from 5% to over 9.5% [24]. The findings from the survey also revealed for the first time that adolescent boys carry a greater burden of malnutrition—underweight, stunting, overweight and obesity—as compared to girls. Modelling estimates show that obesity in children aged 5–19 years was relatively rare in the 1970s but has risen steadily, particularly among adolescents in Pakistan [24]. Unregulated consumption of sugary drinks and high-calorie snacks, lack of nutrition counselling, increasing social media use, and diminishing physical space for exercise within schools and neighbourhoods are noted to be key attributes of rising obesity among adolescents [9]. Poor diet is also documented as a cause of unwanted weight gain—the Cost of Diet Analysis of 2016 shows that 67% of the households in Pakistan are unable to afford a nutritionally adequate diet and substitute routine diets with high-calorie, poorly nutritious foods [25].

Governance and decision-making architecture are complex in Pakistan, as health and other social sectors are devolved from central to provincial governments. This results in a multiplicity of national and provincial stakeholders within each sector, with national policy coordination undertaken by the central government, whereas legislation, resourcing, and service delivery design are done by the provincial governments. Despite recent progress in national policy commitments to nutrition with adults, policy and programming for adolescents remain largely neglected [26].

4.2 Pakistan's Unfolding Nutrition Policy Landscape

Nutrition was historically framed as a multi-sectoral subject in Pakistan to be delivered across relevant sectors. It was nested in the National Planning Commission within the Ministry of Planning and Development having authority to oversee its integration in planning and resourcing across sectors. The operationalisation of nutrition has periodically swung from a 'hunger' lens underwritten by poverty and food security imperatives to a 'health' lens driven by a focus on maternal-child health.

Economists and planners within the government have historically associated nutrition with 'Hunger' with a primary focus on sufficient wheat production, market supply of food supplies at affordable costs for the poor, and links to social protection programmes. Projects such as 'ration stores' for subsidised food supplies in cities, wheat flour bags distribution in disaster-affected regions, and 'Sasti roti' (subsidised flatbread) and 'sarkari kitchen' (Government Kitchen) schemes to supply prepared food at low cost have been used by many parliamentarians to gain political mileage.

Nutrition gained momentum as a health issue in the 1990s with a focus on breastfeeding and infant nutrition, in a movement led by paediatricians and UNICEF. Key interventions included the establishment of Baby-Friendly Hospitals for promoting newborn breastfeeding, nutrition corners at health facilities for nutrition-related advice, distribution of vitamin A supplements to children and iron and folic acid supplements to pregnant women, and the management of acute malnutrition. In 2005, a Nutrition Wing was established in the Federal Ministry of Health (MoH) initially focusing on micronutrient supplementation in children and pregnant mothers and later expanding to interventions across the first 1000 days of life for pregnant women, lactating women, and children under two. Nutrition programming lacked meaningful resourcing by the state and was supported by small-scale projectised funds contributed by donor agencies. It was not successful in translating into funding within the operational budgets of relevant sectors.

The global Scaling Up Nutrition (SUN) Movement helped reinstate the multi-sectoral reliance on nutrition and propel it to the central policy discourse. Pakistan became a signatory to the SUN movement in 2012 and subsequent SUN support for Pakistan helped establish a dedicated SUN secretariat for multi-sector programming. The Secretariat was deliberately housed at the National Planning Commission by development partners and politicians to ensure effective convening of nutrition across sectors and pre-empt efforts at siloed programming within the health sector. Counterpart subnational nutrition secretariats were established within the Planning & Development Departments (P&DD) in the provinces. Service-related sectors of Health, WASH, Education, and Food, as well as poverty-focused sectors of Agriculture, Social Protection along with more than a hundred Civil Society Organisation (CSO) and close to 50 universities, were brought together under a nutrition-poverty framing [12].

As a result of this multi-sectoral emphasis, nutrition interventions were programmed for mothers and children under two years through supplementation programmes, school curricula, and cash transfer initiatives, as well as for the general population through national food fortification and village-based Water, Sanitation, and Hygiene (WASH) interventions [27]. However, adolescents have had marginal inclusion within nutrition programming until recently.

4.3 The Incremental Policy Shift Towards Adolescent Nutrition

Within the programming of nutrition in Pakistan, adolescent nutrition interventions implemented have tended to focus on undernutrition rather than obesity, in late teens as compared to the younger age bracket of 10–14 years, and centred on girls overlooking boys. Geographical coverage remains very limited even for female undernutrition intervention.

Adolescent nutrition was spotlighted after the National Nutrition Survey of 2017–2018, the first of Pakistan's periodic nutrition surveys that provided findings specific to the adolescent age group. Survey findings highlighted the nutritional status of both adolescent boys and girls aged 10–19 years. At the same time, the Global Nutrition Report was published in 2018, [28] spotlighting adolescent nutrition. Pakistan's newly released data on rising obesity in adolescents and high undernutrition in boys were well advocated by converted nutrition champions within the SUN coalition comprising government technocrats, donors, media, experts, and NGOs. Development partners, including GAIN, UNICEF, WHO, and World Bank, joined by academia pushed the momentum in highlighting critically missing components of adolescents within existing health programmes. The construct was widened from undernutrition to include obesity, the addition of boys, and the inclusion of the overlooked 10–14-years age group.

Consequently, adolescent-focused interventions were consolidated into a multi-sector Pakistan Adolescent Nutrition Strategy (PANS) in 2020, led by the Federal Ministry of Health [29]. PANS importantly recognised adolescence as the second window of opportunity to break the vicious cycle of intergenerational malnutrition and proposed strategies that included sports in schools, physical activity in communities, and advertisement control of sugary beverages and crisps, alongside more traditional measures such as iron–folic acid supplementation in adolescent girls [30]. This was followed by detailed Adolescent Nutrition Supplementation Guidelines released by the Federal Health Ministry in 2020.

4.4 Ideologies, Leadership, and Coalitions in Programming Adolescent Nutrition Across Sectors

Despite a broad mandate for adolescent nutrition provided by PANS, the programming gravitated to undernutrition for teenage girls. Old ideologies, loss of nutrition leadership, and a narrow coalition [31] contributed to almost non-existent programming for obesity and males.

Adult nutrition had relied on political championing to provide a directional mandate and unlock resources and accountability across multiple sectors. The framing of adult nutrition with poverty and rural disadvantaged populations had powerful resonance with political leaders, and spearheading was directly provided by the Minister of Planning and Development as well as cross-party support from parliamentary leaders across two successive political governments.

Noticeably, adolescent nutrition gained policy limelight in Pakistan when a newly elected government came to power but missed the opportunity to mobilise political championing.

The new government claimed youth as a critical constituency, creating a Youth Affairs Wing within the Prime Minister's Secretariat and a Youth Affairs Initiative within the Ministry of Planning and Development. The new political government also had a markedly urban constituency that could have resonated with urban issues of obesity-related lifestyle changes and physical spaces within cities. However, the policy discourse for adolescent nutrition continued siloed and parallel to youth initiatives. A National Youth Development Framework [32] was launched in 2019 focusing on Education, Employment, and Engagement with health and well-being identified as one of the core components, but adolescent nutrition did not feature within the framework, continuing as a parallel discourse.

Adolescent nutrition without the support of political champions became confined to a technocratic agenda pushed by development partners and academia [33]. Dwindling of donor-provided SUN resources eroded the planning commission's coordination ability to sensitise and co-opt new constituencies such as local government, industry, media, sports, and youth affairs in the development of PANS. Efforts to sensitise and support the provincial counterpart Planning and Development Departments remained feeble with little bottom-up multi-sector programming contribution by provinces, in contrast to considerable provincial convening seen for adult undernutrition in the preceding years. Hence leadership of adolescent nutrition gravitated towards the better-staffed Health Ministry and its counterpart provincial health departments. The Federal Health Ministry has historically been home to several micronutrient supplementation and fortification projects and long-standing competitor with planning and development for leadership of national nutrition. With adolescent nutrition leadership gravitating to the Health Ministry, the programming was framed by long-standing ideologies of mother–child health and population control and defined by the associated coalitions of fortification technocrats, reproductive health NGOs, paediatrics, gynaecologists, UNICEF, and WHO. Funding was created within ongoing nutrition programmes for iron–folic acid supplementation for young girls and provision of WASH support within secondary girls' schools for countering undernutrition. The more politically contested area of industrial and media regulation for sugary drinks and junk food became side-lined from nutrition programming alongside the more complex social, cultural, and built environment perspectives necessary to support lifestyle changes for obesity [32].

4.5 Navigating Governance Architecture for Horizontal Coordination for Programming

The social sector governance architecture with its distribution of authority, power, and accountability needs to be understood for programming interventions where the health sector may not always be the lead actor. The Health Ministry often has limited legitimacy to convene sectors for several adolescent health interventions. Each sector is organised in federal ministries and counterpart provincial health departments with separate planning, operational budgets, new development initiatives, staffing, and monitoring systems. Sectors often compete for funds, are administratively overstretched in meeting key responsibilities, and are vertically accountable to planning, finance, and political executives for key targets. Even on issues where sectors may be aligned, actively supporting the Health Ministry in achieving its targets has obvious disincentives, including limited time and resources to divert from sector-specific goals to meeting health targets, as well as ownership and credit sharing issues. In other cases, sectors may have opposing interests such as curtailing commercial interests for health benefits. Adult nutrition was successful in mainstreaming nutrition-sensitive targets and monitoring within the working of relevant sectors while providing additional resources to each sector for delivery and a sector-specific plan led by each sector but converging into a joint plan which had inputs and ownership of all sectors. Hence, accountability accompanied by resources, leadership, and recognition created ownership and healthy competition for delivery. Horizontal platforms of planning and development, supported by political executives, ensured joint planning and joint recognition, but separate resourcing and delivery [31].

With the shift in focus to adolescents, the sector had already co-opted into nutrition planning such as health, education, and WASH moved to programming new activities within existing budgetary resources [33]. Within the health sector, iron and folic acid supplementation for adolescent girls and nutrition awareness activities were added within child ongoing stunting programmes. Education departments refreshed school curricula to incorporate awareness content on adolescent nutrition, as well as undertaking small-scale adolescent nutrition-focused advocacy activities through walks, seminars, and talks. The WASH sector introduced hygiene-related behavioural change activities for adolescents in schools alongside activities being undertaken for younger school-going children. In addition, social welfare departments enacted laws on teen marriages as part of measures to control teen pregnancies. However, sectors relevant to lifestyle and regulatory interventions that were not part of the earlier nutrition coalition were not co-opted due to weak convening leadership and misaligned ideological framing. Hence, communal spaces for exercise, sports in schools, and encouraging physical activity in a socially restrictive society did not get ideated, planned, and resourced by relevant sectors [33]. A health levy on sugary drinks was drafted by the Health Ministry but did not get tabled in parliament. Health levies on products are better received by the public than general sales tax; however, the decision to introduce levies lies with finance and commerce ministries who must buy into the underlying ideology, be convinced of its benefits, and take the lead in the design. Sharing the proceeds of the levy across health and finance has worked at least in the case of tobacco levies to curb sales in the Philippines and Iran. Media regulation for carbonated drinks and crisps advertisements, although advocated by the National Heart Association, did not translate into a broader coalition of media affairs, media groups, the youth affairs department, and local government and hence could not be legislated and programmed within the communication sector. There was an attempt at geographical restriction on the sale of carbonated and sugary drinks in the vicinity of schools but confined to one province that had established a food regulatory authority but faced uneven enforcement.

In Pakistan's case, the devolution of considerable power and resourcing for social subjects to the provinces has created a further layer of coordination, co-option, and ownership to be undertaken at the provinces for programming of nutrition strategies. Donor-supported technical assistance through staff, monitoring systems, and small-scale coordination funds to provinces and central government was catalytic for provincial multi-sector programming during the earlier SUN movement for adult nutrition. Although much smaller in dollar value compared to funding for nutrition projects, this ongoing technical support was perceived to be of critical value in supporting a platform for joint deliberations, contextualisation, support, and accountability across sectors. Erosion of technical assistance for horizontal coordination and lapse of donor financing to projectised funds delivered through NGO and UN parts dented the capability to steer adolescent nutrition.

5 Conclusion

Interventions for adolescent nutrition can run the risk of remaining siloed and public health-focused with limited delivery unless the political economy of leading and resourcing by sectors is addressed. Successful multi-sector governance is now recognised to be a managed process in response to a challenge or opportunity, aimed at disrupting business-as-usual arrangements and replacing these with intentional, innovative actions framed in a way that multiple sectors can contribute [26]. Global findings highlight missed constituencies of boys within adolescent nutrition, overlooking the representation of youth groups in policy discourse, the importance of ideologies, and insufficient attention and understanding of national contexts.

In Pakistan's context, adult nutrition befitted from strong championing tied to a pro-poor agenda, resourcing, and multi-sector programming, but adolescent nutrition efforts floundered and failed to take off across multiple sectors. Obesity interventions particularly did not find a solid foothold within programming. Leadership erosion of converted champions, failure to convert new political champions, dominance of old public health and pro-poor ideologies, and institutional polarisation preventing adolescent nutrition from being joined up with youth-centric policies constrained inclusive framing and powerful steering across sectors. Hence, coalitions remained narrowly confined to the converted sectors already working on undernutrition, and while these incrementally expanded to include few adolescent health measures, a widened coalition for social-behavioural, built environment, and regulatory interventions was essentially missing.

The Pakistan findings underscore that careful efforts are required to convert and build leadership within a convening agency that has the mandate to oversee planning and resourcing accountability across health and other sectors. Second, it cautions against the danger of dominance of old ideologies that entrench path dependency on past practices, allowing little space for fresh framing that is inclusive of the interests of other sectors. Third, the incentives and disincentives within the governance architecture need to be understood for forging effective collaborative programming and moving beyond short-term funding to unlock resources held by other sectors. Finally, horizontal coordination cannot be taken for granted unless there is dedicated, even modest, support for staff, systems, and tools to convene, oversee, and monitor across sectors.

In conclusion, the process of how multi-sector programming for adolescent nutrition is brought about within countries is perhaps even more important than the prescriptive content of globally advocated interventions. Inclusive framing with a social-behavioural ideology to build diversity within core coalitions, an organisational home outside the health sector for programming across sectors, leadership-building efforts, and technical assistance for convening can have a domino effect on building collaborative governance for adolescent nutrition.

Acknowledgement Technical inputs from Asha George, the South African Research Chair in Health Systems, Complexity and Social Change (SARChI) based at the University of Western Cape South Africa, are gratefully acknowledged.

References

1. Sheehan P, Sweeny K, Rasmussen B, Wils A, Friedman HS, Mahon J, Patton GC, Sawyer SM, Howard E, Symons J, Stenberg K. Building the foundations for sustainable development: a case for global investment in the capabilities of adolescents. Lancet. 2017;390(10104):1792–806. https://doi.org/10.1016/S0140-6736(17)30872-3.
2. Patton GC, Sawyer SM, Santelli JS, Ross DA, Afifi R, Allen NB, Arora M, Azzopardi P, Baldwin W, Bonell C, Kakuma R. Our future: a lancet commission on adolescent health and wellbeing. Lancet. 2016;387(10036):2423–78. https://doi.org/10.1016/S0140-6736(16)00579-1.

3. WHO. Global accelerated action for the health of adolescents (AA-HA!): guidance to support country implementation. Geneva: World Health Organization; 2017. p. 2017. https://iris.who.int/bitstream/handle/10665/255415/9?sequence=1.
4. George A, Jacobs T, Ved R, Jacobs T, Rasanathan K, Zaidi SA. Adolescent health in the sustainable development goal era: are we aligned for multisectoral action? BMJ Glob Health. 2021;6(3):e004448. https://doi.org/10.1136/bmjgh-2020-004448.
5. Rasanathan K, Bennett S, Atkins V, Beschel R, Carrasquilla G, Charles J, Dasgupta R, Emerson K, Glandon D, Kanchanachitra C, Kingsley P. Governing multisectoral action for health in low-and middle-income countries. PLoS Med. 2017;14(4):e1002285. https://doi.org/10.1371/journal.pmed.1002285.
6. Bennett S, Glandon D, Rasanathan K. Governing multisectoral action for health in low-income and middle-income countries: unpacking the problem and rising to the challenge. BMJ Glob Health. 2018;3(Suppl 4):e000880. https://doi.org/10.1136/bmjgh-2018-000880. PMID: 30364411; PMCID: PMC6195144
7. Shiffman J, Shawar YR. Framing and the formation of global health priorities. Lancet. 2022;399(10339):1977–90. https://doi.org/10.1016/s0140-6736(22)00584-0. Epub 2022 May 17
8. Jacobs T, George A, De Jong M. Policy foundations for transformation: a gender analysis of adolescent health policy documents in South Africa. Health Policy Plan. 2021;36(5):684–94. https://doi.org/10.1093/heapol/czab041. PMID: 33852727; PMCID: PMC8248976
9. Warraitch A, Wacker C, Bruce D, Bourke A, Hadfield K. A rapid review of guidelines on the involvement of adolescents in health research. Health Expect. 2024;27(3):e14058. https://doi.org/10.1111/hex.14058.
10. Acosta AM, Fanzo J. Fighting maternal and child malnutrition: analysing the political and institutional determinants of delivering a national multisectoral response in six countries. Brighton: Institute of Development Studies. 2012 Apr. Available from: DFID_ANG_Synthesis_April2012.pdf (publishing.service.gov.uk)
11. Zaidi S, Bhutta Z, Hussain SS, Rasanathan K. Multisector governance for nutrition and early childhood development: overlapping agendas and differing progress in Pakistan. BMJ Glob Health. 2018;3(Suppl 4):e000678. https://doi.org/10.1136/bmjgh-2017-000678.
12. Zaidi S, Mohmand SK, Hayat N, Acosta AM, Bhutta ZA. Nutrition policy in the post-devolution context in Pakistan: an analysis of provincial opportunities and barriers. IDS Bull. 2013;44:86–93. https://doi.org/10.1111/1759-5436.12035.
13. Akwara E, Idele P. The moral and social narratives of sexual and reproductive health in Kenya: a case of adolescents and young people pre- and within the MDG era. Reprod Health. 2020;17(1):75. https://doi.org/10.1186/s12978-020-00930-x. PMID: 32456657; PMCID: PMC7249422
14. Roy K, Shinde S, Sarkar BK, Malik K, Parikh R, Patel V. India's response to adolescent mental health: a policy review and stakeholder analysis. Soc Psychiatry Psychiatr Epidemiol. 2019;54(4):405–14. https://doi.org/10.1007/s00127-018-1647-2. Epub 2019 Jan 3. PMID: 30607452; PMCID
15. Robinson RS, Kunnuji M, Shawar YR, Shiffman J. Glob. Public Health. 2018;13(12):1807–19. https://doi.org/10.1080/17441692.2018.1449000. Epub 2018 Mar 20.PMID: 29557293 PMC6443608
16. Di Cesare M, Sorić M, Bovet P, Miranda JJ, Bhutta Z, Stevens GA, Laxmaiah A, Kengne AP, Bentham J. The epidemiological burden of obesity in childhood: a worldwide epidemic requiring urgent action. BMC Med. 2019;17(1):212. https://doi.org/10.1186/s12916-019-1449-8. PMID: 31760948; PMCID: PMC6876113
17. Kiendrébéogo JA, Sory O, Kaboré I, Kafando Y, Kumar MB, George AS. Form and functioning: contextualising the start of the global financing facility policy processes in Burkina Faso. Glob Health Action. 2024;17(1):2360702. https://doi.org/10.1080/16549716.2024.2360702. Epub 2024 Jun 24. PMID: 38910459; PMCID: PMC11198144

18. Roche ML, Bury L, Yusadiredja IN, Asri EK, Purwanti TS, Kusyuniati S, Bhardwaj A, Izwardy D. Adolescent girls' nutrition and prevention of anaemia: a school based multisectoral collaboration in Indonesia. BMJ. 2018;363:k4541. Yusadiredjai IN [corrected to Yusadiredja IN]. PMID: 30530813; PMCID: PMC6282733
19. Moise N, Cifuentes E, Orozco E, Willett W. Limiting the consumption of sugar sweetened beverages in Mexico's obesogenic environment: a qualitative policy review and stakeholder analysis. J Public Health Policy. 2011;32(4):458–75. https://doi.org/10.1057/jphp.2011.39. Epub 2011 Jun 9. PMID: 21654826
20. Renzaho AMN, Dachi G, Ategbo E, Chitekwe S, Doh D. Pathways and approaches for scaling-up of community-based management of acute malnutrition programs through the lens of complex adaptive systems in South Sudan. Arch Public Health. 2022;80(1):203. https://doi.org/10.1186/s13690-022-00934-y. PMID: 36064608; PMCID: PMC9442594
21. GoP 2023. Announcement of Results of 7th Population and Housing Census-2023 'The Digital Census.' Pakistan Bureau of Statistics 2023. Available from https://www.pbs.gov.pk/sites/default/files/population/2023/Press%20Release.pdf
22. WHO 2023. UHC service coverage index—South Asia. Global Health Observatory. Geneva: World Health Organization; 2023. [cited 2023 Aug 29]. Available from: who.int/data/gho/data/themes/topics/service-coverage
23. World Bank 2022. School enrollment, primary (% gross)—South Asia. World Bank Data. 2022. [cited 2023 Aug 29]. Available from: School enrollment, primary (% gross)—South Asia | Data (worldbank.org)
24. Pakistan National Nutrition Survey 2018: Key Findings Report. Ministry of National Health Services Coordination and Regulation, UNICEF, UKAID: Islamabad, Pakistan. 2018. [cited 2023 Aug 29]. Available from: Final Key Findings Report 2019.pdf (unicef.org)
25. Pakistan Cost of Diet analysis Ministry of National Health Services Coordination and Regulation, UNICEF, UKAID: https://www.unicef.org/pakistan/media/1506/file/Cost%20of%20Diet%20Report%20-%20Pakistan.pdf
26. Zaidi SA, Bigdeli M, Langlois EV, Riaz A, Orr DW, Idrees N, Bump JB. Health systems changes after decentralisation: progress, challenges and dynamics in Pakistan. BMJ Glob Health. 2019;4(1):e001013. https://doi.org/10.1136/bmjgh-2018-001013.
27. Ministry of Planning, Development and Reform and World Food Programme (2018) Pakistan multi sectoral nutrition strategy (PMNS 2018–2025)-Pakistan, Islamabad, 2018.
28. Global Nutrition Report, Global Nutrition Report 2018. https://globalnutritionreport.org/reports/global-nutrition-report-2018/
29. Government of Pakistan. Nutrition wing, Ministry of National Health Services, Regulation and Coordination, Govt of Pakistan. Pakistan Adolescent Nutrition Strategy and Operational Plan. 2020. https://www.unicef.org/pakistan/media/2846/file/Pakistan%20Adolescent%20Nutrition%20Strategy.pdf
30. GAIN 2021. The Global Alliance for Improved Nutrition Adolescent Nutrition Project Team. Working Paper Number18. https://www.gainhealth.org/sites/default/files/publications/documents/gain-working-paper-series-18-raising-the-profile-of-adolescent-nutrition-in-pakistan-learnings-on-the-journey-from-policy-to-action.pdf
31. Zaidi S, Najmi R, Habib SS, Memon Z, George A. Applying a multi-sectoral approach for programming of health interventions: comparative analysis of nutrition and tobacco control amongst adolescents in Pakistan. Med Res Archiv. 2024;12(9)
32. GoP. National Youth Development Framework 2019. Prime Minister's Office, Government of Pakistan; 2019. https://pmyp.gov.pk/KJAssets/img/docs/NYDF.pdf
33. Zaidi S, Najmi R, Habib S, Memon Z, George A. Applying a multi-sectoral approach for programming of health interventions: comparative analysis of nutrition and tobacco control amongst adolescents in Pakistan. Medical Research Archives, [S.l.]. 2014;12(9) Oct. 2024. ISSN 2375-1924. Available at: https://esmed.org/MRA/mra/article/view/5525

Emerging Challenges

Nutrition in Conflict and Humanitarian Settings

Nadia Akseer, Hana Tasic, Sama El Baz, and Shelley Walton

1 Introduction

Across the globe today, a record 406 million people from across 82 countries live in a humanitarian setting and require humanitarian assistance [1]. This represents a nearly 400% increase from 2010, when 74 million people needed humanitarian assistance. These numbers reflect record highs and an unabating trend given a global context of protracted conflicts, complex crises, rapidly increasing numbers of climate-related disasters, rising inflation, and the residual impacts of the COVID-19 pandemic [2]. These trends signal a reality in which increasingly more of the world's population will be born into, spend their critical developing years, and live much, if not all, of their lives in a humanitarian setting. Within these settings, severe disruptions to the functioning of often already weak structures, systems, and services further expose populations to a wide range of vulnerabilities, depriving many of their basic survival needs and human rights [3]. In particular, food, agricultural, and health systems often collapse in the face of such crises, leaving populations without

N. Akseer (✉)
Department of International Health, Institute for International Programs, Johns Hopkins University, Baltimore, MD, USA

Modern Scientist Global, Toronto, ON, Canada
e-mail: nakseer1@jhu.edu; nakseer@modernscientistglobal.com

H. Tasic
Modern Scientist Global, Toronto, ON, Canada
e-mail: htasic@modernscientistglobal.com

S. El Baz · S. Walton
Department of International Health, Institute for International Programs, Johns Hopkins University, Baltimore, MD, USA
e-mail: selbaz@jh.edu; swalton9@jhu.edu

© The Author(s), under exclusive license to Springer Nature Switzerland AG 2025
Z. S. Lassi, R. A. Salam (eds.), *Nutrition Across Reproductive, Maternal, Neonatal, Child, and Adolescent Health Care*,
https://doi.org/10.1007/978-3-031-95721-5_19

access to adequate and affordable food and essential nutrients and quality, lifesaving healthcare [3]. Subsequent food insecurity and malnutrition result, leading to serious health complications and, for many, death [3]. Globally, levels of hunger were on a downward trend from 2005 to 2017 but have been on the rise since 2017, leaving 9.2% of the world's population facing hunger [4]. Countries in crises, particularly those that are protracted, are most vulnerable [5]. Nearly half of countries with humanitarian crises have populations experiencing at least crisis-level acute food insecurity [5].

In this chapter, key information on nutrition in humanitarian settings is presented with a particular focus on those most vulnerable to malnutrition—women, adolescent girls, and children. The lifecycle approach to malnutrition is utilized as a guiding framework when presenting and understanding risk factors associated with malnutrition at key developmental periods in an individual's life. Data are presented from the largest and most protracted humanitarian crises around the world in terms of numbers of people in need of aid, centering on ten illustrative countries: Somalia, Afghanistan, the Democratic Republic of the Congo, Yemen, Syria, South Sudan, Haiti, Myanmar, Ukraine, and Libya [5]. This chapter concludes with a review of nutrition interventions implemented to prevent and treat malnutrition in humanitarian settings, their implementation challenges, and recommendations for improvement.

2 Burden of Malnutrition and Food Insecurity in Humanitarian Settings

Box 1 Definitions

Types of Humanitarian Settings: Man-made emergencies (e.g., armed conflict, plane or train crashes), natural disasters and climate shocks (e.g., earthquakes, tsunamis, volcanic eruptions, epidemics and pandemics, droughts, famines) [6], or complex emergencies [7].

Humanitarian Setting: One in which an event or series of events result in a critical threat to the health, safety, security, or well-being of a community or other large group of people. The capacity of affected communities is typically overwhelmed and requires substantial external support [7].

Complex Emergency: A country, region, or society where there is a total or considerable breakdown of authority resulting from internal or external conflict and which requires a multi-sectoral, international response that goes beyond the mandate or capacity of any single agency and/or the ongoing United Nations country program [7].

Malnutrition: Deficiencies or excesses in nutrient intake, an imbalance of essential nutrients, or impaired nutrient utilization resulting in stunting, wasting, underweight, micronutrient deficiencies/insufficiencies, overweight, obesity, or diet-related non-communicable diseases [7].

2.1 Malnutrition in Humanitarian Settings

Humanitarian crises weaken already fragile health, social, and other structures necessary for the survival of populations and expose them to devastating and long-lasting impacts. In Table 1, data are presented on key demographic, nutrition, health, and mortality indicators from ten countries experiencing the largest and most protracted humanitarian crises across the world [5].

Within these countries, maternal mortality, neonatal mortality, and under-5 mortality are some of the highest around the world ranging from 17 to 1223 maternal deaths per 100,000 live births, 5 to 40 neonatal deaths per 100,000 live births, and 8 to 112 child deaths per 1000 births, respectively (Table 1). The Sustainable Development Goals aim for a global reduction to less than 70 deaths per 100,000 live births for maternal mortality, 12 deaths per 1000 live births for neonatal mortality, and 25 deaths per 1000 live births for under-5 mortality; however, most of these countries have significantly higher mortality rates than the global targets [37]. As illustrated in Table 1, 8 of these 10 countries have a maternal mortality ratio greater than 70 and 7 countries have neonatal and under-5 mortality rates well above global targets (Table 1). It is critical to note that estimates from these countries, as well as across humanitarian settings generally, are likely to be underestimates given the well-documented challenges in data collection [38].

Several factors contribute to these alarming mortality rates including limited access to routine and lifesaving health services, low health worker density, and low breastfeeding rates, among many others (Table 1). Arguably, the most critical contributing factor to these high mortality rates is malnutrition, inclusive of both undernutrition and overweight/obesity [39]. Undernutrition is the leading cause of ill health and death around the world, particularly for children under 5 years, where it underlies 45% of all deaths [40]. As illustrated in Table 1, malnutrition is rampant in countries experiencing humanitarian crises. The most common forms of malnutrition among children in humanitarian settings include acute malnutrition or *wasting* (inclusive of both moderate acute malnutrition (MAM) and severe acute malnutrition [SAM]), chronic malnutrition or *stunting*, underweight (a composite indicator reflecting both acute and chronic malnutrition), and micronutrient deficiencies, which can occur concurrently with stunting, wasting, and underweight. Overweight and obesity are other forms of malnutrition found in humanitarian settings [41].

While malnutrition impacts entire emergency-afflicted populations, women, adolescent girls, and children are at a much greater morbidity and mortality risk due to their elevated nutritional needs required for growth and development as well as socio-political and cultural practices that can impact accessibility and experiences related to food and healthcare [42, 43].

Table 1 Most recent and best estimates of key demographic, contextual, nutrition, and mortality statistics from chronic humanitarian settings as of 2023, rounded to the nearest whole number

	Somalia	Afghanistan	Democratic Republic of the Congo	Yemen	Syria	South Sudan	Haiti	Myanmar	Ukraine	Libya
Total population in millions (2023) [8–17]	18.1	42.2	102.3	34.4	23.2	11.1	11.7	54.6	36.7	6.9
Conflict										
Years as a Fragile and Conflict-Afflicted State (2010 and beyond) [18]	14	14	14	14	11	11	14	14	1	11
Refugee population by country or territory of origin (total in most recent estimate available) [19]	786,794	5,661,717	932,680	40,147	6,559,736	2,295,082	30,307	1,251,618	5,684,177	17,811
Internally displaced persons, total displaced by conflict and violence (total in most recent estimate available) [19]	3,864,000	4,394,000	5,686,000	4,523,000	6,865,000	1,475,000	171,000	1,498,000	5,914,000	135,000
Gender inequalities										
Gender Inequality Index Value (ranges from 0 to 1) [20]	0.78	0.68	0.60	0.82	0.48	0.59	0.64	0.50	0.20	0.26
Health system										
Density of physicians (per 10,000 population) [21]	0.23	3	4	3	12	0.4	2	8	30	22
Density of nurses and midwives (per 10,000 population) [21]	1	5	11	7	14	4	4	11	67	67

Antenatal care coverage—at least four visits (%) [22, 23]	24	33.4	56	25	64[a]	17	67	59	87	81[a]
Economy										
Poverty headcount ratio at national poverty lines (% of population) [24]	54	55	64	49	35[a]	82	59	25	2	No data available
Current health expenditure (% of GDP) [25]	No data available	17	4	4	3	5	3	5	8	6
Environment										
Incidents of drought, flood, and other natural disasters (2013–2023) [26]	27	58	40	27	12	19	33	31	10	2
Food insecurity and nutrition										
Prevalence of severe food insecurity in population (%) [27]	33	46	26	55	55	63	48	27	25	21
Number of people in IPC Phase 3 or above (as of 2023) [28]	6,500,000 (33%)	19,900,000 (46%)	26,500,000 (26%)	17,370,000 (55%)	12,060,000 (55%)	7,800,000 (63%)	4,700,000 (48%)	15,200,000 (27%)	(25%)	No data available
Prevalence of wasting (% of children under 5 years) [23, 29]	14[a]	4	6	16	12	23	4	7	8[a]	10
Prevalence of stunting (% of children under 5 years) [23, 30]	25	45	42	46	28	31	22	29	23[a]	38
Prevalence of anemia among pregnant women (%) [31]	49	37	47	58	33	40	49	48	23	29

(continued)

Table 1 (continued)

	Somalia	Afghanistan	Democratic Republic of the Congo	Yemen	Syria	South Sudan	Haiti	Myanmar	Ukraine	Libya
Early initiation of breastfeeding (%) [32]	23	41	52	53	46[a]	50	47	67	66	No data available
Infants exclusively breastfed for the first 6 months of life (%) [33]	34	58	54	10	29	45	40	51	20	No data available
Mortality										
Maternal mortality ratio (maternal deaths per 100,000 live births) [34]	621	620	547	183	30	1223	350	179	17	72
Neonatal mortality rate (deaths per 1000 live births) [23, 35]	36	24	26	28	11	40	24	22	5	6
Under-5 mortality rate (deaths per 1000 live births) [23, 36]	112	55	79	62	22	99	59	42	8	11

United Nations Population Fund, 2023; United Nations Refugee Agency, 2023; World Bank Open Data, 2022; United Nations Development Programme, 2023; World Health Organization, 2023; EM-DAT, 2023; United Nations Children's Fund, 2023; International Disaster Database, 2023

[a]Estimates ranging from 1999 to 2010

2.2 Nutrition of Children Under 5 Years in Humanitarian Settings

With nearly 20% of children around the world living in conflict zones and about 50% of children living in countries extremely vulnerable to the impacts of climate change, children across the globe are increasingly exposed to grave nutritional risks [39, 44]. Both acute and chronic malnutrition can negatively impact all children, but the effects are most notable for children under 5 years, particularly in humanitarian settings where the malnutrition burden is both rising and becoming more concentrated [40]. For purposes of this chapter, this review focuses on malnutrition among children under 5 years given the importance of this developmental period and younger children's increased susceptibility to malnutrition and death.

2.2.1 Wasting

Acute malnutrition, or *wasting*, is a critical condition defined by low weight for height and characterized by a recent and moderate-to-severe loss of weight and muscle mass. This condition often results from inadequate food intake, frequent or prolonged illness, suboptimal maternal and childcare practices, and poor sanitation [45]. Of the current 45.4 million children under 5 years suffering from acute malnutrition, 30 million children, or two-thirds of the world's wasted children, come from 15 countries experiencing humanitarian emergencies [46]. Of all those with acute malnutrition, almost 14 million children are experiencing the most dangerous form of malnutrition, severe acute malnutrition (SAM) [28, 46, 47].

Conflict, displacement, and natural disasters exacerbate the risk of acute malnutrition as access to key resources, healthcare, food, and other systems essential to living a healthy life are compromised [40]. The prevalence of wasting among children under 5 years in low- and middle-income countries is 7.3%; the burden is significantly higher in humanitarian settings, where it can affect up to 30% of children under 5 years [28]. This burden of acute malnutrition has historically been concentrated geographically, with South Asia and Sub-Saharan Africa bearing a disproportionate share [48]. Around 70% of all children under 5 years are affected by wasting live in Asia, and 27% live in Africa [48]. Like the geographic disparities observed for wasting, a similar uneven distribution of wasting is seen across the under-5 age span. The highest rates of wasting occur in children aged 6–23 months, typically attributed to the transition from exclusive breastfeeding to complementary feeding where nutritional gaps can exist. This is particularly exacerbated in humanitarian settings where access to nutritious foods and proper sanitation are limited.

2.2.2 Stunting

Stunting, or *chronic* malnutrition, is characterized by impaired linear growth in children, resulting in low height for age. The condition is indicative of chronic or recurrent undernutrition and is typically associated with poverty, poor maternal health and nutrition outcomes, suboptimal growth in utero, regular bouts of illnesses, and inappropriate feeding in early childhood [45].

Despite the steady progress over the past two decades, with global reductions in child stunting from 33% to 22.3%, the prevalence in conflict and humanitarian settings is as high as 57.5% [48, 49]. Furthermore, the proportion of children suffering from stunting in conflict-afflicted countries has risen from 46% of all stunted children in 2015 to up to 75% of all stunted children [4, 48, 50]. Similar to the wasting distribution, Sub-Saharan Africa and South Asia carry the greatest burden of stunting; 37.4% and 30.5% of children under 5 years are stunted in Sub-Saharan Africa and South Asia, respectively [48].

2.2.3 Concurrent Stunting and Wasting

While both stunting and wasting detrimentally impact a child's health and development individually, concurrent wasting and stunting put a child at 12 times greater risk of death than a child neither wasted nor stunted [51]. A study of 84 countries' Demographic and Health Surveys (DHSs) and Multiple Indicator Cluster Surveys (MICSs) revealed that conflict-afflicted or fragile countries have a significantly higher prevalence of concurrent wasting and stunting (3.6%) as compared to stable countries (2.2%), further indicating a higher risk of malnutrition and its adverse consequences for children living in these settings [51].

2.3 Women and Adolescent Girl's Nutrition in Humanitarian Settings

Across the globe, more than 1 billion adolescent girls and women of reproductive age (15–49 years) are malnourished [52] with those living in conflict and humanitarian settings being disproportionately impacted. This group is nutritionally at risk due to a combination of exacerbated pre-existing vulnerabilities, disruptions in service provision, and security-related and other barriers to accessing health and nutrition services. This is alongside the naturally increased nutrient requirements that are needed to support healthy growth and pregnancy [38, 52–54]. Women's and girls' health and nutrition are integral for supporting strong families and communities, as malnutrition tends to be intergenerational. Poor maternal nutrition is a major driver of maternal health risks, adverse birth outcomes, newborn morbidity, and mortality as well as poor postnatal growth and cognition [40, 54].

The most common forms of malnutrition found in women and adolescent girls in humanitarian settings are undernutrition, micronutrient deficiencies, and anemia. While overweight is increasingly becoming more common in low- and middle-income countries, including in humanitarian settings [38], this review focuses on undernutrition and anemia.

2.3.1 Undernutrition

Compared with children under 5 years, there are limited data on girls' and women's nutrition in emergencies, particularly for adolescent girls and non-pregnant women [38, 52]. On a global scale, data reveal that 8% of adolescent girls (49 million) and 10% of women (154 million) are underweight, defined as having a body mass index

(BMI) of less than 18.5 kg/m^2 [52]. Where reliable data exist in humanitarian settings, trends paint a grim picture of rapidly increasing rates of undernutrition, particularly for pregnant or lactating women and adolescent girls (PLW/G) [38, 52]. From 2020 to 2022, underweight increased by 25% among PLW/G in the 12 countries most impacted by the global food crisis and also experiencing a humanitarian crisis, from 5.5 million to 6.9 million PLW/G, respectively [52].

2.3.2 Anemia

Anemia is a condition in which the number of red blood cells, or the hemoglobin concentration within the blood cells, is lower than normal [55]. For women of reproductive age, and pregnant women in particular, anemia is associated with poor maternal and birth outcomes, reduced school performance, reduced productivity, and a lower quality of life [55]. The global prevalence of anemia among non-pregnant women in humanitarian settings is around 30% [56], ranging from 23% (in Ukraine) to 58% (in Yemen) (Table 1).

3 Malnutrition Risk Factors

Within humanitarian settings, certain individuals face a greater risk of becoming malnourished depending upon a myriad of complex and interrelated factors. The MQ-SUN life cycle approach to wasting framework outlines risks at key developmental periods of an individual's life, acknowledging both the cyclical nature of malnutrition as well as the chronic, environmental risk factors that impact malnutrition susceptibility [57]. As shown in the MQ-SUN Life Cycle Framework figure, the cyclicality of malnutrition may begin as early as adolescence, in the pre-pregnancy and pregnancy periods, highlighting the importance of pre-conception and prenatal care in mitigating the cycle. Once born, a child is at greater risk depending upon their exposure to certain risk factors in their infancy (0–6 months) and in their childhood (6–59 months).

3.1 Food Security in Conflict and Humanitarian Settings

A critical risk factor inextricably linked to malnutrition in humanitarian settings is food insecurity. The number one driver of food insecurity is conflict, with 75% of the world's malnourished living in conflict zones [58]. Food security, or the state in which "all people, at all times, have physical, social, and economic access to sufficient, safe, and nutritious food that meets their food preferences and dietary needs for an active and healthy life," [59] plummets as a result of multiple complex drivers in humanitarian settings [60]. During both conflict and natural disasters, food systems are disrupted as crop production is reduced, supply chains are interrupted, and connections with global markets and trade can be severed [61]. Livelihoods are destroyed as systems become less or non-functional, making it challenging for families to sell or purchase food [58]. Furthermore, in conflict settings, hunger is often used as a weapon of war, where warring factions directly cut off food supplies from reaching populations, blocking food aid and humanitarian access, or purposefully destroying agricultural systems and infrastructure [54, 61]. In the context of climate change, extreme weather events, such as droughts, floods, and extreme heat among countless others, often compounded by ongoing conflict, reduce harvest yields, agricultural productivity, and livestock populations, driving dire levels of food insecurity [28, 61]. These severe disruptions result in both food scarcity and inaccessible or unaffordable nutritious foods, ultimately leading to high levels of food insecurity [61].

The number of people affected by conflict- and extreme weather-driven food crises has seen a dramatic increase in recent years, with a 33% increase from 2021 to 2022 alone [28, 61]. According to the 2023 Global Report on Food Crises, of the 58 countries experiencing food crises resulting in an Integrated Food Security Phase Classification (IPC) of 3 or above (i.e., crisis levels), 19 of those countries were affected by conflict, in particular Afghanistan, Burkina Faso, Nigeria, Somalia, South Sudan and Yemen, where populations were facing catastrophic levels of food insecurity as of 2022 (Fig. 1) [28]. Across conflict-afflicted settings, the total population impacted over the past 5 years has been rising substantially, from 73.9 million in 2018 to 117.1 million in 2022 (Fig. 1) [28]. Similarly, the number of people impacted by extreme weather-driven food crises has doubled, from 28.8 million in 2018 to 56.8 million across 12 countries in 2022.

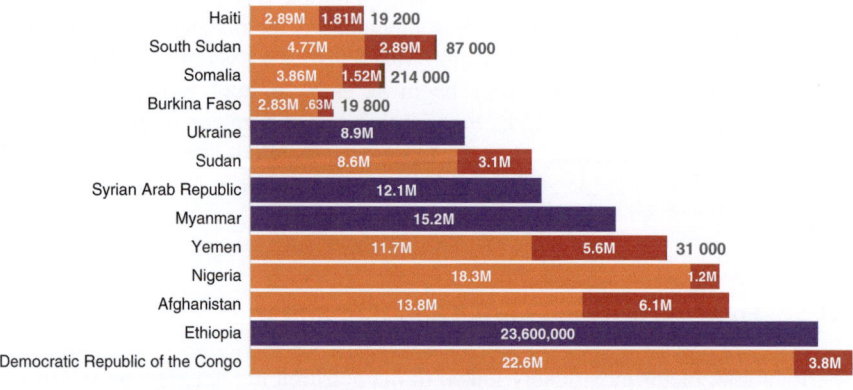

Fig. 1 Countries with the highest numbers of people in IPC/CH Phase 3 or above or equivalent in 2022. (Food Security Information Network, 2023) [28]

> **Box 2 Integrated Food Security Phase Classification Definitions**
>
> **Phase 1 (None/Minimal):** Households are able to meet essential food and non-food needs without engaging in atypical and unsustainable strategies to access food and income. Action is required to build resilience and for disaster risk reduction.
>
> **Phase 2 (Stressed):** Households have minimally adequate food consumption but are unable to afford some essential non-food expenditures without engaging in stress-coping strategies. Action is required for disaster risk reduction and to protect livelihoods.
>
> **Phase 3 (Crisis):** Households are unable to meet their minimum food needs or are compelled to protect food consumption by engaging in coping strategies that will harm their future ability to access food and sustain their livelihoods. Urgent action is required to protect livelihoods and reduce food consumption gaps.
>
> **Phase 4 (Emergency):** Households face large food gaps, which are either reflected in high acute malnutrition levels and excess mortality or mitigated by using emergency coping strategies that severely corrode their well-being and livelihoods. Urgent action is required to save lives and livelihoods.
>
> **Phase 5 (Catastrophe/Famine):** Households have an extreme lack of food and/or other basic needs even after full employment of coping strategies. Starvation, death, destitution, and extremely critical acute malnutrition levels are evident. (For famine classification, the area needs to have extremely critical levels of acute malnutrition and mortality.) Urgent action is required to revert/prevent widespread death and total collapse of livelihoods [28].

4 Interventions to Address Malnutrition in Humanitarian Settings

In humanitarian settings, interventions aimed at improving nutrition outcomes can be either preventative or curative and nutrition-specific or nutrition-sensitive and have evolved over time. The Sphere movement was initiated by humanitarian professionals in 1997 who developed a Humanitarian Charter and a set of humanitarian standards which have since become a primary reference tool for organizations [62]. The Sphere handbook covers key areas including water, sanitation and hygiene promotion, food security and nutrition, shelter and settlement, and health. It is intended to be used by practitioners involved in humanitarian responses and for humanitarian advocacy work [62]. The food security and nutrition interventions in the handbook will be presented in this chapter. While this chapter does not go into detail on interventions related to health, water, sanitation, and hygiene, early childhood development, maternal mental health, child protection, and family planning services, it is important to note that these are nutrition-sensitive interventions that have also been implemented in humanitarian settings [62–66].

> **Box 3 The Food Security Cluster (FSC), the Global Nutrition Cluster (GNC), and Organizations Supporting the Provision of Nutrition Interventions in Humanitarian Settings**
>
> The Food Security Cluster (FSC) and the Global Nutrition Cluster (GNC) coordinate responses to address food availability, access, and utilization in humanitarian crises and to protect or improve the nutritional status of populations impacted by emergencies [67, 68]. The FSC is co-led by the Food and Agriculture Organization (FAO) and the World Food Programme (WFP) and coordinates a network of partners, including UN agencies, international non-governmental organizations (INGOs), and NGOs, in 30 countries [67]. The WFP was established in 1961 and is the world's largest humanitarian organization with a presence in over 120 countries. WFP provides food to people displaced by conflict and disasters, supports women's and children's nutrition, and leads capacity and resilience-building activities in vulnerable communities [69]. The FAO was established by the UN in 1945 with the goal of achieving food security for all. It works in over 130 countries around the world, setting global standards to ensure food quality and safety and supporting member countries to devise national strategies to achieve rural development and hunger alleviation goals [70]. Operating at the local and global levels, the FSC provides guidance to country clusters and sectors and coordinates with other global clusters such as the water, sanitation, and hygiene cluster [67].
>
> The GNC is led by the United Nations Children's Fund (UNICEF). UNICEF was established in 1946 and works in over 190 countries to help save children's lives and protect their rights, including through humanitarian action and the provision of a multitude of interventions in emergencies and for migrant and refugee children [71]. Established as part of the Humanitarian Reform process in 2006, the GNC aims to improve the efficiency of programs responding to humanitarian issues by supporting country coordination mechanisms [68]. The GNC supports strategic decision-making, planning and strategy development, capacity strengthening, advocacy, monitoring and reporting, and contingency planning and preparedness [68].
>
> Though these clusters comprise many large and influential organizations, this is by no means an exhaustive list of the myriad actors working to deliver nutrition interventions in humanitarian crises.

4.1 Assessment

Food security and nutrition assessments are necessary within humanitarian settings to understand the needs of a given population and to adjust interventions appropriately [62]. Food security assessments, which assess livelihood, asset, and coping strategies altered by the crisis, and nutrition assessments, which capture data on malnutrition prevalence and nutrition practices, can overlap as they address access to and use of food. Conducting them jointly can increase cost-effectiveness [62]. Objectives of these assessments include: (1) understanding the current situation and needs, (2) estimating the number of people requiring assistance, (3) identifying groups at the highest risk, and (4) providing a baseline to monitor the impact of humanitarian response [62]. Assessments ideally take place at the start of intervention implementation, with rapid assessments occurring within a few weeks, and detailed assessments within 3–12 months.

4.2 Prevention

Table 2 provides an overview of nutrition interventions and commodities used in humanitarian settings. The following section outlines the interventions aimed at the prevention of malnutrition while Sect. 4.3 describes those used in the treatment of SAM and MAM.

Table 2 Key nutrition-related interventions and commodities used in humanitarian settings

Interventions	
Food assistance	Food assistance programs in humanitarian settings can consist of a range of tools including general food distribution (GFD), blanket supplementary feeding (BSF) programs, targeted supplementary feeding (TSF) programs, and the provision of services and inputs related to food/agriculture such as skill and knowledge transfers [62]. GFD provides in-kind food or cash transfers for the purchase of food, typically supporting those who are most in need within a humanitarian setting. It is meant to be discontinued once people can produce or access food via other means, with transitional arrangements to bridge the interim between GFD and more independent means of obtaining food. These transitional arrangements can include supporting livelihoods or providing conditional cash transfers [62]. BSF programs aim to prevent acute malnutrition and are implemented in humanitarian settings where food insecurity is high. These should be implemented alongside GFD and should target affected households [62]. In order to account for the specific nutritional needs of vulnerable groups, such as children aged 6–59 months and pregnant or breastfeeding women, TSF can be necessary in addition to the general food ration provided [62].
Infant and Young Child Feeding in Emergencies (IYCF-E)	IYCF programs include a multitude of interventions that aim to protect children's nutrition and prevent malnutrition and micronutrient deficiencies. Specifically, these can include capacity building for health workers, education for mothers, community networking, forming mother and baby friendly spaces, lactation support, the baby friendly hospital initiative, and the provision of breastmilk substitutes [72–74]. IYCF-E is specific to emergency situations, comprising priority interventions such as breastfeeding protection and support, appropriate and safe complementary feeding, and management of artificial feeding for infants who cannot breastfeed [62]. Importantly, especially in the context of humanitarian settings, violations of the International Code of Marketing of Breastmilk Substitutes can occur; thus, a significant component of IYCF-E is to ensure that marketing, procurement, and distribution of breastmilk substitutes is restricted [62].

(continued)

Table 2 (continued)

Community Management of Acute Malnutrition (CMAM)	CMAM is the globally endorsed approach for the treatment of malnutrition in children under 5 years. It involves four elements: (i) community outreach, (ii) outpatient care, (iii) inpatient care, and (iv) management of MAM [75]. In CMAM, community health workers screen for malnutrition and initiate the treatment of children with acute malnutrition. If malnutrition is medically uncomplicated; caregivers are responsible for providing the specially formulated food. In the case of medically complicated acute malnutrition, children are referred for inpatient treatment [76]. Supplementary feeding programs (SFPs) fall under the umbrella of CMAM and are used to treat MAM in outpatient settings [77–80]. They target moderately malnourished children and pregnant and lactating people using commodities such as fortified blended foods (FBFs), vegetable oil, high-energy and high-protein biscuits, ready-to-use supplementary food (RUSF), and powdered milk mixed with FBF [81]. CMAM also includes outpatient therapeutic programs (OTPs) that provide home-based treatment to children with uncomplicated SAM. Ready-to-use therapeutic food (RUTF) is used during the rehabilitation phase of SAM. Home-based treatment is more cost-effective and accessible compared to inpatient treatment [82]. In cases where outpatient treatment is not applicable, children are referred to inpatient centers called therapeutic feeding centers (TFC). Children with complicated SAM are treated at TFCs where they are stabilized using therapeutic milks and then referred to outpatient treatment with RUTF.
Commodities	
Fortified blended foods (FBFs)	FBFs include corn-soy blends, wheat-soy blends, and other nutritional blends with added vitamins and minerals to improve their nutritional value [81]. They are used to both prevent and treat acute malnutrition and micronutrient deficiencies in humanitarian settings, including in SFPs to prevent and treat MAM.
Ready-to-use supplementary food (RUSF)	RUSF is a commodity used to manage MAM in the context of CMAM. RUSF is a food product with a high energy and nutrient density, and it can be delivered in a crushable or soft lipid-based form. This commodity is designed for supplementary feeding of the diet and is not meant to be a child's exclusive source of food [81]. Small-quantity lipid-based nutrient supplements (SQ-LNS) can be used in humanitarian emergencies as part of a preventative package of interventions where access to nutritious foods is limited [83].
Ready-to-use therapeutic food (RUTF)	RUTF is used at home during the rehabilitation phase of SAM and has been deemed a more cost-effective and accessible solution when compared to inpatient treatment [82]. RUTF contains peanut paste, powdered milk, vegetable oil, sugar, and a mixture of vitamins and minerals for a total of 500 kilocalories. It does not require any preparation and has a 2-year shelf life [84, 85] RUTF allows children to gain weight quickly in order to recover from malnutrition.
Therapeutic milk (F-75 and F-100)	F-75 and F-100 are therapeutic milk formulas used during the inpatient treatment of complicated SAM [86]. These therapeutic milks are predominantly used by health workers in humanitarian settings to stabilize nutritional deterioration. After stabilization, children are transferred to outpatient treatment using RUTF, with the goal of having them eventually return to a normal diet following treatment. Although RUTF has been increasingly used as it does not require mixing with water, F-75 and F-100 are still essential for inpatient treatment of complicated SAM [86].

4.2.1 Food Distribution and Assistance

Food distribution interventions provide free food assistance directly to individuals or households to ensure food security; they can either be targeted (e.g., to children under 5 years or pregnant women) or cover all the households in a particular geographic region [87]. General food distribution (GFD) in conflict settings can include take-home rations, hot-cooked meal provision, or cash and/or vouchers for food [78]. Evidence has shown that both in-kind and cash-based options should be considered for a food basket to promote and restore food security and nutritional well-being, and where cash-based assistance is used, complementary food distribution should also be considered [62, 88, 89]. The delivery of assistance to those in need is complex and involves many political and logistical considerations. For example, food aid is vulnerable to looting in conflict situations whereas cash assistance can be a more efficient and effective method of assistance that targets a range of people's needs [90]. Implementation of cash-based assistance instead of in-kind assistance depends on numerous factors including local capacity, resources, recipients' preferences, the political environment, and historical lessons [91]. Save the Children (STC), WFP, UNICEF, and the World Bank have all delivered cash-based transfers to millions of households in humanitarian settings [3, 92–94].

The WFP's food basket program is designed to meet the nutritional requirements of populations in humanitarian settings. The size and composition of the basket are tailored to local preferences, demographics, activity levels, climatic conditions, coping capacity, and existing prevalence of malnutrition and disease [95]. This program can provide enough food to cover an individual's basic energy needs (i.e., 2100 kcal per person) or supplement the diet. WFP often tops up the general food distribution ration for all pregnant or lactating people with Super Cereal to improve its nutritional value [95, 96]. Blanket supplementary feeding (BSF) is a measure to prevent acute malnutrition and is recommended where food insecurity is high [62]. BSF should be accompanied by GFD, targeting households that have been affected by the humanitarian crisis and are at risk of malnutrition. It is important to monitor coverage, adherence, and acceptability of the rations that are provided [62].

The WFP has reported that GFD improves nutrition outcomes for those at risk in humanitarian settings and that food transfers have a protective effect on food insecurity among populations in conflict settings [97, 98]. Aid is positively associated with increased household non-food and food expenditures, food consumption, and children's height [98]. However, food distribution can be hindered in crisis settings by limited resources (including commodities and program funding), movement restrictions, physical barriers, security issues, distance to distribution points, food pantry location and hours of operation, and limited eligibility in the case of targeted programs [99, 100]. Factors that can ensure successful food distribution interventions include context awareness, management and coordination, training and support for implementation, a decentralized general food distribution system, timing of the intervention, and women's involvement [101].

4.2.2 Infant and Young Child Feeding: Emergencies (IYCF-E)

IYCF-E consists of priority interventions including breastfeeding protection and support, appropriate and safe complementary feeding, and management of artificial feeding for infants who cannot breastfeed within emergency settings [62]. Organizations including STC, UNICEF, and UNHCR have all provided IYCF-E support [93, 94, 102, 103]. Within IYCF-E, the International Code of Marketing of Breastmilk Substitutes must be followed to ensure that marketing, procurement, and distribution of breastmilk substitutes is restricted to promote breastfeeding, where appropriate. In crisis situations, violations of the Code typically result from issues of labeling and untargeted distribution of breastmilk substitutes [62].

In conflict settings, health worker capacity along with designated places, such as feeding tents, and provision of clean utensils and water for those preparing complementary feeds should be ensured [104]. IYCF interventions are hindered by high health worker turnover, a lack of funds, poor multisectoral coordination, poor monitoring and evaluation, a focus on treatment versus prevention, and marketing efforts for breastmilk substitutes [104]. Delivery of IYCF interventions in humanitarian settings can be improved through increased capacity building of health workers, more accessible services and improved infrastructure, a lack of discrimination, and the use of local languages to deliver services [105].

4.2.3 Micronutrient Supplementation and Fortification

Preventing and alleviating micronutrient deficiencies can be done through micronutrient supplementation, fortification, or food-based approaches [62, 106]. Food-based approaches involve policies and programs to support the consumption of adequate varieties and quantities of good quality micronutrient-rich foods.

Micronutrient supplementation interventions, the most commonly used approach, have been undertaken by numerous international organizations including UNICEF [107], WFP [108], and Action Against Hunger/Action Contre la Faim (ACF) [63]. Supply shortages, insufficient resources, including human resources, limited funding, and ongoing conflict situations, are barriers to delivering micronutrient supplementation interventions [78]. Multiple micronutrient supplementation can be cost-effective when produced locally, which can make supplementation more affordable while simultaneously helping local economies [109].

Controlling micronutrient deficiencies can also be done through fortification of staple foods or other food products with micronutrients. Some common examples of staple food fortification include iodized salt, vegetable oil fortified with vitamin A or D, and wheat and maize flour fortified with iron, folic acid, and often other micronutrients [62, 110]. Fortified blended foods (FBFs) are a type of specialized nutritious food that typically blends cereals, soya, beans, and pulses with a micronutrient mix. Including FBFs in a basic ration in a humanitarian situation is an important way to help vulnerable populations, such as children, pregnant and lactating women, and the elderly, meet their micronutrient needs [110]. The WFP's food basket provides fortified vegetable oil and iodized salt, and, in the case of supplementary rations, FBFs or ready-to-eat foods fortified with vitamins and minerals [95]. This is a cost-effective way to reach many recipients and can be implemented rapidly; however, it is limited to food commodities that can be fortified and needs to be sustained until populations have access to fresh foods [110].

4.3 Treatment

4.3.1 Community Management of Acute Malnutrition (CMAM)

CMAM is a model of treatment for acute malnutrition through outpatient instead of inpatient care that has been shown to improve coverage of services [111]. CMAM evolved from the Community-based Therapeutic Care (CTC) approach, which demonstrated that treatment of SAM and MAM during emergency situations was possible through a decentralized approach implemented through outpatient services and outreach posts [112].

In a 2013 Lancet review of the evidence, CMAM was one of the ten nutrition interventions with the greatest impact on reducing child mortality [113]. Some of the barriers to effective CMAM include limited human and other resources, disjointed planning between government partners, other partners and communities, community outreach being constrained by insufficient assessment, planning and funding, poor monitoring, inadequate support for community health workers (CHWs), high opportunity costs for families, and high program dropout rate [111, 114]. Successful implementation of CMAM requires a sufficient number of trained health and nutrition staff, a reliable source of RUTF and medications, sustainability through the incorporation of CMAM into the health system, and adequate financial resources [115].

There exist also a variety of simplified approaches to CMAM intended to increase coverage and decrease costs, and these can include using a single product for treatment (of MAM and SAM), modified dosing of RUTF, reduction in frequency of health worker visits, using only mid-upper arm circumference (MUAC) for admission, and discharge based on MUAC [116]. These approaches have been evaluated in a variety of settings, and evidence is still being gathered though is promising for some simplifications both alone and combined [116, 117].

4.3.2 Supplementary Feeding Programs (SFPs)

Supplementary feeding is an aspect of CMAM that typically targets children under 5 years to prevent acute malnutrition, or it is used for the management of children or pregnant and lactating women who are moderately malnourished [78] [80]. Several commodities are used to manage MAM in the context of CMAM, including FBF, vegetable oil, high-energy and high-protein biscuits, ready-to-use supplementary food (RUSF), and powdered milk mixed with FBF [81]. RUSF is a food product with high energy and nutrient density that comes in a crushable or soft lipid-based form. It is designed for supplementary feeding and is not meant to be a child's exclusive source of food [81]. FBFs include corn-soy blends, wheat-soy blends, and other nutritional blends that have an added vitamin and mineral mix [81]. There are some issues with using FBFs for the treatment of MAM given that they are not energy-dense, they require cooking, and the prevalence of intra-household sharing of foods is high in many contexts, which could reduce access to the child in need [81].

A review of nutritional interventions targeted at children under 5 years following natural disasters found that food supplementation was effective at reducing wasting, underweight, stunting, and anemia, though the overall evidence quality was weak to moderate [77]. A systematic review of nutrition interventions for women and children in conflict settings found that targeted supplementary feeding led to recovery, but with varying rates, from SAM and MAM [78]. UNHCR's Emergency Handbook includes SFPs as one of the means to manage acute malnutrition in refugee settings [80]. Barriers to implementing supplementary feeding include insufficient coordination, insufficient resources, ongoing conflict, poor outcome reporting, and limited adherence by the population [78].

4.3.3 Outpatient Therapeutic Programs (OTPs)

OTPs are an aspect of CMAM established to provide home-based treatment of children with uncomplicated SAM. Home-based RUTF is used during the rehabilitation phase of SAM and has been deemed a more cost-effective and accessible solution when compared to inpatient treatment [82]. A Cochrane review of RUTF for home-based nutritional rehabilitation of SAM children aged 6–59 months found that standard RUTF, compared to alternative dietary approaches, probably improves recovery and could increase weight gain rate, though effects on relapse and mortality are unknown [82]. A Lancet review found no difference in mortality between RUTF and standard inpatient care in community settings; however, faster weight gain was observed for those who received RUTF accompanied by a greater likelihood of recovery [113, 118].

UNICEF procures nearly 80% of RUTF globally and distributes it widely, including to nearly 250,000 children in South Sudan annually [84]. The use of RUTF for SAM treatment does have some drawbacks. It needs to be combined with complementary foods for children aged 6–23 months. Some children refuse to eat it, some report diarrhea and vomiting after consumption, and some caregivers find it difficult to maintain the recommended serving of RUTF at home when compared to outpatient program sites [119]. There can also be sharing and selling of RUTF in the marketplace, supply shortages, and insufficient funding and human resources for its distribution [78]. For locally sourced RUTF, technical knowledge, financing, and sustainability of production (without donor funding) need to be ensured [120].

4.3.4 Therapeutic Feeding Centers (TFCs)

TFCs provide management for complicated SAM on an inpatient basis with specialized diets, medical treatment, and follow-up [121–123]. SAM is treated in two phases: stabilization and rehabilitation, the latter involving rapid weight gain for the patient [82, 123]. Therapeutic milk formulas F-75 and F-100 are products used by UNICEF and partners for inpatient treatment of complicated SAM, ultimately aimed at decreasing related mortality [86]. In emergency settings, these therapeutic milks are used by health workers to stabilize nutritional deterioration, aiming to return the child to a normal diet after treatment. Although RUTF has been increasingly used as it does not require mixing with water, F-75 and F-100 are still essential for inpatient treatment of complicated SAM [86].

Inpatient treatment at TFCs was found to be effective at reducing the case fatality rate for children who completed the 30-day program, but it was also associated with malnourished children presenting late, cross-infection due to crowding in the centers, high default rates, and high opportunity costs for caregivers [112]. TFCs continue to be a part of strategies to treat childhood malnutrition [124]. In 2023, the WHO supported local authorities in Yemen to provide nutritional care through TFCs to reduce under-5 mortality [125]. TFCs are resource-intensive, and barriers to their implementation can include high financial and opportunity costs for families and limited bed availability in the centers, which constrains the number of children who can be treated [111].

5 Recommendations and Conclusions

5.1 Overarching Challenges

Several overarching issues exist that can be addressed to support the effective delivery and implementation of nutrition interventions in humanitarian settings. Available funds are not sufficient to meet the needs of vulnerable populations, and often political and financial commitment to address undernutrition in these contexts is lacking. Today, approximately 30% of the required funding has been received, presenting an alarming situation for those in need [126]. Food crises and famines are increasingly viewed as economic and political failures as food access, instead of food availability, is the main driver.

Additionally, several cross-cutting challenges to implementation must be acknowledged and understood. This includes a lack of resources, including financial resources, human resources, products, and medications [78, 99, 100, 104, 111, 114, 127–130]. In addition, there are often issues of program accessibility in humanitarian situations that are due to physical barriers, movement restrictions, inadequate roadwork, dangers due to conflict, and the high cost of travel [78, 99, 100, 104, 127–129]. As the delivery of nutrition interventions in crisis settings often involves multiple organizations working together, poor coordination has been cited as a challenge as well [78, 104, 131]. Despite the difficulty in gathering information in emergency situations, it is important to effectively monitor and evaluate nutrition programming to inform future endeavors, as a dearth of this information poses challenges to intervention implementation [78, 104, 111, 114]. Finally, high opportunity costs for recipients and caregivers have been identified as barriers to the uptake and success of some nutrition interventions [111, 114].

5.2 Recommendations and Conclusions

Recommendations to improve the nutrition situation in conflict-affected areas include the expansion of geographic coverage, access, and equitable distribution of nutrition interventions. Tailoring interventions to meet the unique social contexts in areas experiencing conflict, as well as intervention sustainability, food safety, and recipient security, is also recommended in conflict situations [122]. Advance emergency planning can serve to prevent stockouts and supply issues in crisis settings. In addition, a holistic approach to public health, including community engagement and community preventive activities, could accelerate the uptake of nutrition interventions in humanitarian settings [2].

Malnutrition in conflict and humanitarian settings is widespread and increasing amidst a global context of unabated conflicts, displacement, climate change, and extreme weather events. Not all populations are impacted equally; women, adolescent girls, and children bear the brunt of the malnutrition burden in these settings due to interrelated biological, social, and cultural factors. Many interventions have been developed and have evolved over the years to address malnutrition; however, implementation challenges and barriers have limited the potential impact of such efforts. Looking ahead, sustainable, coordinated, evidence-based, and data-driven actions can ensure malnutrition is effectively addressed across humanitarian settings.

References

1. UN Office for the Coordination of Humanitarian Affairs (OCHA). Global Humanitarian Overview; 2023 [Internet]. [cited 2023 Jul 22]. Available from: https://humanitarianaction.info/document/global-humanitarian-overview-2023.
2. Rodo M, Singh L, Russell N, Singh NS. A mixed methods study to assess the impact of COVID-19 on maternal, newborn, child health and nutrition in fragile and conflict-affected settings. Confl Health [Internet]. 2022;16(1):30. https://doi.org/10.1186/s13031-022-00465-x.
3. UNICEF. Leveraging nutrition and social protection programming to address malnutrition and poverty, including in fragile and humanitarian contexts [Internet]. New York; 2023 [cited 2023 Jul 9]. Available from: https://www.unicef.org/documents/leveraging-nutrition-and-social-protection-programming.
4. Food and Agricultural Organization (FAO), International Fund for Agricultural Development. The state of food security and nutrition in the world 2023 [Internet]; 2023 [cited 2023 Aug 20]. Available from: https://www.fao.org/3/cc3017en/online/state-food-security-and-nutrition-2023/global-nutrition-targets-trends.html.
5. Development Initiatives. Global humanitarian assistance report 2023 [Internet]; 2023. Available from: https://devinit.org/resources/global-humanitarian-assistance-report-2023.
6. United Nations Human Rights Office of the High Commissioner. OHCHR and protecting human rights in humanitarian crises [Internet]; 2023 [cited 2023 Jul 22]. Available from: https://www.ohchr.org/en/humanitarian-crises.
7. Office for the Coordination of Humanitarian Affairs (OCHA). Glossary of Humanitarian Terms in relation to the Protection of Civilians in Armed Conflict [Internet]; 2003 [cited 2023 Jul 22]. Available from: https://inee.org/sites/default/files/resources/OCHA_2003_Glossary_of_Humanitarian_Terms_in_relation_to_the_Protection_of_Civilians_in_Armed_Conflict.pdf.

8. United Nations Population Fund (UNFPA). World Population Dashboard Somalia [Internet]; 2023 [cited 2023 Aug 22]. Available from: https://www.unfpa.org/data/world-population/SO.
9. United Nations Population Fund (UNFPA). World Population Dashboard Afghanistan [Internet]; 2023 [cited 2023 Aug 22]. Available from: https://www.unfpa.org/data/world-population/AF.
10. United Nations Population Fund (UNFPA). World Population Dashboard Congo, the Democratic Republic of the [Internet]; 2023 [cited 2023 Aug 22]. Available from: https://www.unfpa.org/data/world-population/CD.
11. United Nations Population Fund (UNFPA). World Population Dashboard Yemen [Internet]; 2023 [cited 2023 Aug 22]. Available from: https://www.unfpa.org/data/world-population/YE.
12. United Nations Population Fund (UNFPA). World Population Dashboard Syrian Arab Republic [Internet]; 2023 [cited 2023 Aug 22]. Available from: https://www.unfpa.org/data/world-population/SY.
13. United Nations Population Fund (UNFPA). World Population Dashboard South Sudan [Internet]; 2023 [cited 2023 Aug 22]. Available from: https://www.unfpa.org/data/world-population/SS.
14. United Nations Population Fund (UNFPA). World Population Dashboard Haiti [Internet]; 2023 [cited 2023 Aug 22]. Available from: https://www.unfpa.org/data/world-population/HT.
15. United Nations Population Fund (UNFPA). World Population Dashboard Myanmar [Internet]; 2023 [cited 2023 Aug 22]. Available from: https://www.unfpa.org/data/world-population/MM.
16. United Nations Population Fund (UNFPA). World Population Dashboard Ukraine [Internet]; 2023 [cited 2023 Aug 22]. Available from: https://www.unfpa.org/data/world-population/UA.
17. United Nations Population Fund (UNFPA). World Population Dashboard Libya [Internet]; 2023 [cited 2023 Aug 22]. Available from: https://www.unfpa.org/data/world-population/LY.
18. World Bank. Classification of Fragile and Conflict-Affected Situations [Internet]; 2023 [cited 2023 Aug 12]. Available from: https://www.worldbank.org/en/topic/fragilityconflictviolence/brief/harmonized-list-of-fragile-situations.
19. United Nations Refugee Agency (UNHCR). Refugee Data Finder [Internet]; 2023 [cited 2023 Aug 12]. Available from: https://www.unhcr.org/refugee-statistics/download/?url=Tv8X1a.
20. United Nations Development Programme. Gender Inequality Index [Internet]; 2021 [cited 2023 Aug 12]. Available from: https://hdr.undp.org/data-center/thematic-composite-indices/gender-inequality-index#/indicies/GII.
21. World Health Organization (WHO). Global Health Workforce statistics database [Internet]; 2020 [cited 2023 Aug 22]. Available from: https://www.who.int/data/gho/data/themes/topics/health-workforce.
22. World Health Organization (WHO). Antenatal care coverage - at least four visits (%) [Internet]; 2020 [cited 2023 Aug 22]. Available from: https://www.who.int/data/gho/data/indicators/indicator-details/GHO/antenatal-care-coverage-at-least-four-visits.
23. UNICEF. Afghanistan Multiple Indicator Cluster Survey (MICS) Summary Findings Report, 2022–2023 [Internet]; 2023 [cited 2023 Aug 27]. Available from: https://www.unicef.org/afghanistan/reports/afghanistan-multiple-indicator-cluster-survey-mics-2022-2023.
24. World Bank. Poverty headcount ratio at national poverty lines (% of population) [Internet]; 2022 [cited 2023 Aug 22]. Available from: https://data.worldbank.org/indicator/SI.POV.NAHC.
25. World Bank. Current health expenditure (% of GDP) [Internet]; 2021 [cited 2023 Aug 22]. Available from: https://data.worldbank.org/indicator/SH.XPD.CHEX.GD.ZS.
26. Centre for Research on the Epidemiology of Disasters. EM-DAT The International Disaster Database [Internet]; 2023 [cited 2023 Aug 22]. Available from: https://www.emdat.be/.
27. World Bank. Prevalence of severe food insecurity in the population (%) [Internet]; 2020 [cited 2023 Aug 22]. Available from: https://data.worldbank.org/indicator/SN.ITK.SVFI.ZS.
28. Food Security Information Network (FSIN). Global Report on Food Crises 2023 [Internet]; 2023 [cited 2023 Aug 20]. Available from: www.fsinplatform.org/sites/default/files/resources/files/GRFC2023-hi-res.pdf.

29. World Bank. Prevalence of wasting, weight for height (% of children under 5) [Internet]; 2022 [cited 2023 Aug 27]. Available from: https://data.worldbank.org/indicator/SH.STA.WAST.ZS.
30. World Bank. Prevalence of stunting, height for age (% of children under 5) [Internet]; 2022 [cited 2023 Aug 22]. Available from: https://data.worldbank.org/indicator/SH.STA.STNT.ZS.
31. World Bank. Prevalence of anemia among pregnant women (%) [Internet]; 2019 [cited 2023 Aug 22]. Available from: https://data.worldbank.org/indicator/SH.PRG.ANEM.
32. World Health Organization (WHO). Early initiation of breastfeeding (%) [Internet]; 2023 [cited 2023 Aug 22]. Available from: https://www.who.int/data/gho/data/indicators/indicator-details/GHO/early-initiation-of-breastfeeding-(-).
33. World Health Organization (WHO). Infants exclusively breastfed for the first six months of life (%) [Internet]; 2023 [cited 2023 Aug 22]. Available from: https://www.who.int/data/gho/data/indicators/indicator-details/GHO/infants-exclusively-breastfed-for-the-first-six-months-of-life-(-).
34. World Health Organization. Maternal mortality [Internet]; 2023 [cited 2023 Aug 22]. Available from: https://data.unicef.org/topic/maternal-health/maternal-mortality/#data.
35. UNICEF. UNICEF Data Warehouse - Neonatal Mortality Rate [Internet]; 2021 [cited 2023 Aug 22]. Available from: https://data.unicef.org/resources/data_explorer/unicef_f/?ag=UNICEF&df=GLOBAL_DATAFLOW&ver=1.0&dq=.CME_TMM0+CME_PND+CME_MRM0..&startPeriod=2021&endPeriod=2022.
36. UNICEF. UNICEF Data Warehouse - Infant Mortality Rate [Internet]; 2021 [cited 2023 Aug 22]. Available from: https://data.unicef.org/resources/data_explorer/unicef_f/?ag=UNICEF&df=GLOBAL_DATAFLOW&ver=1.0&dq=.CME_TMY0+CME_MRY0+CME_MRY0T4+CME_TMY0T4+CME_TMY1T4+CME_MRY1T4..&startPeriod=2016&endPeriod=2022.
37. World Health Organization. Goal 3: Ensure healthy lives and promote well-being for all at all ages [Internet]; 2023 [cited 2023 Aug 27]. Available from: https://sdgs.un.org/goals/goal3.
38. Lelijveld N, Brennan E, Akwanyi B, Wrottesley VS, James TP. Nutrition of women and adolescent girls in humanitarian contexts: current state of play. [Internet]. Kidlington, Oxford; 2022 [cited 2023 Jun 8]. Available from: https://www.ennonline.net/attachments/4608/ENN_State-of-Play_Humanitarian-Womens-Nutrition_FINAL.pdf.
39. United Nations Children's Investment Fund (UNICEF). UNICEF Humanitarian Action for Children 2023 Overview [Internet]; 2023 [cited 2023 Aug 20]. Available from: www.unicef.org/media/131491/file/%20Humanitarian%20Action%20for%20Children%202023.pdf.
40. Black RE, Victora CG, Walker SP, Bhutta ZA, Christian P, de Onis M, et al. Maternal and child undernutrition and overweight in low-income and middle-income countries. Lancet. 2013;382(9890):427–51.
41. Shortland T, McGranahan M, Stewart D, Oyebode O, Shantikumar S, Proto W, et al. A systematic review of the burden of, access to services for and perceptions of patients with overweight and obesity, in humanitarian crisis settings. PLoS One. 2023;18(4):e0282823.
42. Agabiirwe CN, Dambach P, Methula TC, Phalkey RK. Impact of floods on undernutrition among children under five years of age in low- and middle-income countries: a systematic review. Environ Health [Internemt]. 2022;21(1):98. Available from: https://ehjournal.biomedcentral.com/articles/10.1186/s12940-022-00910-7
43. Nisbett N, Harris J, Backholer K, Baker P, Jernigan VBB, Friel S. Holding no-one back: The nutrition equity framework in theory and practice, vol. 32. Global Food Security. Elsevier B.V; 2022.
44. Save the Children. Stop the War on Children Let Children Live in Peace [Internet]; 2023 [cited 2024 Jan 10]. Available from: https://www.stopwaronchildren.org/.
45. World Health Organization. Malnutrition [Internet]; 2023 [cited 2023 Aug 12]. Available from: https://www.who.int/health-topics/malnutrition#tab=tab_1.
46. World Food Programme. WFP Global Operational Response Plan 2023 Update #7 [Internet]; 2023 [cited 2023 Aug 20]. Available from: https://executiveboard.wfp.org/document_download/WFP-0000146953.

47. United Nations Children's Fund (UNICEF). Severe Wasting An Overlooked Child Survival Emergency [Internet]; 2022 [cited 2023 Aug 20]. Available from: https://www.unicef.org/media/120346/file/Wasting%20child%20alert.pdf.
48. World Health Organization, United Nations Children's Fund (UNICEF), & International Bank for Reconstruction and Development/The World Bank. Levels and trends in child malnutrition: UNICEF/WHO/World Bank Group joint child malnutrition estimates: key findings of the 2023 edition; 2023.
49. Khara T, Dolan C, Shoham J. Stunting in protracted emergency contexts [Internet]; 2015 [cited 2023 Aug 22]. Available from: https://www.ennonline.net/stuntinginprotractedemergencycontextsennbriefingnote.
50. Emergency Nutrition Network. Time for a change: Can we prevent more children from becoming stunted in countries affected by crisis? A briefing note for policy-makers and programme implementers; 2019.
51. Khara T, Mwangome M, Ngari M, Dolan C. Children concurrently wasted and stunted: a meta-analysis of prevalence data of children 6–59 months from 84 countries. Matern Child Nutr. 2018;14(2)
52. United Nations Children's Fund (UNICEF). Undernourished and overlooked: a global nutrition crisis in adolescent girls and women [Internet]; 2023 [cited 2023 Aug 21]. Available from: https://www.unicef.org/media/136876/file/Full%20report%20(English).pdf.
53. Save the Children, Oxfam International. Dangerous Delay 2 The Cost of Inaction [Internet]; 2022 [cited 2023 Aug 21]. Available from: https://www.savethechildren.ca/wp-content/uploads/2022/05/Dangerous-Delay-2-the-Cost-of-Inaction_2022.pdf.
54. Corley AG. Linking armed conflict to malnutrition during pregnancy, breastfeeding, and childhood. Glob Food Sec [Internet]; 2021 [cited 2023 Aug 20];29:100531. https://doi.org/10.1016/j.gfs.2021.100531.
55. WHO. Anaemia [Internet]; 2023 [cited 2023 Aug 17]. Available from: https://www.who.int/health-topics/anaemia#tab=tab_1.
56. World Bank. Prevalence of anemia among non-pregnant women (% of women ages 15-49) [Internet]; 2019 [cited 2024 Jan 10]. Available from: https://data.worldbank.org/indicator/SH.ANM.NPRG.ZS.
57. Emergency Nutrition Network. The Current State of Evidence and Thinking on Wasting Prevention [Internet]; 2018 [cited 2023 Aug 20]. Available from: https://mqsunplus.path.org/wp-content/uploads/2020/06/MQSUN_State-of-Evidence-and-Thinking-on-Wasting_18Jun20_disseminated.pdf.
58. Vos R, Jackson J, James S, Sanchez M. 2020 Global food policy report: building inclusive food systems [Internet]; 2020. Available from: https://ebrary.ifpri.org/digital/collection/p15738coll2/id/133646.
59. International Food Policy Research Institute (IFPRI). Food security [Internet]. [cited 2023 Aug 20]. Available from: https://www.ifpri.org/topic/food-security.
60. Devakumar D, Birch M, Osrin D, Sondorp E, Wells JC. The intergenerational effects of war on the health of children. BMC Med [Internet]. 2014;12(1):57. Available from: http://bmcmedicine.biomedcentral.com/articles/10.1186/1741-7015-12-57
61. Kemmerling B, Schetter C, Wirkus L. Addressing food crises in violent conflicts. In: Science and innovations for food systems transformation. Cham: Springer; 2023. p. 217–28.
62. Sphere Association. The sphere handbook: humanitarian charter and minimum standards in humanitarian response, fourth edition [Internet]. Geneva, Switzerland; 2018 [cited 2023 Dec 17]. Available from: www.spherestandards.org/handbook.
63. Action Against Hunger. Health approach: The fundamentals of the health and nutrition alignment [Internet]; 2017 [cited 2023 Jun 4]. Available from: https://knowledgeagainsthunger.org/wp-content/uploads/2018/11/Health-Approach.pdf.
64. IRC. International Rescue Committee; 2022 [cited 2023 Jul 14]. Family Planning in Humanitarian Settings: the Right to Choose Matters Most in the Hardest of Times. Available from: https://reliefweb.int/report/world/family-planning-humanitarian-settings-right-choose-matters-most-hardest-times.

65. WHO. World Health Organization; 2022 [cited 2023 Jul 14]. WHO guide for integration of perinatal mental health in maternal and child health services. Available from: https://www.who.int/publications/i/item/9789240057142.
66. Inter-Agency Working Group on Reproductive Health in Crises. Collaborating for maternal mental wellbeing: technical brief on perinatal mental health in humanitarian settings [Internet]; 2023 [cited 2023 Jul 14]. Available from: https://iawg.net/resources/collaborating-for-maternal-mental-wellbeing.
67. World Food Programme. WFP; 2023 [cited 2023 Dec 26]. Food Security Cluster. Available from: https://www.wfp.org/food-security-cluster.
68. Global Nutrition Cluster. Nutrition Cluster; 2023 [cited 2023 Dec 26]. About Us. Available from: https://www.nutritioncluster.net/about-us-0.
69. WFP. World Food Programme; 2023 [cited 2023 Jul 4]. Who we are. Available from: https://www.wfp.org/who-we-are.
70. Food and Agriculture Organization. FAO; 2023 [cited 2023 Dec 26]. About FAO. Available from: https://www.fao.org/home/en/.
71. UNICEF. United Nations Children's Fund; 2023 [cited 2023 Jul 4]. What We Do. Available from: https://www.unicef.org/what-we-do.
72. UNHCR. UNHCR Global Public Health Strategy 2021–2025 [Internet]; 2021 [cited 2023 May 14]. Available from: https://www.unhcr.org/media/39417.
73. UNHCR. Global strategy for public health: a UNHCR strategy 2014-2018 public health – HIV and reproductive health – food security and nutrition – water, sanitation and hygiene (WASH) [Internet]; 2014. Available from: https://www.unhcr.org/media/global-strategy-public-health-unhcr-strategy-2014-2018-public-health-hiv-and-reproductive.
74. Kavle JA, Ahoya B, Kiige L, Mwando R, Olwenyi F, Straubinger S, et al. Baby-friendly community initiative—from national guidelines to implementation: a multisectoral platform for improving infant and young child feeding practices and integrated health services. Matern Child Nutr. 2019;15(S1)
75. World Vision. World Vision; 2012 [cited 2023 Jul 4]. Community Management of Acute Malnutrition (CMAM). Available from: https://www.wvi.org/nutrition/project-models/cmam.
76. Global Database on the Implementation of Nutrition Action (GINA). World Health Organization; 2012 [cited 2023 Jul 4]. Action - Community-based Management of Acute Malnutrition (CMAM) Programme in Niger - Prevention or treatment of moderate malnutrition - MAM child. Available from: https://extranet.who.int/nutrition/gina/en/node/17821.
77. Pradhan PMS, Dhital R, Subhani H. Nutrition interventions for children aged less than 5 years following natural disasters: a systematic review. BMJ Open. 2016;
78. Shah S, Padhani ZA, Als D, Munyuzangabo M, Gaffey MF, Ahmed W, et al. Delivering nutrition interventions to women and children in conflict settings: a systematic review. BMJ Glob Health [Internet]. 2021;6(4):e004897. Available from: https://gh.bmj.com/lookup/doi/10.1136/bmjgh-2020-004897
79. Mohmand N. UNHCR experiences of enabling continuity of acute malnutrition care in the East, Horn of Africa and Great Lakes region. Emergency Nutrition Network [Internet]; 2019 [cited 2023 Jul 9];(Field Exchange issue 60):101. Available from: www.ennonline.net/fex/60/unhcrexperiences.
80. UNHCR. UNHCR; 2020 [cited 2023 Jul 4]. Nutrition programme performance standards. Available from: https://emergency.unhcr.org/emergency-assistance/health-and-nutrition/nutrition/nutrition-programme-performance-standards.
81. FHI 360. Training Guide for Community-Based Management of Acute Malnutrition (CMAM) Module 6 [Internet]; 2008 [cited 2023 Dec 20]. Available from: https://www.fhi360.org/resource/training-guide-community-based-management-acute-malnutrition-cmam-pdf-english.
82. Schoonees A, Lombard MJ, Musekiwa A, Nel E, Volmink J. Ready-to-use therapeutic food (RUTF) for home-based nutritional rehabilitation of severe acute malnutrition in children from six months to five years of age. Cochrane Database Syst Rev. 2019;2019(5)
83. UNICEF. Small supplements for the prevention of malnutrition in early childhood: small quantity lipid-based nutrient supplements brief guidance note. New York; 2023.

84. UNICEF. Saving lives with RUTF (ready-to-use therapeutic food). UNICEF [Internet]; 2022 [cited 2023 Jul 9]. Available from: https://www.unicef.org/supply/stories/saving-lives-rutf-ready-use-therapeutic-food.
85. UNICEF USA Staff. What is ready-to-use therapeutic food? UNICEF [Internet]; 2023 [cited 2023 Jun 19]. Available from: https://www.unicefusa.org/stories/what-ready-use-therapeutic-food.
86. UNICEF Supply Division. Therapeutic Milk Market and Supply Update [Internet]; 2018 [cited 2023 Dec 19]. Available from: https://www.unicef.org/supply/media/521/file/therapeutic-milk-market-note-April-2018.pdf.
87. CARE International [Internet]; 2023 [cited 2023 Jun 19]. Emergency Toolkit: Food Distribution and Nutritional Support. Available from: https://www.careemergencytoolkit.org/core-sectors/1-food-security-and-livelihoods/3-what-to-do-response-options/3-2-types-of-activities/3-2-1-food-distribution-and-nutritional-support/..
88. Farr E, Finnegan L, Grace J, Truscott M. Dangerous Delay 2: The Cost of Inaction; 2022 [cited 2023 Jun 19]. Available from: https://www.oxfam.org/en/research/dangerous-delay-2-cost-inaction.
89. Harman L. The Role of Cash Transfers in Improving Child Outcomes: The importance of child-sensitivity and taking a "Cash Plus" approach. Save the Children UK [Internet]; 2018 [cited 2023 Jul 9]. Available from: https://resourcecentre.savethechildren.net/document/role-cash-transfers-improving-child-outcomes-importance-child-sensitivity-and-taking-cash/.
90. Elayah M, Gaber Q, Fenttiman M. From food to cash assistance: rethinking humanitarian aid in Yemen. J Int Humanit Action. 2022;7(1):11.
91. Doocy S, Tappis H, Lyles E. Are cash-based interventions a feasible approach for expanding humanitarian assistance in Syria? J Int Humanit Action. 2016;1(1):13.
92. World Food Programme. Regional drought response plan for the horn of Africa: 2023 [Internet]. Addis Ababa; 2023 [cited 2023 Jul 9]. Available from: https://www.wfp.org/publications/regional-drought-response-plan-horn-africa-2023.
93. Save the Children. Nutrition at Save the Children 2022 [Internet]; 2022 [cited 2023 May 10]. Available from: https://resourcecentre.savethechildren.net/pdf/Nutrition-at-Save-the-Children-2022.pdf/.
94. UNICEF. Humanitarian action global annual results report 2020 [Internet]. New York; 2021 [cited 2023 Jul 9]. Available from: https://www.unicef.org/reports/global-annual-results-2020-humanitarian-action.
95. WFP. World Food Programme; 2023 [cited 2023 Jul 4]. The World Food Programme Food Basket. Available from: https://www.wfp.org/wfp-food-basket.
96. WFP. Technical Specifications for the manufacture of: Super Cereal [Internet]. World Food Programme; 2013 [cited 2023 Jul 4]. Available from: https://documents.wfp.org/stellent/groups/public/documents/manual_guide_proced/wfp251114.pdf.
97. Kaul T, Husain S, Tyrell T, Gaarder M. Synthesis of impact evaluations of the World Food Programme's nutrition interventions in humanitarian settings in the Sahel [Internet]. Relief Web; 2018 [cited 2023 Jul 4]. (3ie Working Paper). Report No.: 31. Available from: https://www.3ieimpact.org/evidence-hub/publications/working-papers/synthesis-impact-evaluations-world-food-programmes.
98. Tranchant JP, Gelli A, Bliznashka L, Diallo AS, Sacko M, Assima A, et al. The impact of food assistance on food insecure populations during conflict: evidence from a quasi-experiment in Mali. World Dev. 2019;119:185–202.
99. Larson N, Alexander T, Slaughter-Acey JC, Berge J, Widome R, Neumark-Sztainer D. Barriers to accessing healthy food and food assistance during the COVID-19 pandemic and racial justice uprisings: a mixed-methods investigation of emerging adults' experiences. J Acad Nutr Diet. 2021;121(9):1679–94.
100. Anthem P. WFP and FAO sound the alarm as global food crisis tightens its grip on hunger hotspots. World Food Programme [Internet]. 2022 [cited 2023 Jul 3]. Available from: https://www.wfp.org/stories/wfp-and-fao-sound-alarm-global-food-crisis-tightens-its-grip-hunger-hotspots.

101. Emergency Nutrition Network. General Food Distribution Fact Sheet [Internet]; 2011 [cited 2023 Jul 4]. Available from: https://www.ennonline.net/attachments/2023/HTP-v2-module-11-fact-sheet.doc.
102. UNICEF. Middle East and North Africa Humanitarian Situation Report [Internet]; 2022 [cited 2023 May 11]. Available from: https://www.unicef.org/media/136961/file/MENA-Humanitarian-SitRep-(End-of-Year),-31-December-2022.pdf.
103. Save the Children [Internet]; 2023 [cited 2023 Jul 9]. Our emergency health and nutrition work. Available from: https://www.savethechildren.org/us/what-we-do/health/health-and-nutrition-emergencies.
104. Rabbani A, Padhani ZA, Siddiqui A, F, Das JK, Bhutta Z. Systematic review of infant and young child feeding practices in conflict areas: what the evidence advocates. BMJ Open. 2020;10(9):e036757.
105. UNICEF. Evaluation of the Infant and Young Child Feeding Programme: how has UNICEF reflected on and responded to the ongoing nutrition needs of infants and young child in Syria [Internet]. Damascus, Syria; 2022 [cited 2023 Jul 9]. Available from: https://www.unicef.org/syria/reports/evaluation-infant-and-young-child-feeding-programme.
106. Emergency Nutrition Network. Module 14: Micronutrient interventions [Internet]; 2011 [cited 2023 Dec 18]. Available from: https://www.ennonline.net/attachments/2054/HTP-v2-module-14-fact-sheet.pdf.
107. UNICEF. South Asia Regional Humanitarian Situation Report No.3 [Internet]; 2022 [cited 2023 May 11]. Available from: https://www.unicef.org/media/137396/file/ROSA-Humanitarian-Situation-Report-No.3-January-December-2022.pdf.
108. WFP. World Food Programme. [cited 2023 Jun 4]. Specialized nutritious food. Available from: https://www.wfp.org/specialized-nutritious-food.
109. Multiple micronutrient supplementation: an approach to improving the quality of nutrition care for mothers and preventing low birthweight [Internet]. UNICEF; 2022 [cited 2023 Jul 17]. Available from: https://www.unicef.org/media/123271/file.
110. UNHCR, UNICEF, WFP, WHO. Food and nutrition needs in emergencies [Internet]. Geneva, Switzerland; 2004 [cited 2023 Dec 18]. Available from: https://www.who.int/publications/i/item/food-and-nutrition-needs-in-emergencies.
111. Rogers E, Myatt M, Woodhead S, Guerrero S, Alvarez JL. Coverage of community-based management of severe acute malnutrition programmes in twenty-one countries, 2012–2013. PLoS One. 2015;10(6):e0128666.
112. Anopheles and Nutrition working group of Technical Assistants of DG ECHO. Community-based Management of Acute Malnutrition (CMAM) [Internet]. Europa; 2011 Nov [cited 2023 Jul 4]. (Nutrition Working Group Technical Paper). Report No.: 1. Available from: https://ec.europa.eu/echo/files/policies/sectoral/TIP%20CMAM.pdf.
113. Bhutta ZA, Das JK, Rizvi A, Gaffey MF, Walker N, Horton S, et al. Evidence-based interventions for improvement of maternal and child nutrition: what can be done and at what cost? Lancet. 2013;382(9890):452–77.
114. UNICEF. Evaluation of Community Management of Acute Malnutrition (CMAM): global synthesis report. New York; 2013.
115. World Vision International. Project Model: Community-Based Management of Acute Malnutrition (CMAM) [Internet]; 2017 [cited 2023 Jul 17]. Available from: https://www.wvi.org/sites/default/files/Community_Based_Management_of_Acute_Malnutrition_Project_Model%20%281%29.pdf.
116. UNICEF. Treatment of wasting using simplified approaches: a rapid evidence review [Internet]; 2020 [cited 2024 Jan 15]. Available from: https://www.unicef.org/documents/rapid-review-treatment-wasting-using-simplified-approaches.
117. Doocy S, King S, Ismail S, Leidman E, Stobaugh H. A prospective comparison of standard and modified acute malnutrition treatment protocols during COVID-19 in South Sudan. Nutrients. 2023;15(23):4853.

118. Lenters LM, Wazny K, Webb P, Ahmed T, Bhutta ZA. Treatment of severe and moderate acute malnutrition in low- and middle-income settings: a systematic review, meta-analysis and Delphi process. BMC Public Health. 2013;13(S3):S23.
119. Puett C, Guerrero S. Barriers to access for severe acute malnutrition treatment services in Pakistan and Ethiopia: a comparative qualitative analysis. Public Health Nutr. 2015;18(10):1873–82.
120. Van Pelt S, Newton S, Twiss C. Ready-to-use therapeutic food feasibility study final report [Internet]. Nigeria; 2015 [cited 2023 Jul 17]. Available from: https://resourcecentre.savethechildren.net/pdf/ready-to-use_therapeutic_food_feasibility_study_nigeria_2015-1.pdf/.
121. UNHCR, WFP. Guidelines for selective feeding: The management of malnutrition in emergencies [Internet]. Geneva; 2011 [cited 2023 Jul 9]. Available from: https://www.unhcr.org/media/guidelines-selective-feeding-management-malnutrition-emergencies.
122. Carroll GJ, Lama SD, Martinez-Brockman JL, Pérez-Escamilla R. Evaluation of nutrition interventions in children in conflict zones: a narrative review. Adv Nutr. 2017;8(5):770–9.
123. MSF. Medecins Sans Frontieres; 2000 [cited 2023 Jun 18]. MSF therapeutic feeding programmes. Available from: https://www.msf.org/msf-therapeutic-feeding-programmes.
124. UNHCR. Bangladesh refugee emergency factsheet - nutrition [Internet]. UNHCR; 2019 [cited 2023 Jun 19]. Available from: https://reliefweb.int/report/bangladesh/bangladesh-refugee-emergency-factsheet-nutrition-april-2019.
125. WHO. WHO in Yemen: Nutrition. World Health Organization Regional Office for the Eastern Mediterranean [Internet]; 2022 [cited 2023 Jun 19]. Available from: https://www.emro.who.int/yemen/priority-areas/therapeutic-feeding-centres.html.
126. UNOCHA. Global humanitarian overview 2023, October update (snapshot as of 31 October 2023) [Internet]. Geneva, Switzerland; 2023 [cited 2024 Jan 15]. Available from: https://www.unocha.org/publications/report/world/global-humanitarian-overview-2023-october-update-snapshot-31-october-2023.
127. Freccero J, Taylor A, Ortega J, Buda Z, Awah PK, Blackwell A, et al. Safer cash in conflict: exploring protection risks and barriers in cash programming for internally displaced persons in Cameroon and Afghanistan. Int Rev Red Cross. 2019;101(911):685–713.
128. Sibson VL, Grijalva-Eternod CS, Noura G, Lewis J, Kladstrup K, Haghparast-Bidgoli H, et al. Findings from a cluster randomised trial of unconditional cash transfers in Niger. Matern Child Nutr. 2018;14(4):e12615.
129. Mangasaryan N, Arabi M, Schultink W. Revisiting the concept of growth monitoring and its possible role in community-based nutrition programs. Food Nutr Bull. 2011;32(1):42–53.
130. Noznesky EA, Ramakrishnan U, Martorell R. A situation analysis of public health interventions, barriers, and opportunities for improving maternal nutrition in Bihar, India. Food Nutr Bull. 2012;33(2_suppl1):S93–103.
131. Als D, Meteke S, Stefopulos M, Gaffey MF, Kamali M, Munyuzangabo M, et al. Delivering water, sanitation and hygiene interventions to women and children in conflict settings: a systematic review. BMJ Glob Health. 2020;5(Suppl 1):e002064.

Climate Change and Nutrition

Amira M. Khan and Zulfiqar A. Bhutta

1 Introduction

Climate change is a driver and at the same time an outcome of the food system. Nutrition is an outcome of the food system, and dietary patterns determine the food-production systems. Climate mitigation and adaptation measures, in turn, impact nutrition outcomes. [1]

Termed the "greatest health threat facing humanity" [2], climate change is a global threat that transcends borders. The term climate change refers to long-term shifts in temperatures and weather patterns [3]. The Oxford Dictionary defines it as "a change in global or regional climate patterns, in particular, a change apparent from the mid to late 20th century onwards and attributed largely to the increased levels of atmospheric carbon dioxide produced by the use of fossil fuels" [4]. Research estimates that nearly 80% of the earth's area, where 85% of the global population resides, is impacted by climate change effects [5].

Climate change, health, and nutrition are inextricably linked. An estimated five million extra deaths a year are attributable to non-optimal temperatures [6]. In addition to other climate change-related factors, global warming, disruption of habitat, and human displacement can exacerbate food insecurity and the transmission of pathogenic diseases among humans [7]. Scientists and advocacy groups are striving to limit the rise in global temperature to no more than 1.5 °C, with the adverse impact on human health and nutrition estimated to be considerably greater if the

A. M. Khan
Centre for Global Child Health, Hospital for Sick Children, Toronto, ON, Canada
e-mail: amira.khan@sickkids.ca

Z. A. Bhutta (✉)
Centre for Global Child Health, Hospital for Sick Children, Toronto, ON, Canada

Centre of Excellence in Women and Child Health, Aga Khan University, Karachi, Pakistan
e-mail: zulfiqar.bhutta@sickkids.ca

temperature increase is 2 °C. Projections estimate that the global undernourished would increase to 530–550 million at a 1.5 °C increase compared to 540–590 million at 2 °C [8].

The Sustainable Development Goal (SDG) 2 to "end hunger, achieve food security and improved nutrition, and promote sustainable agriculture" and SDG 13 to "take urgent action to combat climate change and its impacts" are much more closely related than was predicted and planned for [9]. While achieving one could positively impact the other, the reverse is also possible, with increasing food production leading to a potential increase in carbon emissions. Given the many linkages, the 2015 Global Nutrition Report highlighted the urgent need for the climate change and nutrition communities to collaborate effectively in a manner that is advantageous for both climate adaptation and the nutritional well-being of the global population [10]. Notably, countries already burdened with poverty, conflict, and an agriculture-dependent economy are at the highest risk of climate change's impact on population nutrition.

2   Climate Change and the Unequal Impact in Low- and Middle-Income Countries

The world's poorest countries are located in the tropics and are, thus, also the warmest (Fig. 1) [11]. Given their location and weaker economies, the impact of climate change on daily lives is excessive while the adaptive capacity is the lowest. These

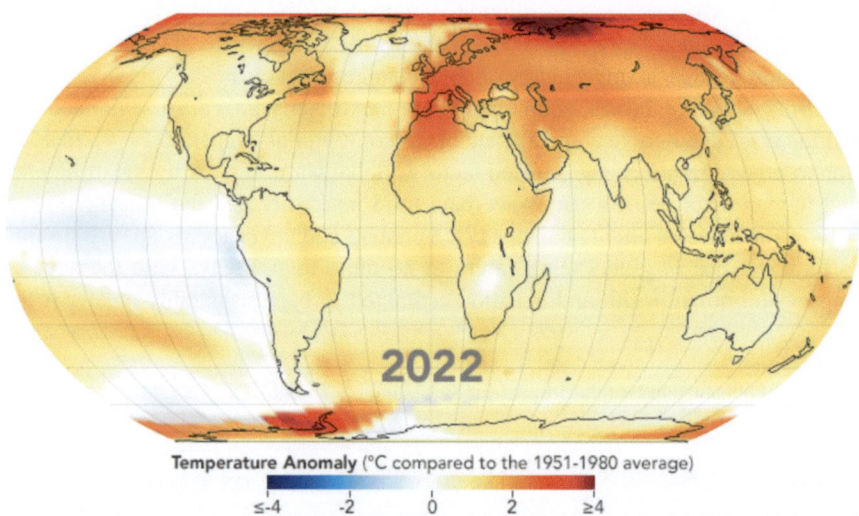

Fig. 1 Heat map showing temperature anomaly for the year 2022, compared to the 1951–1980 average. (Reproduced from NASA Earth Observatory. World of Change: Global temperatures [Internet]. Available from: https://earthobservatory.nasa.gov/world-of-change/global-temperatures)

low- and middle-income countries (LMICs) already struggle with low agricultural productivity and food shortages, while being disproportionately affected by climate-related effects and environmental changes. Despite the least contributions to global emissions, LMICs and tropical countries bear the greatest brunt of climate change.

It is, thus, not surprising that the gross domestic product (GDP) per capita of LMICs is adversely affected by climate change. Recent evidence indicates that owing to global warming the world's economy lost between 5 trillion and 29 trillion US dollars from 1992 to 2013; while low-income tropical nations saw an average reduction of 6.7% in their GDP, owing to heat waves, high-income countries only faced an average 1.5% decrease (Fig. 2).

Nearly two-thirds of the total population of low- and lower-middle-income countries live in rural areas. Close to 70% of the global rural population lives in low or lower-middle-income countries, making up nearly two-thirds of the total population in those settings [12]. The livelihoods of these communities depend on agricultural yield which is greatly disrupted by extreme weather events, such as droughts and floods, leading to lower incomes and worsening food insecurity. Such extreme weather events are also capable of disaster and devastation leading to injuries and death. In turn, these environmental and social conditions have the potential to cause conflict and massive displacements, both of which also affect health and nutrition

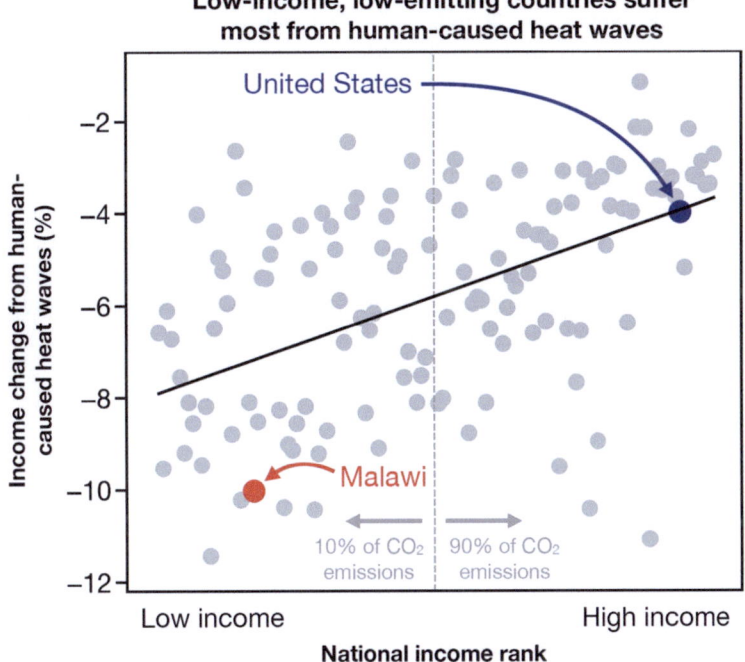

Fig. 2 Unequal burden of climate change. (Reproduced from Callahan CW, Mankin JS. Globally unequal effect of extreme heat on economic growth. Science Advances [Internet]. 2022 Oct 28;8(43). Available from: https://doi.org/10.1126/sciadv.add3726)

adversely. With rising temperatures, increased population movement, and urbanization, vector-borne and waterborne diseases such as dengue, malaria, and cholera are on the rise. A recent literature review concluded that 58% of all known infectious diseases (218/375) can be aggravated by climate hazards linked to rising greenhouse gas emissions [7].

Notably, hazardous air quality and pollution increase the risk of ischemic heart disease, lung cancer, chronic respiratory conditions, neurological disorders, and strokes. It is estimated that in 2020, nearly 4.2 million deaths globally were attributable to ambient particulate matter, of which approximately 35% of deaths were associated with the combustion of fossil fuels [13]. Additionally, in low-resource settings, the use of solid fuels for household cooking contributed to nearly 3.8 million deaths in 2016 [14].

2.1 Climate Change and Disproportionate Impact on Vulnerable Populations Within LMICs

Even within these countries, climate change is not experienced equally by all. Women remain more vulnerable to climate change owing to multiple social, economic, and cultural factors. Women often have less access to education and economic opportunities and bear the burden of household cooking and water supply while also contributing substantially to the agricultural workforce. In sub-Saharan Africa, 66% of all employed women work in agrifood systems [15]. However, the women and children in these communities face structural hindrances that curtail their access to adaptive resources, technologies, and social support, rendering them more vulnerable to climate change [16]. In fact, health constraints, childcare responsibilities, and sociocultural barriers often prevent these women from moving or seeking shelter when extreme weather events hit. The devastating floods in Pakistan left one million homes destroyed and at least 650,000 pregnant women without access to healthcare and safe delivery spaces [17]. Women caught in natural disasters or exposed to extreme heat are more likely to experience adverse pregnancy outcomes [18]. As well, during droughts or food insecure situations, women, especially adolescent girls, are more likely to go hungry than men [19, 20]. Evidence indicates that intimate partner violence, rape, and human trafficking incidents increase during such disasters [21, 22].

Nearly 90% of the world's 1.2 billion adolescents live in LMICs [23]. This generation of adolescents is facing unprecedented challenges at an extremely vulnerable period of their lives. The combined crises of climate change, conflict, and rising cost of living have exposed this young generation to extraordinary adversities. In addition to the direct impact of climate change on their health and nutrition, many school-age children and adolescents are faced with food insecurity and poverty leading to forced migration or the need to support their families by earning an income [24]. Importantly, many adolescents drop out of school as a consequence of climate-related infrastructure destruction or economic losses [25, 26].

3 Climate Change and the Impact on Nutrition

The consequences of rising greenhouse gas emissions and climate change, including rising temperatures, unpredictable rainfall patterns, and an increase in extreme weather events, influence food availability, food systems, care environments, and overall population health, and consequently impact the nutritional status of the population. The 2015 Global Nutrition Report presented a conceptual framework outlining the linkages between the climate crisis and nutrition and highlighted potential adaption and mitigation strategies (Fig. 3). Although simply presented for clarity, the interrelationships between climate change and nutrition are multi-directional and complex [10]. These linkages will be discussed considering the various pathways climate change and nutrition intersect, including the food environment, the social and living environment and the health environment.

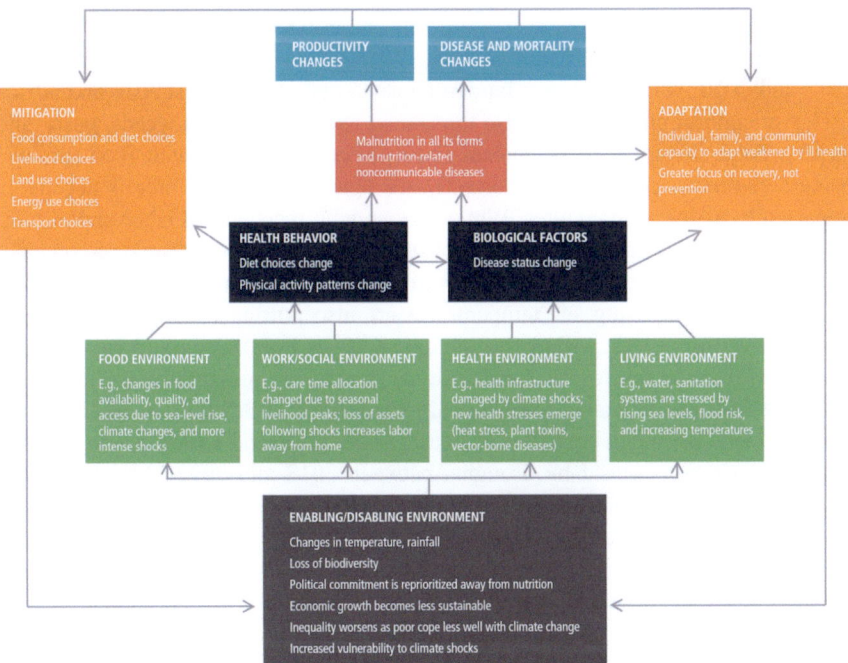

Fig. 3 Conceptual links between climate change and nutrition. (Reproduced with permission from the International Food Policy Research Institute (IFPRI) www.ifpri.org. The original figure is available online at https://doi.org/10.2499/9780896298835)

3.1 Food Environment

The discussion around the impact of climate change on the food environment will focus on agricultural production, crop quality, livestock, and aquatic food sources, all of which are critical for the global nutrition supply.

Weather and atmospheric changes including temperature increase, variable rainfall, frequent extreme weather events, and rise in atmospheric carbon dioxide levels adversely affect crop yield, increase pests and pathogens, and postharvest losses. It is estimated that the adverse impact of climate change on crop yield by 2100 will be approximately between −20% and −45% for maize, −20% and −30% for rice, −5% and −50% for wheat, and between −30 and −60% for soybean [27, 28]. Notably, rising carbon dioxide levels not only impact crop yield but also the nutritional quality of food crops. Experiments have shown that elevated atmospheric carbon dioxide levels can cause a 7–15% reduction in protein content in rice, wheat, barley, and potatoes. It can also lead to a 3–11% decrease in zinc and iron content of cereals and grains, and a 5–10% decrease in potassium and calcium, along with even greater reductions at higher levels [29, 30]. A simulation modeling study estimated that with increasing carbon dioxide concentration, decreasing zinc and iron levels in crops could cause an additional 125.8 million disability-adjusted life years (DALYs) globally between 2015 and 2050, with the largest burden concentrated in Southeast Asia and Africa [31]. Agricultural production is also threatened by an increase in weeds, pests, and insects. Food storage is more challenging in extreme weather, with food spoilage being a common occurrence. Importantly, the agricultural labor force is negatively impacted by rising temperatures. While regions with mechanized labor and/or temperate climates may be less affected, tropical, low-resource settings are more severely impacted, especially when adaptive measures are costly and not readily available.

Heat stress and rising sea temperatures are also putting livestock and aquatic food production at risk. Vulnerable regions such as South Asia and sub-Saharan Africa, with underdeveloped water systems, have seen massive losses in animal numbers owing to repeated droughts [32]. A staggering 3.5 million head of livestock and wild animals were lost in pastoral regions of Ethiopia, Kenya, and Somalia due to devastation caused by droughts between 2018 and 2022 [33]. Also, with declining marine fish numbers and reduced fishery production, researchers estimate that nearly 1.4 billion people globally are at risk of multiple micronutrient deficiencies as fish make up nearly 20% of their food intake [30]. Most of the at-risk populations are those in low-latitude LMICs where communities are dependent on wild fish and adaptive strategies and mitigation measures are scarce [34].

Importantly, the detrimental impact on and reduction in food production, seasonality, and the cost of mitigation strategies drive up food prices. Models estimate that by 2050, rice, wheat, and maize will cost an additional 31–106% more owing to climate change, depending on mitigation measures, population growth, and the increase in income [35]. An increase in food prices will predispose to food insecurity, especially for the poorest populations. A recent analysis of 1.25 million preschool children from 44 LMICs showed that a 5% increase in the price of food increased the risk of wasting and severe wasting by 9% and 14%, respectively [36].

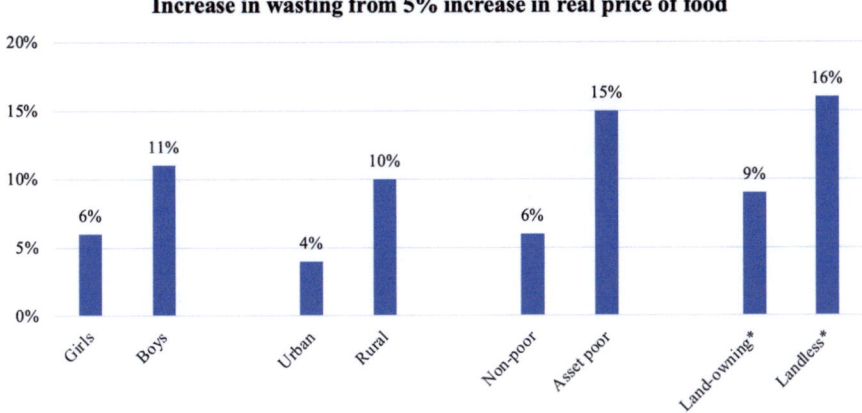

Fig. 4 Predicted impact of food inflation on wasting risk, by gender, location, poverty status, and land ownership. (Reproduced from Headey D, Ruel M. IFPRI Blog: Research Post The global food price crisis threatens to cause a global nutrition crisis: New evidence from 1.27 million young children on the effects of inflation [Internet]. International Food Policy Research Institute. 2022. Available from: https://www.ifpri.org/blog/global-food-price-crisis-threatens-cause-global-nutrition-crisis-new-evidence-127-million). Published under the terms of the Creative Commons Attribution (CC BY 4.0) license https://creativecommons.org/licenses/by/4.0/deed.en

It showed that the risk was higher for male children, rural residents, and those from asset-poor, landless households (Fig. 4). They also found that food price increase was associated with a reduction in dietary diversity [36].

Thus, as illustrated in Fig. 5, the food environment involves multiple linkages between climate, land, food production, storage, transportation, and consumption, i.e., "farm to table," which are all being affected by increasing carbon dioxide in the environment and changing weather patterns. These in turn impact the nutrition and health outcomes of the population.

It is critical to recognize that while climate change impacts food systems, in turn, food production and what populations eat also impact the climate. As per estimates, the production of food has led to 70% and 50% loss of biodiversity on land and in freshwater, respectively. Importantly, nearly 30% of all greenhouse gas emissions are secondary to food systems [37].

3.2 Social and Living Environment

Households and communities, globally, are affected directly and indirectly by climate shocks. With rising food insecurity, threatened livelihoods, infrastructure destruction, climate-related displacement, conflict, and insufficient water resources, people around the world are facing heightened levels of social and economic stress secondary to climate change.

A staggering 345 million people around the world faced food insecurity in 2023, an alarming increase from the pre-pandemic number of 200 million [38, 39].

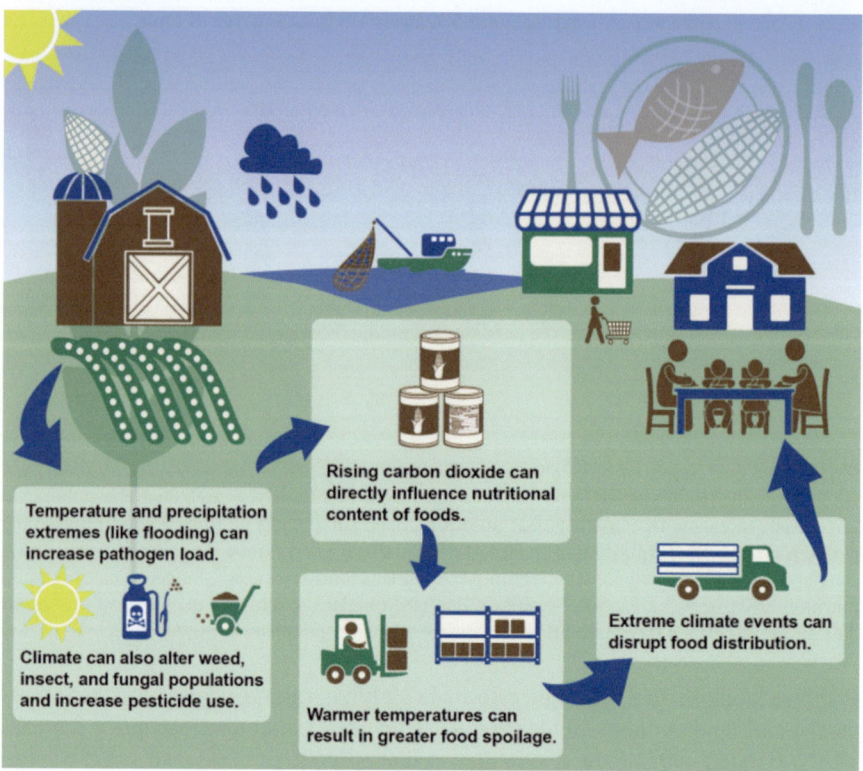

Fig. 5 Farm to table: the potential interactions of climate change with food production, food safety, and nutrition. (Reproduced from U.S. Federal Government. Food- and Water-Related Threats. U.S. Climate Resilience Kit. https://health2016.globalchange.gov/low/ClimateHealth2016_07_Food_small.pdf)

Conflict, COVID-19, and the climate crisis have exacerbated the food and cost-of-living crisis. Extreme weather is estimated to be the primary driving factor of acute food insecurity for nearly 57 million people in 12 countries in 2023, nearly a 100% increase from 23.5 million in 2021 [38]. In such challenging environments, family dynamics and childcare practices can be impacted and compromised.

Climate change sequelae can lead to an increase in female workload, household disruption, and poor maternal physical and mental health, all of which can affect a mother's ability to care for her children (Fig. 6) [40]. Breastfeeding, optimal complementary feeding, and appropriate hygiene practices may be disrupted given the circumstances, thus impacting infant and child nutrition [41]. Moreover, in hot weather, caregivers may tend to give more formula milk and/or water, under the false impression that the infant needs extra fluids [42]. Diminished access to clean water and poor hygiene can heighten the risk of waterborne and foodborne diseases for the entire family. Furthermore, in such environments, women, an already vulnerable population, are at greater risk of nutritional deficits especially if pregnant or lactating [43, 44].

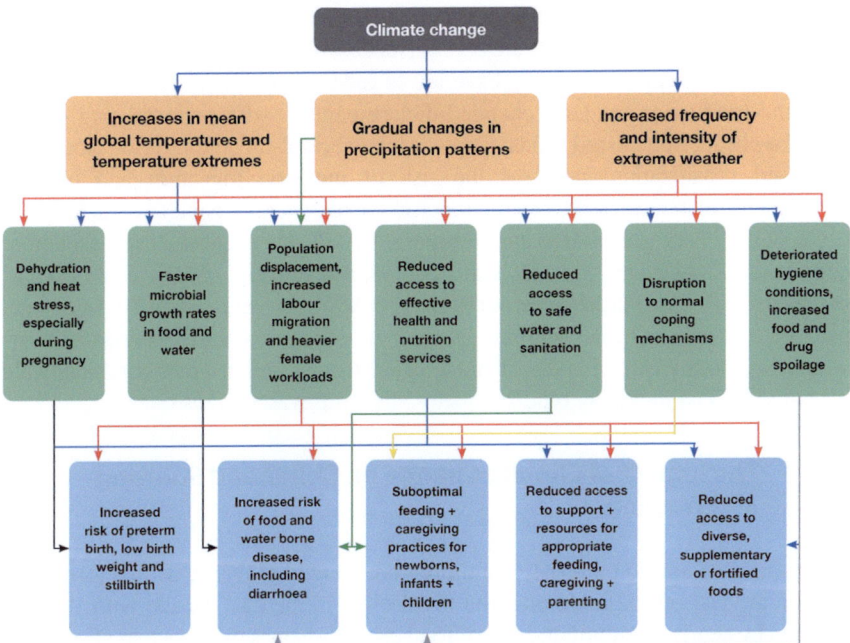

Fig. 6 Impacts of climate change on care and feeding practices, and resulting consequences for human health and nutrition. (Reproduced from Bush A, Wrottesley S, Mates E, Fenn B. Nutrition and Climate Change – Current State of Play: Scoping Review [Internet]. Emergency Nutrition Network; 2021. Available from: https://www.ennonline.net/nutritionandclimatechange)

3.3 Health Environment

Extreme weather events, in particular, floods, cyclones, droughts, and wildfires can impact people directly and/or by the destruction of health and communication infrastructures. Air pollution has also led to an increase in chronic respiratory conditions among other diseases, all of which can affect nutrition as well. Additionally, rising global temperatures and changing precipitation patterns have indirectly increased the transmission of many vector-borne, waterborne, and foodborne diseases.

Many waterborne diseases such as diarrhea and cholera can exacerbate undernutrition and heighten the risk of wasting [45]. Conversely, undernutrition can increase the risk of infection thus triggering a vicious cycle of morbidity and disease [28]. Research indicates that maternal health is also adversely affected by climate change, heat exposure, and pollution, which may lead to an increase in preterm birth and low birth weight incidence [46, 47]. Displaced populations are at greater risk of morbidity given reduced access to food and clean water and disrupted healthcare.

In terms of nutrition, the Lancet Obesity Commission recommends framing the three pandemics of climate change, obesity, and undernutrition together as the "Global Syndemic" [48]. The Commission affirmed that as the three pandemics had "common underlying societal drivers" [48], it would be effective and prudent to address these challenges in an integrated manner. While the linkages between climate change and undernutrition are certain, those with obesity are less obvious [49]. Increasing temperatures globally have led to reduced physical activity, and rising crop and produce prices have changed dietary patterns with an increasing preference for cheaper processed foods. Climate-related rural-urban migration leading to increased urbanization increases the risk of nutrition transition and obesity. Conversely, increased food production for an overweight population's growing needs will escalate greenhouse gas emissions. In fact, it is estimated that agriculture and livestock contribute 15–23% and 12–19%, respectively, of all greenhouse gas emissions [50, 51]. Furthermore, as more people prefer vehicles for transport, the use and cost of fossil fuels increase. As climate change increases the risk of overweight and obesity, it is also associated with a rise in diet-related non-communicable diseases (NCDs) including type 2 diabetes and cardiovascular diseases.

3.4 The Impact of Climate Change on Childhood Stunting and Wasting

More than 148 million under-five children are stunted globally, while close to 45 million are wasted [52]. Although on the decline in the past decade with stunting reduced by nearly one-third, the global food crisis threatens this progress. The world is not on track to meet the global target of reducing under-five stunting numbers to 89 million by 2030 and is predicted to miss it by 40 million children, 80% of whom are in Africa. Climate change, poverty, and conflict are some of the drivers of this slow progress in LMICs. In fact, models estimate that between 2000 and 2050, there will be an additional 25.2 million malnourished children globally owing to climate change [53, 54]. Notably, the adverse impact of climate change on childhood growth remains more in rural vs. urban settings and in regions with low incomes and high food prices [55]. Importantly, erratic rainfall patterns, droughts, and flooding have been associated with food insecurity, reduced dietary diversity, and hunger leading to childhood underweight and wasting [53, 56, 57].

4 Strategies and Policies

Most strategies, policies, and mitigation measures center solely on climate, and collaboration is limited between climate and nutrition initiatives. However, there is a notable increase in the consultations, evidence-building, and collaboration interlinking the two.

4.1 Governance and Leadership

Historically, it was the declaration at the first Earth Summit in Stockholm, Sweden in 1972 that drew attention to the matter of climate change [58]. In the two decades that followed, the global community gradually turned its focus toward climate, and in 1992, the United Nations Framework Convention on Climate Change was adopted and signed by 158 states. Following that, the Kyoto Protocol, the Paris Agreement, and the annual COP summit have worked toward stabilizing greenhouse gas emissions, reducing the rise in global average temperatures, addressing drivers of climate change, and facilitating mitigation measures.

While integrated action is limited, there are a growing number of forums leading efforts regarding climate change and its impact on nutrition. These are summarized in Table 1.

Table 1 Governance and leadership initiatives for climate change and nutrition

Forum	Notable activities
Initiative on nutrition and climate change (I-CAN)	Multisectoral, multi-stakeholder global flagship program launched COP27 in Egypt in 2022 Partners include WHO, FAO, GAIN, SUN, and UN-nutrition secretariat To accelerate progress on both climate change and nutrition issues and provide support to all member states for integrated action The focus of the initiative is on implementation and action; capacity building, data and knowledge transfer; policy and strategy; and investments
UNFCCC/conference of parties (COP)	Owing to active advocacy efforts, the COP27 emphasized on nutrition and food systems transformation COP27 was the first to host a food systems pavilion, a special adaptation and agriculture thematic day, and the launch of the I-CAN
World Health Organization (WHO)	Core partner in I-CAN WHO UNFCCC health and climate change country profile project: Monitoring of health sector response to climate change, in collaboration with national governments. Initiatives include global surveys, country profiles, and a dynamic dashboard Developed technical series on adapting to climate-sensitive health impacts: Undernutrition: Guidelines on how to conduct a vulnerability and adaptation assessment The WHO climate and WHO nutrition teams are actively involved in COP summits and the food systems summit
Food and agriculture organization (FAO)	Hosts the Office of Climate Change, biodiversity and environment (OCB) focusing on food and agricultural sustainability Produced key strategy and technical documents including the FAO Strategy on Climate Change 2022–2031 and Climate Change and Food Security: Risks and Responses Key partner for COP, I-CAN, and the UNFCCC
Scaling up nutrition (SUN)	Attended the COP25 in 2019 and brought forward the nutrition agenda at the climate change forum for the first time Core partners of the I-CAN
Global Alliance for improved nutrition (GAIN)	Core partner of I-CAN Partnered with the worldwide Fund for Nature (WWF) to stop the degradation of the natural environment and to develop "nature-positive" food systems

Adapted from: Bush A, Wrottesley S, Mates E, Fenn B. Nutrition and Climate Change—Current State of Play: Scoping Review [Internet]. Emergency Nutrition Network; 2022. Available from: www.ennonline.net/nutritionandclimatechange; Haddad L. Why Are WWF and GAIN Teaming up on food? [Internet]. GAIN. 2021 [cited 2023 Oct 29]. Available from: https://www.gainhealth.org/media/news/why-are-wwf-and-gain-teaming-food; Lina M. Initiative on Climate Action and Nutrition (I-CAN) - Member States Briefing [Internet]. World Health Organization; 2023. Available from: https://apps.who.int/gb/MSPI/pdf_files/2023/09/Item4_28-09.pdf

4.2 Sustainable Food Systems

Adaptive and resilient agrifood systems are an urgent requirement to combat climate change and provide healthier, accessible diets for all. In each of the food systems categories, such as food supply chains, the food environment, consumer behavior, and dietary choices, it is possible to identify double- or triple-duty actions that serve multiple purposes, potentially multiplying their impact on climate change and nutritional outcomes of the food system. The food system includes production, processing, transport, and consumption and is impacted notably by climate, governance, and economics.

At government and international levels, policies that should be prioritized to facilitate climate change adaptation of food producers toward sustainable and resilient food systems include those to support food producers, especially small-scale producers, promote collaboration and collective efforts, and enable prediction, prevention, and control of climate-related risks [27]. There needs to be an investment in climate risk and impact assessment tools such as the Modelling System for Agricultural Impacts of Climate Change (MOSAICC) developed by FAO—an integrated set of models that helps to assess the impact of climate change on agriculture [59]. Additionally, investments are needed in environmental monitoring systems, vulnerability assessment tools, and early warning systems. Such early warning systems not only forecast and warn against weather events but also pests and diseases such as the FAO's Desert Locust Information System (DLIS), which monitors and warns countries globally of the locust threat [60].

Adaptive measures at the farm level include introducing new, resilient crop varieties that can endure climatic shocks such as heat shocks and droughts [61]. Altering the use of fertilizers, modifying irrigation timings, and changing the timing or location of cropping are strategies that are effective. Water management strategies are key including conserving soil moisture or transporting water better in areas with less rainfall or preventing water logging and nutrient leaching in areas with greater rainfall. Experts also recommend the use of effective pest and weed management solutions [61].

A risk-minimizing and climate-secure intervention is to adopt integrated agricultural systems where rather than focusing on only one kind of farming activity, farmers focus on combinations such as crops and livestock raising or livestock and forestry, and so on. An example is from Brazil, where INOCAS (Innovative Oil and Carbon Solutions) has integrated palm tree plantations with livestock pastures, where the trees improve the soil and provide vegetable oil while providing shade and a healthier land for the livestock [62]. Biofortification, i.e., breeding of staple crop varieties richer in micronutrients and agronomic fortification where fertilizers or irrigation water are enriched with minerals such as zinc, iodine, or selenium are strategies recommended for LMICs to enhance the nutritional value of the crops and improve human nutrition and growth outcomes [63]. Such strategies have been successfully used in several high-income countries such as China and Finland. Protection from extreme temperatures (indoor systems or trees), water management, changing species/breeds, and disease control are key measures that can be taken for climate change adaptation for livestock.

Table 2 Social protection for mitigating climate change impacts

Social protection strategy	Potential impact	Challenges
Conditional and unconditional cash transfer In-kind transfers Agricultural subsidies Commercial disaster insurance schemes Unemployment insurance Employment programs Public works approach Incentivizing technological and infrastructural adaptation Training and education on adaptive measures	Reduce income poverty and increase capacity to cope Maintain income in conditions of climactic shock Improve access to food Support sustainable food systems transformation Enhance women's empowerment and their ability to care for children and households Help increase "ecological resilience" and reduce environmental degradation Increases social inclusion of often marginalized populations facing inequitable impacts of climate change Employment for those impacted by climate change mitigation measures	Effective targeting Lower coverage in rural areas Feasibility in slow-onset events Limited anticipatory action based on forecasting Alignment required with disaster risk management, agriculture, and climate change policies

Adapted from: Climate change and food security: risks and responses. FAO, and Can social protection tackle emerging risks from climate change, and how? A framework and a critical review Cecilia Costella. 2023. Climate Risk Management.

Technological advances including solar energy to provide temperature-controlled storage facilities or digital connections for farmers to access knowledge and climatic forecasting information can help mitigate climatic stress [64]. Mutual learning between farmers, sharing of best practices and lessons learned, and participation in risk monitoring systems are imperative for building agricultural resilience [27].

Enhancing resilience at the household level is especially important for agriculture-dependent livelihoods which are widespread in LMICs. As per FAO, 45% of the labor force in LMICs, including paid and unpaid workers, are employed in agriculture. Predictably, this group would be most affected by the impact of climate change on agricultural systems and would thus require assistance and adaptation to prevent food insecurity and hunger. A key strategy governments employ is social protection, a policy instrument to assist households and individuals in mitigating risks associated with income and food insecurity. A summary of social protection interventions, their potential impact in mitigating climate change impact, and associated challenges are summarized in Table 2.

Gender-equitable strategies are critical in the context of climate change, whether it is for social protection or reducing household vulnerabilities. Recognition of gender-specific impacts of climate change and gender roles in earning livelihoods, agricultural activities, household decision-making, and purchasing is imperative in designing gender-sensitive adaptations [27].

Altering consumer behavior and diets, leading to changes in food production practices could potentially reduce greenhouse gas emissions in 2050 by almost

10%, and adopting plant-based diets could reduce them by up to 80% as per the EAT-Lancet Commission [65]. Consuming plant-based diets and cutting back on meat intake contributes to the reduction of methane emissions from livestock. Much of the production and consumption of greenhouse gas-intensive foods takes place in high-income countries with beef production leading in emissions, primarily secondary to livestock methane production and land conversion. At an individual and household level, eating more plant-based diets and reducing food waste could play a critical role in reducing greenhouse gas emissions.

5 Intervention Success Stories

Below are some climate mitigation stories from around the world that have successfully helped communities adapt to climate-induced stress and sustain livelihoods and food security.

5.1 Climate-Adaptive Agriculture in Zimbabwe

Zimbabwe's economy relies largely on rain-fed agricultural systems, which are increasingly being impacted by erratic rainfall patterns, frequent dry spells, and rising temperatures. Mitigation strategies are central to maintaining food systems and preventing food insecurity [66]. At the ground level, smallholder farmers are seeing the benefits of climate adaptation measures that have been taken as part of the "Building Climate Resilience of Vulnerable Agricultural Livelihoods in Southern Zimbabwe Project." Notably, farmers have been provided with improved, more resilient varieties of cereal crops including sorghum and pearl millet and seed inputs, which have led to an increase in crop yields and a greater variety of food production. Importantly, the project has also implemented practical, hands-on "Farmer Field School" approaches, where government extension officers teach farmers about climate-resilient measures including small grain production, appropriate land preparation and planting, and water and soil conservation [66]. A farmer from Chipenge district, who adopted early land preparation and planting, summed up the project impact well, "This is why my crop is thriving despite the erratic rains" [66].

5.2 Social Protection in Bangladesh

Bangladesh is at high risk for climate-related hazards, especially floods, cyclones, landslides, and erosions. Datinkhali, a small village in Satkhira District of southwest Bangladesh faces frequent, extreme climatic events including cyclones, floods, and river erosions, given its risky geographical location [67]. Such events have left the residents with no long-term assets, food insecurity, and financial uncertainty. To improve the climate resilience of the community, World Vision introduced the

Samabay Samiti, a cooperative fund committee, formed of eight groups, each with 20–25 female members. The group members add money to the fund weekly and the saved amount is used to provide microloans to those in need. Additionally, the members are trained in the diversification of livelihoods and in starting new businesses. The success of the initiative has led to the expansion of the fund and the involvement of Building Resources Across Communities (BRAC), a global pioneer in microcredit [67].

5.3 Sustainable Ecosystem in Nicaragua

Climate variability, shrimp fisheries, urban waste, deforestation, increased use of pesticides, and mining threaten the tropical mangrove estuary located in northern Nicaragua [68]. Loss of mangrove forests and poor watershed management have also threatened fisheries and biodiversity in the area. The FAO-led ecosystem approach to fisheries and aquaculture (EAFA) is supporting and training fish farmers to farm successfully while sustaining the ecosystem and enhancing community climate resilience [68]. The intervention based on strategies, including a robust aquatic environment monitoring system, capacity building of small-scale fishermen to adopt additional livelihood opportunities so as to discourage negative fishing practices, and improved communication and collaboration between fisheries and institutions, has been successful in supporting livelihoods of these fishermen and promoting a sustainable environment.

6 Conclusion

Climate change and nutrition are fundamentally linked and impacted by one another. Globally, the adverse impacts of the climate crisis are felt most by the least resilient countries. Political commitment and multi-sectoral partnerships are critical for the successful implementation of climate-adaptive strategies, such as resilient agricultural systems, altered diets, and social protection schemes, that can ultimately combat climate change and improve population health and nutrition.

References

1. Bakker S, Macheka L, Eunice L, Koopmanschap E, Bosch D, Hennemann I, et al. Food-system interventions with climate change and nutrition co-benefits: a literature review [Internet]; 2021. https://doi.org/10.18174/547743
2. World Health Organization: WHO. Climate change [Internet]; 2023. Available from: https://www.who.int/news-room/fact-sheets/detail/climate-change-and-health
3. United Nations. What is climate change? | United Nations [Internet]. United Nations. Available from: https://www.un.org/en/climatechange/what-is-climate-change
4. The Oxford English Dictionary | Oxford Languages [Internet]; 2024. Available from: https://languages.oup.com/research/oxford-english-dictionary/

5. Callaghan M, Schleußner CF, Nath S, Lejeune Q, Knutson TR, Reichstein M, et al. Machine-learning-based evidence and attribution mapping of 100,000 climate impact studies. Nat Clim Change [Internet]. 2021;11(11):966–72. https://doi.org/10.1038/s41558-021-01168-6.
6. Zhao Q, Guo Y, Ye T, Gasparrini A, Tong S, Overcenco A, et al. Global, regional, and national burden of mortality associated with non-optimal ambient temperatures from 2000 to 2019: a three-stage modelling study. Lancet Planet Health [Internet]. 2021;5(7):e415–25. https://doi.org/10.1016/s2542-5196(21)00081-4.
7. Mora C, McKenzie T, Gaw IM, Dean JM, Von Hammerstein H, Knudson TA, et al. Over half of known human pathogenic diseases can be aggravated by climate change. Nat Clim Change [Internet]. 2022;12(9):869–75. https://doi.org/10.1038/s41558-022-01426-1.
8. World Health Organization. The 1.5 Health Report – Synthesis on Health & Climate Science In the IPCC SR1.5 [Internet]. WHO. World Health Organization; 2016. Available from: https://apo.who.int/publications/i/item/the-1.5-health-report
9. Overcoming the world's challenges – the global goals [Internet]. The Global Goals; 2024. Available from: https://www.globalgoals.org/
10. International Food Policy Research Institute. Global nutrition report 2015: actions and accountability to advance nutrition and sustainable development. Washington, DC; 2015. https://doi.org/10.2499/9780896298835.
11. Why tropical countries are underdeveloped – summary of working paper 8119 [Internet]. National Bureau of Economic Research National Bureau of Economic Research; 2001. Available from: https://www.nber.org/digest/jun01/why-tropical-countries-are-underdeveloped
12. United Nations Department of Economic and Social Affairs. World social report 2021 – reconsidering rural development [Internet]. United Nations; 2021. Available from: https://www.un-ilibrary.org/content/books/9789216040628
13. Romanello M, Di Napoli C, Drummond P, Green C, Kennard H, Lampard P, et al. The 2022 report of the Lancet Countdown on health and climate change: health at the mercy of fossil fuels. Lancet [Internet]. 2022;400(10363):1619–54. https://doi.org/10.1016/s0140-6736(22)01540-9.
14. World Health Organization. Data/GHO/indicators household air pollution attributable death rate (per 100 000 population) [Internet]. World Health Organization; 2024. Available from: https://www.who.int/data/gho/data/indicators/indicator-details/GHO/household-air-pollution-attributable-death-rate-(per-100-000-population)
15. Food and Agriculture Organization. The status of women in agrifood systems. In: FAO eBooks [Internet]; 2023. https://doi.org/10.4060/cc5343en.
16. United Nations. Eradicating rural poverty to implement the 2030 agenda for sustainable development – report of the secretary-general [Internet]. United Nations: United Nations Digital Library; 2020. Available from: https://digitallibrary.un.org/record/3879212?ln=en&v=pdf
17. Women and girls bearing the brunt of the Pakistan Monsoon floods [Internet]. UNFPA Pakistan; 2022. Available from: https://pakistan.unfpa.org/en/news/women-and-girls-bearing-brunt-pakistan-monsoon-floods
18. Ha S. The changing climate and pregnancy health. Curr Environ Health Rep [Internet]. 2022;9(2):263–75. https://doi.org/10.1007/s40572-022-00345-9.
19. Keshavarz M, Karami E, Vanclay F. The social experience of drought in rural Iran. Land Use Policy [Internet]. 2013;30(1):120–9. https://doi.org/10.1016/j.landusepol.2012.03.003.
20. Oxfam, United Nations Vietnam. Responding to climate change in Viet Nam: opportunities for improving gender equality. United Nations Vietnam and Oxfam; 2009.
21. Epstein A, Bendavid E, Nash D, Charlebois ED, Weiser SD. Drought and intimate partner violence towards women in 19 countries in sub-Saharan Africa during 2011–2018: a population-based study. PLOS Med [Internet]. 2020;17(3):e1003064. https://doi.org/10.1371/journal.pmed.1003064.
22. Sanz-Barbero B, Linares C, Vives-Cases C, González JL, López-Ossorio JJ, Díaz J. Heat wave and the risk of intimate partner violence. Sci Total Environ [Internet]. 2018;644:413–9. https://doi.org/10.1016/j.scitotenv.2018.06.368.

23. Shinde S, Harling G, Assefa N, Bärnighausen T, Bukenya J, Chukwu A, et al. Counting adolescents in: the development of an adolescent health indicator framework for population-based settings. EClinicalMedicine [Internet]. 2023;61:102067. https://doi.org/10.1016/j.eclinm.2023.102067.
24. McGushin A, Gasparri G, Graef V, Ngendahayo C, Timilsina S, Bustreo F, et al. Adolescent wellbeing and climate crisis: adolescents are responding, what about health professionals? BMJ [Internet]. 2022:e071690. https://doi.org/10.1136/bmj-2022-071690.
25. Nauges C, Strand J. Water hauling and girls' school attendance: some new evidence from Ghana. Environ Resour Econ [Internet]. 2015;66(1):65–88. https://doi.org/10.1007/s10640-015-9938-5.
26. Save the Children. Born into the climate crisis: why we must act now to secure children's rights [Internet]. Save the Children; 2021. Available from: https://www.savethechildren.net/news/climate-crisis-%E2%80%93-children-face-life-far-more-heatwaves-floods-droughts-and-wildfires
27. Food and Agriculture Organization of the United Nations. Climate change and food security: risks and responses [Internet]. FAO. Food and Agriculture Organization; 2015. Available from: https://www.fao.org/3/i5188e/I5188E.pdf
28. Agostoni C, Baglioni M, La Vecchia A, Molari G, Berti C. Interlinkages between climate change and food systems: the impact on child malnutrition—narrative review. Nutrients [Internet]. 2023;15(2):416. https://doi.org/10.3390/nu15020416.
29. Myers SS, Zanobetti A, Kloog I, Huybers P, Leakey ADB, Bloom AJ, et al. Increasing CO2 threatens human nutrition. Nature [Internet]. 2014;510(7503):139–42. https://doi.org/10.1038/nature13179.
30. Loladze I. Hidden shift of the ionome of plants exposed to elevated CO2 depletes minerals at the base of human nutrition. eLife [Internet]. 2014;3:e02245. https://doi.org/10.7554/elife.02245.
31. Weyant C, Brandeau ML, Burke M, Lobell DB, Bendavid E, Basu S. Anticipated burden and mitigation of carbon-dioxide-induced nutritional deficiencies and related diseases: a simulation modeling study. PLOS Med [Internet]. 2018;15(7):e1002586. https://doi.org/10.1371/journal.pmed.1002586.
32. Porter JR, Xie L, Challinor AJ, Cochrane K, Howden SM, Iqbal MM, et al. Food security and food production systems. In: Field CB, Barros VR, Dokken DJ, Mach KJ, Mastrandrea MD, editors. Climate change 2014: impacts, adaptation, and vulnerability part a: global and sectoral aspects contribution of working group II to the fifth assessment report of the intergovernmental panel on climate change. Cambridge, UK\New York, NY: Cambridge University Press; 2014.
33. Kariuki T, Omumbo JA, Ciugu K, Marincola E. The interconnected global emergencies of climate change, food security and health: a call to action by the Science for Africa Foundation. Open Res Africa [Internet]. 2023;6:1. https://doi.org/10.12688/openresafrica.13566.1.
34. Golden CD, Allison EH, Cheung WWL, Dey MM, Halpern BS, McCauley DJ, et al. Nutrition: fall in fish catch threatens human health. Nature [Internet]. 2016;534(7607):317–20. https://doi.org/10.1038/534317a.
35. Nelson GC, Rosegrant MW, Palazzo A, Gray I, Ingersoll C, Robertson RD, et al. Food security, farming, and climate change to 2050: scenarios, results, policy options. RePEc: Research Papers in Economics [Internet]; 2010. Available from: https://econpapers.repec.org/RePEc:fpr:resrep:geraldnelson
36. Headey D, Ruel MT. Food inflation and child undernutrition in low and middle income countries. Nat Commun [Internet]. 2023;14(1):5761. https://doi.org/10.1038/s41467-023-41543-9.
37. World Wide Fund for Nature. Food for thriving biodiversity [Internet]. WWF. Available from: https://wwf.panda.org/discover/our_focus/food_practice/food_for_thriving_biodiversity/
38. Food Security Information Network. Global report on food crises (GRFC) 2023 [Internet]. Food Security Information Network, Global Network against Food Crises; 2025. Available from: https://www.wfp.org/publications/global-report-food-crises-2023

39. A global food crisis | World Food Programme [Internet]. Available from: https://www.wfp.org/global-hunger-crisis
40. Bush A, Wrottesley S, Mates E, Fenn B. Nutrition and climate change – current state of play: scoping review [Internet]. Emergency Nutrition Network; 2022. Available from: https://www.ennonline.net/nutritionandclimatechange
41. Hirani SAA, Richter S, Salami B. Humanitarian aid and breastfeeding practices of displaced mothers: a qualitative study in disaster relief camps. Eastern Mediterr Health J [Internet]. 2021;27(12):1197–202. https://doi.org/10.26719/emhj.20.087.
42. Edney JM, Kovats S, Filippi V, Nakstad B. A systematic review of hot weather impacts on infant feeding practices in low-and middle-income countries. Front Pediatr [Internet]. 2022;10 https://doi.org/10.3389/fped.2022.930348.
43. Blakstad MM, Smith ER. Climate change worsens global inequity in maternal nutrition. Lancet Planet Health [Internet]. 2020;4(12):e547–8. https://doi.org/10.1016/s2542-5196(20)30246-1.
44. GGCA. Gender and climate change: a closer look at existing evidence. Global Gender and Climate Alliance; 2016.
45. Al-Jawaldeh A, Nabhani M, Taktouk M, Nasreddine L. Climate change and nutrition: implications for the Eastern Mediterranean region. Int J Environ Res Public Health [Internet]. 2022;19(24):17086. https://doi.org/10.3390/ijerph192417086.
46. Kuehn L, McCormick S. Heat exposure and maternal health in the face of climate change. Int J Environ Res Public Health [Internet]. 2017;14(8):853. https://doi.org/10.3390/ijerph14080853.
47. Bekkar B, Pacheco SE, Basu R, DeNicola N. Association of air pollution and heat exposure with preterm birth, low birth weight, and stillbirth in the US. JAMA Network Open [Internet]. 2020;3(6):e208243. https://doi.org/10.1001/jamanetworkopen.2020.8243.
48. Swinburn B, Kraak V, Allender S, Atkins V, Baker P, Bogard JR, et al. The global Syndemic of obesity, undernutrition, and climate change: the lancet commission report. Lancet [Internet]. 2019;393(10173):791–846. https://doi.org/10.1016/s0140-6736(18)32822-8.
49. An R, Ji M, Zhang S. Global warming and obesity: a systematic review. Obesit Rev [Internet]. 2017;19(2):150–63. https://doi.org/10.1111/obr.12624.
50. Reisinger A, Clark H. How much do direct livestock emissions actually contribute to global warming? Global Change Biol [Internet]. 2017;24(4):1749–61. https://doi.org/10.1111/gcb.13975.
51. Vermeulen SJ, Campbell BM, Ingram J. Climate change and food systems. Ann Rev Environ Resour [Internet]. 2012;37(1):195–222. https://doi.org/10.1146/annurev-environ-020411-130608.
52. UNICEF/WHO/World Bank Group. Levels and trends in child malnutrition child malnutrition: UNICEF/WHO/World Bank Group joint child malnutrition estimates: key findings of the 2023 Edition [Internet]. WHO. World Health Organization; 2022. Available from: https://www.who.int/publications/i/item/9789240073791
53. Phalkey R, Aranda-Jan CB, Marx S, Höfle B, Sauerborn R. Systematic review of current efforts to quantify the impacts of climate change on undernutrition. Proc Natl Acad Sci USA [Internet]. 2015;112(33) https://doi.org/10.1073/pnas.1409769112.
54. Nelson GC, Rosegrant MW, Koo J, Robertson RD, Sulser TB, Zhu T, et al. Climate change: impact on agriculture and costs of adaptation [Internet]; 2009. https://doi.org/10.2499/089629535.
55. Lloyd SJ, Bangalore M, Chalabi Z, Kovats S, Hallegatte S, Rozenberg J, et al. A global-level model of the potential impacts of climate change on child stunting via income and food price in 2030. Environ Health Perspect [Internet]. 2018;126(9):97007. https://doi.org/10.1289/ehp2916.
56. Rodriguez-Llanes JM, Ranjan-Dash S, Degomme O, Mukhopadhyay A, Guha-Sapir D. Child malnutrition and recurrent flooding in rural eastern India: a community-based survey. BMJ Open [Internet]. 2011;1(2):e000109. https://doi.org/10.1136/bmjopen-2011-000109.
57. Niles MT, Emery BF, Wiltshire S, Brown ME, Fisher B, Ricketts TH. Climate impacts associated with reduced diet diversity in children across nineteen countries. Environ Res Lett [Internet]. 2021;16(1):015010. https://doi.org/10.1088/1748-9326/abd0ab.

58. United Nations. From Stockholm to Kyoto: a brief history of climate change | United Nations [Internet]. United Nations. Available from: https://www.un.org/en/chronicle/article/stockholm-kyoto-brief-history-climate-change
59. Food and Agriculture Organization of the United Nations. The modelling system for agricultural impacts of climate change (MOSAICC) Tool and the Enhanced Transparency Framework (ETF) [Internet]. FAO; 2021. Available from: https://www.fao.org/documents/card/en/c/CB4295EN
60. Food and Agriculture Organization of the United Nations. FAO Desert Information Locust Service (DLIS) helps countries to control locusts [Internet]. FAO; 2014. Available from: https://www.fao.org/3/i4353e/i4353e.pdf
61. Howden M, Soussana J, Tubiello FN, Chhetri N, Dunlop M, Meinke H. Adapting agriculture to climate change. Proc Natl Acad Sci USA [Internet]. 2007;104(50):19691–6. https://doi.org/10.1073/pnas.0701890104.
62. Calmon M. 4 Ways Farmers can adapt to climate change and generate income [Internet]. World Resources Institute. Available from: https://www.wri.org/insights/4-ways-farmers-can-adapt-climate-change-and-generate-income
63. Morton CM, Pullabhotla H, Bevis L, Lobell DB. Soil micronutrients linked to human health in India. Sci Rep [Internet]. 2023;13(1):13591. https://doi.org/10.1038/s41598-023-39084-8.
64. Institute IFPRI. Global food policy report: climate change and food systems [Internet]; 2022. https://doi.org/10.2499/9780896294257.
65. EAT Forum. Summary report of the EAT-lancet commission – healthy diets from sustainable food systems [Internet]. EAT Forum; 2019. Available from: https://eatforum.org/eat-lancet-commission/eat-lancet-commission-summary-report/
66. UNDP. Climate-smart for the future: How smallholder farmers in Zimbabwe are reaping bumper crops by adapting to a changing climate [Internet]; 2023. Available from: https://undp-climate.exposure.co/zimbabwe-smallholder-farmers-adapt
67. Mondal V. From debt cycle to self-resilience: a story from the small village of Datinakhal. Global Resilience Partnership [Internet]. Available from: https://www.globalresiliencepartnership.org/from-debt-cycle-to-self-resilience-a-story-from-the-small-village-of-datinakhali/
68. Food and Agriculture Organization of the United Nations. FAO success stories on climate smart agriculture [Internet]. FAO; 2014. Available from: https://www.fao.org/documents/card/en?details=504ba808-e8cd-4246-8992-e844c1223210

Role of Technologies in Nutritional Advances Along the RMNCAH Continuum of Care

Samra Naz, Asma Zulfiqar, and Ammarah Kanwal

1 Introduction

Nutrition is a cornerstone of Reproductive, Maternal, Newborn, Child, and Adolescent Health (RMNCAH) care, playing a vital role in ensuring the well-being of individuals throughout various life stages. Adequate nutrition is essential for reproductive health, supporting both men's and women's ability to conceive and maintain optimal reproductive capacity. For women, proper nutrition during pregnancy is critical to meet the increased nutritional needs of the developing fetus, reducing the risk of complications such as anemia, gestational diabetes, and preterm delivery. Newborn health is profoundly influenced by nutrition, with breastfeeding providing essential nutrients and antibodies that bolster the immune system and protect against infections. During early childhood, a balanced diet is crucial for growth, cognitive development, and immune function, preventing long-term adverse health consequences such as stunted growth and impaired development. Adolescents, experiencing rapid growth and development, require specific nutritional support to ensure healthy bone development, timely sexual maturation, and reduced risk of chronic diseases. Effective nutrition monitoring is necessary to detect and prevent deficiencies, assess intervention effectiveness, and manage nutrition-related

---

S. Naz (✉)
Australian Institute for Machine Learning, University of Adelaide, Adelaide, SA, Australia
e-mail: samra.naz@adelaide.edu.au

A. Zulfiqar
School of Social and Political Science University of Melbourne/Institute for Social Science Research, University of Queensland, St Lucia, QLD, Australia

A. Kanwal
Pakistan Council of Scientific and Industrial Research Laboratories (PCSIR),
Ministry of Science and Technology, Islamabad, Pakistan

© The Author(s), under exclusive license to Springer Nature Switzerland AG 2025
Z. S. Lassi, R. A. Salam (eds.), *Nutrition Across Reproductive, Maternal, Neonatal, Child, and Adolescent Health Care*,
https://doi.org/10.1007/978-3-031-95721-5_21

complications. By integrating innovative technologies and approaches, healthcare providers can enhance nutrition assessment and monitoring, ultimately improving health outcomes and fostering a healthier future generation. This chapter explores the potential of innovative technologies to optimize nutritional support and health outcomes.

2   Innovations in Nutrition Assessment and Monitoring

Emerging technologies are reshaping the landscape of nutrition assessment, particularly in the domains of nutritional biomarkers and metabolomics. Metabolomics, which involves the comprehensive analysis of metabolites in biological samples, is providing a holistic view of an individual's metabolic profile. Advanced techniques like mass spectrometry and nuclear magnetic resonance spectroscopy are identifying and quantifying metabolites associated with nutrition, offering valuable insights into nutrient intake, metabolism, and metabolic dysregulation. Wearable devices have become increasingly popular for tracking dietary requirements and monitoring nutritional habits [1]. These devices employ a combination of sensors, data analysis algorithms, and user-friendly interfaces to provide real-time insights into an individual's food consumption and dietary choices. One of their primary functions is food tracking and logging, where users can easily record their meals using features like barcode scanning, voice recognition, or image recognition [2]. This data is then processed to offer valuable information such as calorie intake, macronutrient distribution, and other nutritional parameters. Additionally, wearable devices excel at calorie counting by calculating the calorie content of consumed foods and comparing it to estimated energy expenditure, often factoring in individual characteristics like age, gender, weight, and physical activity level [3]. Nutrient tracking is another key feature, allowing users to monitor essential nutrients like vitamins and minerals, as well as macronutrients such as carbohydrates, proteins, and fats [4, 5]. IoT (Internet of Things) sensors and devices are used to monitor the nutrient content of food. These devices can quickly analyze the nutritional composition of meals, providing real-time feedback to healthcare providers and mothers. This technology is particularly useful in addressing malnutrition in children. An example is NutriPhone, a handheld device that can analyze the nutrient content of breast milk to ensure it meets the needs of preterm infants [6]. Personalized nutrient targets and alerts for exceeding or falling short of daily requirements can be integrated into these devices. Moreover, some wearables support meal timing and frequency tracking, helping users establish regular eating patterns with reminders for meals and snacks [7, 8]. They also offer hydration tracking features, encouraging users to maintain proper fluid intake through customized reminders. Users can analyze their dietary patterns over time, utilizing charts, graphs, and reports to gain insights into their nutrition habits. Many wearable devices can seamlessly integrate with health and fitness apps and devices, providing a comprehensive overview of an individual's overall well-being by incorporating data on physical activity and energy expenditure [9]. Additionally, social and community support features enable users to connect with others who share similar dietary goals, fostering motivation, accountability, and a sense of community. These devices prioritize personalization, tailoring recommendations and feedback based on individual characteristics, preferences, and objectives. Wearable devices offer continuous monitoring of dietary habits, empowering users to maintain awareness of their food choices throughout the day and make real-time adjustments to their diet as needed. These devices are valuable tools for enhancing dietary awareness and promoting healthier eating habits, ultimately contributing to improved overall health and well-being. This data can be used in RMNCAH programs to assess the overall health and activity levels of pregnant women and provide personalized dietary recommendations. For example, Fitbit and Garmin devices have been used in research studies to monitor physical activity and calorie expenditure in pregnant women [10, 11].

In the context of body composition analysis, cutting-edge remote sensing and imaging technologies are making significant strides. Prominent among these technologies are dual-energy X-ray absorptiometry (DXA) and bioelectrical impedance analysis (BIA), both of which are non-invasive methods with the capability to deliver highly accurate measurements of various body components, including fat mass, lean mass, and bone density [12]. These measurements are pivotal for assessing an individual's nutritional status and are particularly invaluable in clinical and research environments where precision and reliability are paramount. DXA is an advanced imaging technique that employs low-dose X-rays to differentiate and quantify different body tissues [13]. It can discern not only the total body fat and lean mass but also provide regional insights, allowing for a comprehensive assessment of body composition. Additionally, DXA excels in bone density measurement, making it an essential tool for evaluating skeletal health, especially in conditions such as osteoporosis. Researchers and healthcare professionals rely on DXA to precisely monitor changes in body composition over time, making it indispensable for studies exploring the impact of nutrition, exercise, and medical treatments on an individual's physique. However, bioelectrical impedance analysis (BIA), on the other hand, uses a low-level electrical current to estimate body composition [14–16]. This painless and non-invasive technique relies on the principle that electrical conductivity differs between fat, muscle, and bone. BIA devices can be as simple as handheld devices or as sophisticated as multi-frequency analyzers. While BIA may not offer the same level of precision as DXA, it is a practical and widely accessible method for assessing body composition, making it suitable for routine clinical assessments and large-scale research studies. It is particularly useful in tracking changes in fat and lean mass, which are crucial indicators of nutritional health. In essence, remote sensing and imaging technologies like DXA and BIA represent a vital frontier in body composition analysis. They provide healthcare practitioners and researchers with the tools needed to obtain accurate and detailed information about an individual's fat distribution, muscle mass, and bone density, which in turn enables a comprehensive evaluation of nutritional status. These technologies are particularly valuable in clinical settings, where they can aid in the diagnosis and management of conditions related to body composition, such as obesity, malnutrition, and osteoporosis, and in research environments, where they contribute to a deeper understanding of the effects of nutrition and lifestyle on the human body.

Genomic and epigenomic approaches have emerged as powerful tools in elucidating the intricate genetic underpinnings that influence an individual's nutritional status [17]. Genomic studies delve into an individual's genetic makeup, examining their unique DNA sequences and variations that can impact how the body metabolizes nutrients [18, 19]. This genetic information holds vital clues about an individual's predisposition to nutritional deficiencies and susceptibility to nutrition-related diseases. For instance, certain genetic variants can affect the absorption, utilization, or metabolism of specific nutrients, making individuals prone to deficiencies. Understanding these genetic factors can provide a personalized roadmap for tailoring nutrition recommendations and interventions. Genomic and epigenomic approaches are at the forefront of unraveling the complex genetic factors that influence an individual's nutritional status. These advanced techniques offer profound insights into how an individual's genetic makeup and epigenetic modifications collectively shape their susceptibility to nutritional deficiencies and predisposition to nutrition-related diseases. Collectively, genomic and epigenomic approaches provide a holistic comprehension of an individual's genetic susceptibilities and epigenetic alterations, paving the way for personalized nutrition recommendations. This personalized approach tailors dietary guidance to an individual's unique genetic and epigenetic profile, offering the potential to optimize nutritional outcomes and reduce the risk of diet-related health issues. In essence, genomic and epigenomic approaches represent a transformative shift toward precision nutrition, where dietary interventions are fine-tuned to accommodate genetic predispositions and epigenetic modifications, thereby enhancing the efficacy of nutrition strategies and ultimately improving overall health outcomes. Table 1 summarizes the technologies used for nutritional monitoring:

Emerging technologies are at the forefront of revolutionizing nutrition assessment and dietary behavior monitoring. Nutritional biomarkers, metabolomics, wearable devices, and sensor technology collectively provide a comprehensive toolkit for personalized nutrition management. These innovations empower individuals to gain real-time insights into their dietary habits, metabolic profiles, and body composition, facilitating informed decision-making. Moreover, the integration of sensor data and privacy considerations underscore the need for collaborative efforts among researchers, users, and developers to ensure the seamless and secure use of these technologies. This transformative wave of precision and personalization in nutrition assessment not only holds the promise of improving individual health outcomes but also deepens our comprehension of the intricate interplay between food, metabolism, and overall well-being. As these technologies continue to advance, they have the potential to empower individuals to take charge of their nutrition, promoting healthier lifestyles and contributing to a brighter future for public health and wellness.

Table 1 Summary of devices and their functionality

Device/technology	Functionality
Mass spectrometry	Identifies and quantifies metabolites associated with nutrition, providing insights into nutrient intake, metabolism, and metabolic dysregulation
Nuclear magnetic resonance (NMR)	Analyzes metabolites in biological samples, offering a holistic view of an individual's metabolic profile
Wearable devices	Tracks dietary requirements and monitors nutritional habits using sensors and data analysis algorithms Functions include food tracking, calorie counting, nutrient tracking, meal timing, hydration tracking, and integration with health apps
Dual-energy X-ray absorptiometry (DXA)	Provides accurate measurements of body components, including fat mass, lean mass, and bone density. Used for assessing nutritional status and monitoring changes over time
Bioelectrical impedance analysis (BIA)	Estimates body composition using a low-level electrical current. Tracks changes in fat and lean mass, suitable for routine clinical assessments and large-scale research studies
Genomic approaches	Examines DNA sequences and variations to understand genetic factors influencing nutrient metabolism, predisposition to deficiencies, and nutrition-related diseases
Epigenomic approaches	Studies epigenetic modifications affecting gene expression related to nutrient absorption, utilization, and metabolism. Provides personalized nutrition recommendations

3   Innovations in Nutrition Data

The integration of electronic health records (EHRs) and nutrition data signifies a groundbreaking development in healthcare [20]. Digital technologies, including electronic medical records (EMRs) and EHRs, have become essential tools in modern healthcare, efficiently managing and monitoring patient health data [20, 21]. EHRs, the digital counterparts of traditional paper patient charts, provide a comprehensive overview of a patient's medical journey, enabling seamless data exchange among healthcare providers and organizations. By incorporating dietary supplement (DS) data, EHRs prove invaluable in identifying potential DS-drug interactions, thereby raising the standard of patient care. Registered dietitian/nutritionists (RDNs) are central figures in ensuring the accurate documentation of DS usage in various clinical settings, underscoring the pivotal role of EHRs in their workflow.

Some EHRs offer direct links between pharmacy systems and drug knowledge databases, significantly enhancing the monitoring of DS usage and potential interactions with prescription medications. Nevertheless, challenges persist in implementing DS/drug interaction checks, particularly due to the complex composition of many DS products, which often contain multiple active ingredients. This complexity increases the risk of adverse events when DS is combined with other supplements or medications. The standardization of practices across federal agencies could facilitate more effective monitoring of DS use and interactions. To enhance DS documentation within EHRs and improve patient safety, best practices recommend the use of structured fields for DS information and cross-referencing DS with medications where applicable. Additionally, healthcare providers should be well-versed in the reference literature that supports drug knowledge databases, enabling them to accurately interpret adverse event or allergy flags related to DS use. Access to resources and ongoing education for healthcare providers is vital, ensuring the timely and precise documentation of DS information, ultimately contributing to enhanced patient care.

In parallel, real-time monitoring and data analytics have ushered in transformative approaches to nutrition monitoring, with a specific emphasis on the early detection of malnutrition [22]. These cutting-edge technologies leverage various data sources, including wearable devices, mobile applications, and advanced imaging techniques, to continuously gather and analyze pertinent information related to an individual's nutritional status. This innovative approach empowers healthcare providers to swiftly identify indicators of malnutrition, such as weight loss or dietary imbalances, enabling timely interventions to prevent its progression and associated health complications. Wearable devices and mobile apps are instrumental in enabling users to monitor their dietary habits, physical activity, and calorie expenditure, promoting proactive engagement in their health. In clinical settings, advanced imaging technologies like DXA and BIA provide detailed data on body composition, further enhancing the ability to detect malnutrition-related changes in muscle mass or bone density. The integration of data analytics and artificial intelligence (AI) is pivotal in processing the vast amounts of data generated by these technologies, enabling the identification of trends and risk factors associated with malnutrition. AI is used to analyze large datasets related to maternal and child nutrition, helping healthcare providers identify trends, risk factors, and areas that require intervention. For instance, AI algorithms have been applied to electronic health records to predict which pregnant women are at a higher risk of gestational diabetes, allowing for early intervention and personalized dietary recommendations [38, 39]. Moreover, real-time monitoring extends its benefits to population health management, assisting public health agencies and policymakers in tracking and addressing malnutrition on a broader scale. These innovations collectively empower individuals, healthcare providers, and public health authorities to take proactive measures against malnutrition, resulting in improved health outcomes and overall well-being.

4 Digital Platforms for Delivery of Nutrition-Related Interventions

Digital interventions encompass a broader range of technological tools, including mobile apps, wearable devices, and online platforms, designed to promote healthy eating habits. These interventions offer features like meal planning, real-time nutrient tracking, and personalized recommendations based on an individual's dietary preferences and goals. Users can monitor their food intake, receive instant feedback on their choices, and access educational resources about nutrition. Additionally, these interventions often include behavior change techniques, like goal-setting and self-monitoring, to help individuals establish and maintain healthier eating patterns.

Telemedicine and virtual care have emerged as innovative approaches for nutrition counseling and support, particularly for patients with inherited metabolic disorders during the COVID-19 pandemic [23]. It enables RDNs to conduct remote nutrition assessments, review recent anthropometrics, and assess dietary adherence. The technology allows for the sharing of educational resources, such as charts and videos, to enhance patient understanding and compliance. Furthermore, RDNs can provide real-time nutrition counseling, offer formula/diet prescriptions, and set nutrition goals. These innovative approaches address the critical need for continued healthcare while minimizing the risk of viral transmission. While challenges exist, RDNs have adapted to these new methods, ultimately improving access to care and patient outcomes. As telemedicine continues to evolve, it holds promise for the sustained delivery of nutrition monitoring and support in the post-pandemic era.

Gamification and digital interventions represent an innovative approach to nutrition monitoring, particularly in promoting healthy eating behaviors [24]. These strategies leverage technology and behavioral psychology to engage individuals in making better dietary choices and sustaining healthier lifestyles. Gamification involves incorporating game elements, such as challenges, rewards, and competition, into non-game contexts like nutrition-tracking apps or websites. For instance, individuals can earn points or badges for meeting daily fruit and vegetable consumption goals or for choosing nutritious options over unhealthy ones. These gamified platforms often employ interactive features, progress tracking, and social components, making the process of monitoring and improving one's diet more enjoyable and motivating. The key advantages of gamification and digital interventions for nutrition monitoring are their accessibility and convenience. They can be easily integrated into daily life, enabling users to track their dietary intake and receive support whenever and wherever they need it. Moreover, these approaches are highly adaptable to individual preferences and dietary requirements, ensuring that nutrition monitoring aligns with each person's unique goals. Furthermore, the engagement factor is crucial. Gamification elements tap into intrinsic motivators like achievement and competition, making individuals more committed to monitoring their diet and making healthier food choices. The interactive nature of digital interventions keeps users actively involved in their dietary progress, fostering a sense of empowerment and ownership over their health.

In summary, the integration of EHRs and nutrition data, along with the adoption of real-time monitoring, telemedicine, and gamification-based digital interventions, signifies a profound shift in healthcare toward more innovative and patient-centric approaches to nutrition monitoring and support. These advancements hold great promise in improving patient outcomes, enhancing healthcare provider workflows, and promoting healthier lifestyles. From preventing potential interactions between dietary supplements and medications to early detection of malnutrition and engaging patients with inherited metabolic disorders through telemedicine, these innovations demonstrate the healthcare industry's adaptability and commitment to ensuring the well-being of individuals. Furthermore, gamification and digital interventions offer accessible and convenient tools for promoting healthy eating habits and encouraging individuals to take charge of their nutrition. As we continue to embrace and refine these technologies, we pave the way for a future where personalized, data-driven, and engaging approaches to nutrition monitoring become the norm, ultimately contributing to better health and well-being for all.

5 Implementation Challenges and Considerations

Advancements in technology have paved the way for innovative approaches to nutrition within the RMNCAH continuum, holding promise for improved health outcomes. However, the implementation of these technologies and approaches is accompanied by several multifaceted challenges. The following are key challenges to consider for effective implementation.

5.1 Cost-Effectiveness: Balancing Investment with Impact

The cost-effectiveness of implementing emerging technologies and innovative approaches in RMNCAH nutrition is a critical concern. While these technologies often require substantial initial investments, assessing their long-term cost-effectiveness is essential [25]. It involves analyzing the ratio of benefits to the costs incurred, considering both direct and indirect economic impacts [25].

Direct costs encompass the expenses associated with technology acquisition, development, maintenance, and staff training. These costs need to be balanced against the benefits, such as improved nutritional outcomes, reduced morbidity, and potential long-term healthcare cost savings. It is essential to scrutinize the direct costs involved and weigh them against the tangible health benefits. Ensuring that the cost per unit of health gain justifies the investment is crucial for decision-makers [25].

Indirect costs and benefits encompass broader socioeconomic impacts, including enhanced productivity, reduced absenteeism, and improved quality of life. Quantifying these intangible benefits provides a more comprehensive understanding of the technology's cost-effectiveness. Evaluating the broader socioeconomic implications is essential to assess the true cost-effectiveness. If the technology positively influences societal well-being and the economy, the initial investment may be deemed justified.

Comparing the costs of implementing emerging technologies with existing conventional approaches would allow for a thorough evaluation of cost-effectiveness to ascertain whether these are truly efficient in terms of resources. Rigorous comparative cost analyses are vital to ensure that the investment in emerging technologies aligns with their anticipated benefits, offering a clear justification for their adoption.

5.2   Scalability: Ensuring Widespread Impact and Accessibility

Scalability is a fundamental aspect when considering the implementation of emerging technologies and approaches. An effective intervention should have the potential to be expanded, replicated, and integrated into routine healthcare settings, ensuring widespread reach and impact across diverse populations.

Flexibility and adaptability are key components for achieving broader implementation [26]. Assessing the adaptability of technologies across diverse contexts is crucial. A "one-size-fits-all" approach might hinder scalability, necessitating customization to suit specific local needs and conditions. The seamless integration of emerging technologies into existing healthcare infrastructures and workflows is paramount for scalability. Technologies that can complement and enhance current practices are more likely to be adopted on a broader scale [27]. Examining the compatibility and ease of integration within established healthcare systems is necessary to ensure that the technologies can be adopted without causing disruption or undue burden.

The financial implications of scaling a technology or approach are a crucial consideration. Assessing the costs associated with broader implementation and ensuring they align with available resources is essential for successful scalability [27, 28]. Careful financial planning and analysis are required to determine the feasibility and sustainability of scaling the technology. Overlooking the cost implications can lead to challenges during the scaling process.

Achieving a balance between cost-effectiveness and scalability is imperative. Technologies and approaches that offer an optimal ratio of benefits to costs and can be effectively scaled are more likely to have a transformative impact on nutrition within the RMNCAH continuum. Striking this balance necessitates a pragmatic approach that involves stakeholder engagement, rigorous evaluation, continuous monitoring, and adaptive strategies. Policymakers, healthcare professionals, technology developers, and communities must collaborate to design and implement interventions that achieve the delicate equilibrium between cost-effectiveness and scalability.

5.3   Infrastructure Requirements and Technological Feasibility

Implementing emerging technologies demands a robust digital infrastructure encompassing high-speed, reliable internet connectivity, and EHR systems. Accessible, interoperable, and secure digital platforms are essential for storing and managing vast amounts of health data generated through these technologies [29]. From a critical perspective, the insufficiency of a comprehensive digital infrastructure in many regions poses a significant hindrance [29, 30]. This inadequacy impedes the seamless implementation and integration of emerging technologies into healthcare systems, leading to a digital divide. Governments and healthcare institutions must prioritize substantial investments in digitalization to lay a strong foundation for technological integration, ensuring equitable access and utilization of these technologies across diverse demographics and geographical regions [29].

The digital divide exacerbates existing healthcare disparities, creating a divide between those who have access to advanced healthcare technologies and those who do not. This inequality in access can result in differential health outcomes, perpetuating existing health inequities. Bridging this divide requires concerted efforts, not only in enhancing digital infrastructure but also in addressing socioeconomic and geographical barriers to ensure equal access to the benefits of technological advancements. Additionally, beyond infrastructure, considerations of digital literacy and accessibility become imperative to truly harness the potential of emerging technologies for improved RMNCAH care.

5.4 Inclusivity in Technologies

Implementing targeted interventions, such as subsidies for technological devices and connectivity, can significantly bridge the digital divide. Governments and organizations should collaborate to provide affordable access to devices and internet services [31]. Although subsidies can indeed help make technologies more accessible; however, a comprehensive approach is needed. Simply providing devices and internet access may not be sufficient. While subsidies are a valuable initial step, they should be seen as part of a larger strategy to close the digital divide comprehensively. Education and training play a pivotal role in empowering individuals to utilize technology effectively [32]. Access alone does not guarantee meaningful use; digital literacy is key. Hence, investing in educational initiatives that enhance digital skills, teach responsible and effective technology usage, and encourage critical thinking is imperative. Moreover, tailoring these educational efforts to the specific needs and demographics of the target population is essential for their effectiveness. A holistic approach that encompasses both infrastructure support and digital literacy education is essential to bridge the divide effectively and empower communities to navigate the digital landscape.

6 Future Scope

In an era marked by rapid technological advancements, innovative solutions are reshaping the landscape of maternal and child nutrition within RMNCAH programs. This transformative wave is evident in a multitude of emerging technologies that are revolutionizing nutrition monitoring and counseling. From mobile health applications tailored to low-resource settings, which offer personalized guidance and employ cutting-edge machine learning algorithms, to the repurposing of wearable devices to monitor nutritional status, each innovation is poised to make a substantial impact. Moreover, blockchain's integration into food supply chains ensures the verification of nutritional quality, while IoT-enabled sensors swiftly analyze the composition of meals. AI mines vast datasets for predictive analytics, aiding healthcare providers in identifying trends and intervention areas, and telemedicine empowers remote monitoring and guidance. Lastly, 3D printing is opening new horizons by customizing nutrient-rich foods, particularly vital for resource-constrained regions. In this exploration of these pioneering technologies, we delve into real-world examples that underscore their effectiveness in advancing maternal and child nutrition, offering promising solutions to longstanding challenges. Emerging 3D printing technology is used to create nutrient-rich foods that cater to the specific dietary needs of pregnant women and children [33, 34]. These printed foods can be customized to deliver essential nutrients and calories, addressing malnutrition in resource-constrained settings.

These real-world examples demonstrate how emerging technologies are being leveraged to enhance nutrition monitoring within RMNCAH programs, ultimately improving the health and well-being of mothers and children in various parts of the world. In this rapidly evolving age of technology, we have seen remarkable innovations that are reshaping how we care for the health of mothers and children in RMNCAH programs. These new technologies are changing the way we monitor and provide nutrition guidance. For instance, mobile health apps are tailoring advice to those with limited resources, using advanced computer programs to help. We're also using everyday wearables like fitness trackers to keep an eye on nutrition and health. Even blockchain is being used to make sure the food we eat is nutritious. Smart sensors can quickly tell us what is in our meals, and artificial intelligence helps healthcare providers find trends and areas needing attention. Telemedicine lets us monitor health from afar, which is especially important in remote areas. And the new frontier of 3D printing is giving us the ability to create special foods packed with nutrients. Real-world examples show that these technologies are making a real difference in improving maternal and child nutrition, offering hope for longstanding challenges.

In the realm of maternal and child nutrition within the RMNCAH continuum, the application of emerging technologies has the potential to usher in transformative advancements. To effectively navigate this technological frontier, several future directions should be considered. Firstly, there is a need for longitudinal studies to assess the long-term efficacy of these technologies, focusing on their impact on maternal and child health outcomes over extended periods. Exploring how various emerging technologies can synergize and complement each other is another critical avenue for research. Customization of these technologies to suit diverse populations, with particular attention to cultural and socioeconomic factors, should be a priority. Furthermore, understanding the most effective strategies for enhancing user engagement and behavior change within these technological platforms is essential. Robust research into data privacy and security measures is also imperative to protect sensitive health information.

On the policy front, governments and international bodies should establish clear regulatory frameworks for emerging technologies in RMNCAH nutrition, encompassing data privacy, safety standards, and quality control. Investment in healthcare infrastructure, particularly digital infrastructure, must be prioritized to ensure equitable access to these technologies. Considering insurance coverage for prescribed emerging technologies can reduce financial barriers. Moreover, building the capacity of healthcare professionals through comprehensive training programs is essential to harness the full potential of these tools. Community engagement and awareness campaigns should be leveraged to promote technology adoption and address cultural or social barriers.

Lastly, fostering collaboration among technology developers, healthcare institutions, governments, and NGOs is crucial for a coordinated approach to implementing emerging technologies in RMNCAH nutrition. Feedback mechanisms must be established to collect input from healthcare providers and patients, informing continuous improvement efforts. In summary, the integration of emerging technologies offers promising solutions to longstanding challenges in maternal and child nutrition, but realizing their full potential requires a concerted effort in research, policy development, capacity building, and stakeholder engagement.

7 Conclusion

In conclusion, the integration of EHRs with nutrition data and the adoption of emerging technologies are reshaping the landscape of nutrition monitoring in healthcare. These innovations have profound implications for RMNCAH care.

Firstly, nutrition's pivotal role in RMNCAH care cannot be overstated. Adequate nutrition is fundamental to reproductive health, maternal well-being, healthy pregnancies, newborn development, and the growth of children and adolescents. By integrating nutrition data into EHRs, healthcare providers can enhance patient care by identifying potential interactions between dietary supplements and prescribed medications. This ensures safer and more effective RMNCAH care. Secondly, the emergence of wearable devices, advanced imaging technologies, and real-time monitoring offers unprecedented opportunities for early detection and prevention of malnutrition. These technologies empower individuals and healthcare providers to proactively address nutritional deficiencies, ultimately improving health outcomes and reducing complications.

Thirdly, telemedicine and virtual care have proven invaluable, especially during the COVID-19 pandemic, for providing nutrition counseling and support to vulnerable populations like those with inherited metabolic disorders. These approaches enhance access to care while minimizing health risks. Lastly, gamification and digital interventions are promoting healthier eating behaviors by making nutrition monitoring enjoyable and engaging. These innovative tools can be personalized to individual preferences and dietary requirements, fostering a sense of ownership over one's health. Continuous innovation and collaboration among healthcare providers, researchers, and technology developers are essential to further improve nutrition monitoring. By embracing these advancements, the healthcare industry is poised to deliver more patient-centric, data-driven, and engaging approaches to nutrition monitoring and support, ultimately enhancing the well-being of individuals across various life stages.

References

1. Das SK, Miki AJ, Blanchard CM, Sazonov E, Gilhooly CH, Dey S, et al. Perspective: opportunities and challenges of technology tools in dietary and activity assessment: bridging stakeholder viewpoints. Adv Nutr. 2022;13(1):1–15.
2. Boushey C, Spoden M, Zhu F, Delp E, Kerr D. New mobile methods for dietary assessment: review of image-assisted and image-based dietary assessment methods. Proc Nutr Soc. 2017;76(3):283–94.
3. Lyden K, Swibas T, Catenacci V, Guo R, Szuminsky N, Melanson EL. Estimating energy expenditure using heat flux measured at single body site. Med Sci Sports Exerc. 2014;46(11):2159.
4. Evans K, Hennessy Á, Walton J, Timon C, Gibney E, Flynn A. Development and evaluation of a concise food list for use in a web-based 24-h dietary recall tool. J Nutr Sci. 2017;6:e46.
5. Blanchard CM, Chin MK, Gilhooly CH, Barger K, Matuszek G, Miki AJ, et al. Evaluation of PIQNIQ, a novel mobile application for capturing dietary intake. J Nutr. 2021;151(5):1347–56.
6. Lee S, O'Dell D, Hohenstein J, Colt S, Mehta S, Erickson D. NutriPhone: a mobile platform for low-cost point-of-care quantification of vitamin B12 concentrations. Sci Rep. 2016;6(1):28237.
7. Simpson E, Bradley J, Poliakov I, Jackson D, Olivier P, Adamson AJ, et al. Iterative development of an online dietary recall tool: INTAKE24. Nutrients. 2017;9(2):118.
8. Watkins I, Kules B, Yuan X, Xie B. Heuristic evaluation of healthy eating apps for older adults. J Consum Health Internet. 2014;18(2):105–27.
9. Lemacks JL, Adams K, Lovetere A. Dietary intake reporting accuracy of the bridge2u mobile application food log compared to control meal and dietary recall methods. Nutrients. 2019;11(1):199.
10. Ehrlich SF, Maples JM, Barroso CS, Brown KC, Bassett DR, Zite NB, et al. Using a consumer-based wearable activity tracker for physical activity goal setting and measuring steps in pregnant women with gestational diabetes mellitus: exploring acceptance and validity. BMC Pregnancy Childbirth. 2021;21(1):1–10.
11. Grym K, Niela-Vilén H, Ekholm E, Hamari L, Azimi I, Rahmani A, et al. Feasibility of smart wristbands for continuous monitoring during pregnancy and one month after birth. BMC Pregnancy Childbirth. 2019;19(1):1–9.
12. Marra M, Sammarco R, De Lorenzo A, Iellamo F, Siervo M, Pietrobelli A, et al. Assessment of body composition in health and disease using bioelectrical impedance analysis (BIA) and dual energy X-ray absorptiometry (DXA): a critical overview. Contrast Media & Molecular. Imaging. 2019;2019:1.
13. Mazess RB, Barden HS, Bisek JP, Hanson J. Dual-energy x-ray absorptiometry for total-body and regional bone-mineral and soft-tissue composition. Am J Clin Nutr. 1990;51(6):1106–12.
14. Kyle UG, Bosaeus I, De Lorenzo AD, Deurenberg P, Elia M, Gómez JM, et al. Bioelectrical impedance analysis—part I: review of principles and methods. Clin Nutr. 2004;23(5):1226–43.
15. Foster KR, Lukaski HC. Whole-body impedance--what does it measure? Am J Clin Nutr. 1996;64(3):S388–S96.
16. Matthie J, Zarowitz B, De Lorenzo A, Andreoli A, Katzarski K, Pan G, et al. Analytic assessment of the various bioimpedance methods used to estimate body water. J Appl Physiol. 1998;84(5):1801–16.
17. Dauncey MJ. Genomic and epigenomic insights into nutrition and brain disorders. Nutrients. 2013;5(3):887–914.
18. Bras J, Guerreiro R, Hardy J. Use of next-generation sequencing and other whole-genome strategies to dissect neurological disease. Nat Rev Neurosci. 2012;13(7):453–64.
19. Sullivan PF, Daly MJ, O'donovan M. Genetic architectures of psychiatric disorders: the emerging picture and its implications. Nat Rev Genet. 2012;13(8):537–51.

20. Singh RH, Pringle T, Kenneson A. The use of telemedicine and other strategies by registered dietitians for the medical nutrition therapy of patients with inherited metabolic disorders during the COVID-19 pandemic. Front Nutr. 2021;8:637868.
21. Costello RB, Deuster PA, Michael M, Utech A. Capturing the use of dietary supplements in electronic medical records: room for improvement. Nutr Today. 2019;54(4):144.
22. Stirling E, Willcox J, Ong K-L, Forsyth A. Social media analytics in nutrition research: a rapid review of current usage in investigation of dietary behaviours. Public Health Nutr. 2021;24(6):1193–209.
23. Shima M, Piovacari SMF, Steinman M, Pereira AZ, Dos Santos OFP. Telehealth for nutritional care: a tool for improving patient flow in hospitals. Telemed Rep. 2022;3(1):117–24.
24. Suleiman-Martos N, García-Lara RA, Martos-Cabrera MB, Albendín-García L, Romero-Béjar JL, Cañadas-De la Fuente GA, et al. Gamification for the improvement of diet, nutritional habits, and body composition in children and adolescents: a systematic review and meta-analysis. Nutrients. 2021;13(7):2478.
25. Kagaha A, Manderson L. Power, policy and abortion care in Uganda. Health Policy Plan. 2021;36(2):187–95.
26. Alam N, Mamun M, Dema P. Reproductive, maternal, newborn, child, and adolescent health (RMNCAH): key global public health agenda in SDG era. Good Health Well-Being. 2020:583–93.
27. Morgan R, Garrison-Desany H, Hobbs AJ, Wilson E. Strengthening effectiveness evaluations through gender integration to improve programs for women, newborn, child, and adolescent health. Glob Health Action. 2022;15(sup1):2006420.
28. World Health Organization. Report of the fifth meeting of the South-East Asia regional technical advisory group and first meeting of sexual reproductive health technical subcommittee towards reduction of maternal mortality and stillbirths in the context of universal health coverage New Delhi India, 25–27 November, 2019. World Health Organization. Regional Office for South-East Asia; 2020.
29. Belaid L, Bayo P, Kamau L, Nakimuli E, Omoro E, Lobor R, et al. Health policy mapping and system gaps impeding the implementation of reproductive, maternal, neonatal, child, and adolescent health programs in South Sudan: a scoping review. Confl Heal. 2020;14:1–16.
30. Organization WH. Monitoring and evaluating digital health interventions: a practical guide to conducting research and assessment; 2016.
31. Labrique A, Agarwal S, Tamrat T, Mehl G. WHO digital health guidelines: a milestone for global health. NPJ Digit Med. 2020;3(1):120.
32. Fletcher RR, Nakeshimana A, Olubeko O. Addressing fairness, bias, and appropriate use of artificial intelligence and machine learning in global health. Front Media SA. 2021;3:561802.
33. Guo Z, Arslan M, Li Z, Cen S, Shi J, Huang X, et al. Application of protein in extrusion-based 3D food printing: current status and prospectus. Food Secur. 2022;11(13):1902.
34. Varvara R-A, Szabo K, Vodnar DC. 3D food printing: principles of obtaining digitally-designed nourishment. Nutrients. 2021;13(10):3617.

Conclusion and the Way Forward

Conclusion and Way Forward

Rehana A. Salam, Zahra Ali Padhani, and Zohra S. Lassi

The previous chapters in this book presented challenges associated with nutritional indicators across the continuum of reproductive, maternal, newborn, child and adolescent health, along with the existing evidence-based interventions to overcome these challenges. Interventions like antenatal multiple micronutrient supplementation, provision of supplementary food and utilising locally produced food in food-insecure settings have shown to be effective in reducing the risk of adverse pregnancy outcomes and managing childhood malnutrition [1]. Some emerging interventions, such as preventive small-quantity lipid-based nutrient supplements for children aged 6–23 months, have shown positive effects on child growth. Integrated interventions (e.g. diet, exercise, and behavioural therapy) have shown effectiveness for the prevention and management of childhood obesity [1]. Indirect nutrition strategies, such as malaria prevention, preconception care, water, sanitation, and hygiene promotion, delivered inside and outside the healthcare sector, have also shown to improve nutritional and broad health outcomes [1]. Despite the existence of proven evidence-based interventions, worldwide in 2022, an estimated 148.1 million children under 5 years of age (22.3%) were stunted, 45 million (6.8%) were wasted, and 37 million (5.6%) were overweight [2]. The same year, 735 million people were undernourished, and

R. A. Salam (✉)
The Daffodil Centre, The University of Sydney, a joint venture with Cancer Council NSW, Sydney, NSW, Australia
e-mail: rehana.abdussalam@sydney.edu.au

Z. A. Padhani · Z. S. Lassi
School of Public Health, University of Adelaide, Adelaide, SA, Australia

Robinson Research Institute, Adelaide Medical School, The University of Adelaide, Adelaide, SA, Australia
e-mail: zahraali.padhani@adelaide.edu.au; zohra.lassi@adelaide.edu.au

© The Author(s), under exclusive license to Springer Nature Switzerland AG 2025
Z. S. Lassi, R. A. Salam (eds.), *Nutrition Across Reproductive, Maternal, Neonatal, Child, and Adolescent Health Care*,
https://doi.org/10.1007/978-3-031-95721-5_22

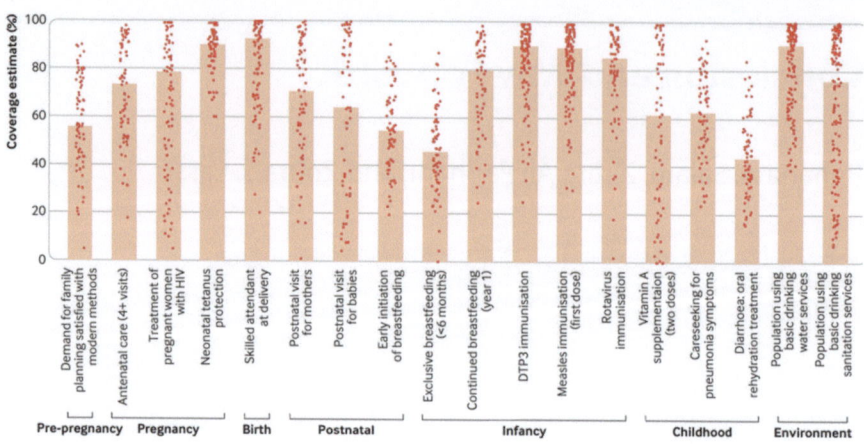

Fig. 1 Median national coverage for selected interventions for women's and child health [4]. (Published under the terms of the Creative Commons Attribution (CC BY 4.0) licence https://creativecommons.org/licenses/by/4.0/deed.en)

2.4 billion were food insecure [3]. Access and coverage of these interventions remain a concern, even though these are not only beneficial but also cost-effective.

Figure 1 depicts the median national coverage for selected interventions for women's and child health using the most recent data from the World Health Organisation (WHO) and the United Nations Children's Fund (UNICEF) for each country [4]. Not only does the coverage of these proven interventions remain low, but there also exist inequities. These inequities not only exist between high-income countries and low- and middle-income countries (LMICs) but also among the vulnerable population groups within the countries.

An analysis of wealth inequalities from 83 LMICs assessed the composite coverage index (CCI), which was a combined measure of coverage with eight key reproductive, maternal, newborn and child health interventions [5]. The study found that in 61 of the 83 countries, the wealthiest decile achieved 70% or higher CCI coverage and that the inequality was mostly driven by coverage among the poor, which is much more variable than coverage among the rich across countries. Well-performing countries were particularly effective in achieving high coverage among the poor, while underperforming countries failed to reach the poorest, despite reaching the better-off. This depicts that huge inequalities exist between the richest and the poorest women and children in most countries. Besides inequality, conflict also poses a major challenge in achieving universal coverage. An analysis reports that inequalities in coverage of reproductive/maternal health and child vaccine interventions are significantly worse in conflict-affected countries [6]. When compared to non-conflict countries, access to essential reproductive and maternal health services for poorer, less educated and rural-based families was several-fold worse in conflict countries [6]. There are gendered dimensions to inequity in access and coverage. These are influenced by factors operating at various levels, e.g. age of marriage, literacy, decision-making capacity, household composition, social norms, and access to services [7]. Hence, there is a need to intervene at multiple levels, including individual, household, and broader communities. Challenges associated with climate change have added another dimension to the already existing inequities. With increasing urbanisation, there is greater availability of cheaper, convenience, pre-prepared and fast foods, often energy dense and high in fats, sugars and/or salt, that can contribute to malnutrition. Loss of land and natural capital due to urbanisation pose potential future challenges like insufficient availability of vegetables and fruits and exclusion of small farmers from formal value chains.

Although proven interventions exist, little is known about the effectiveness of these interventions in various challenging scenarios mentioned above. Moreover, how best to deliver these interventions in these evolving times also remains a black box. These wide-spanning challenges across multiple domains not only require a bird's-eye view of the issue but also appropriate cross-cutting strategies that involve a broader range of stakeholders than previously included (Fig. 2). There are a host of delivery factors that have proven to be enablers in implementing programmes targeting nutrition indicators, and these include community advocacy and social

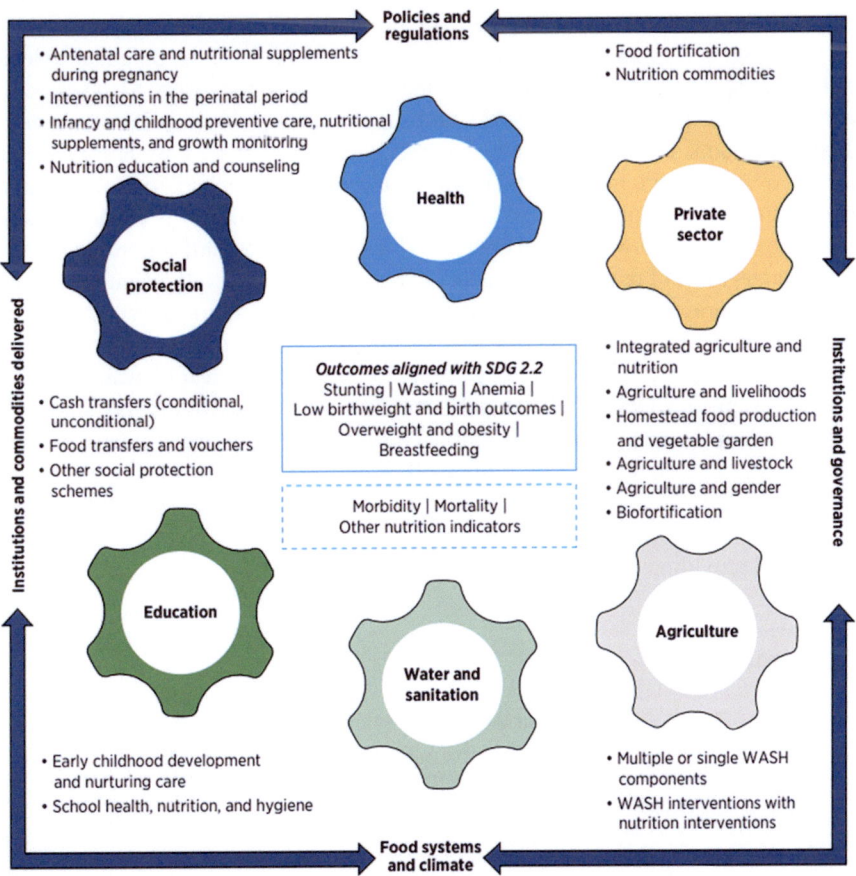

Fig. 2 Nutritional services can be delivered through several sectors [9]

mobilisation, effective monitoring, and integration of nutrition with other sectoral interventions and services [3]. Similarly, some of the major reported barriers include insufficient resources, nutritional commodity shortages, security concerns, poor reporting, limited cooperation, and difficulty accessing and following up with beneficiaries [3]. These challenges require considerations out of the box, e.g. incorporating complex scenarios like gendered dimensions of inequality in designing programmes targeting nutritional indicators or adapting existing delivery platforms to meet the needs of populations residing in conflict settings. These adaptations would require a more comprehensive understanding of the issues underlying the prevalent lack of access and coverage at all levels, and not just the myopic approach taken historically to improve individuals' nutrition status. Broader structural drivers that underpin the political economy of interpersonal relations and conflict scenarios need to be incorporated when designing future programmes [8].

Looking forward, greater effort is required to improve intervention coverage, especially for the most vulnerable, and there is a crucial need to address the growing double/triple burden of malnutrition in LMICs [1]. Primary health care was and remains an important platform to achieve universal health coverage. However, essential nutrition actions are required at multiple levels of health service delivery, including secondary and tertiary care. These investments have the potential to lead to humongous returns that far outweigh the costs of inaction; every $1 invested in addressing undernutrition returns $23, and an estimated $2.4 trillion is being generated in economic benefits [9]. On the contrary, lack of action can cost us around $41 trillion over 10 years, including $21 trillion in economic productivity losses due to undernutrition and micronutrient deficiencies and $20 trillion in economic and social costs from overweight and obesity [9]. Future work towards improving nutritional targets would require investments in the domains of development assistance and domestic resources, innovative financing approaches, empirical research, maximisation of delivery platforms for scaling up, and technical and implementation support to countries to scale up [9]. In order to take a step forward towards achieving the Sustainable Development Goals, concrete measures need to be taken to integrate nutrition-related actions into national health systems, to improve the coverage and quality of essential nutrition actions [9]. A multisectoral plan of action needs to be devised that is coherent and designed to achieve universal health coverage, embodying equity in access to health services, ensuring good quality of health services, and providing protection against financial risks [10].

References

1. Keats EC, Das JK, Salam RA, et al. Effective interventions to address maternal and child malnutrition: an update of the evidence. Lancet Child Adolesc Health. 2021;5(5):367–84.
2. FAO, UNICEF, WFP and WHO. The state of food security and nutrition in the world 2024—financing to end hunger, food insecurity and malnutrition in all its forms. Rome; 2024. https://doi.org/10.4060/cd1254en.
3. The World Health Organization. The state of food security and nutrition in the world 2023: urbanization, agrifood systems transformation and healthy diets across the rural–urban continuum, vol. 2023. Food & Agriculture Org; 2023.

4. Requejo J, Diaz T, Park L, et al. Assessing coverage of interventions for reproductive, maternal, newborn, child, and adolescent health and nutrition. BMJ. 2020:368.
5. Barros AJ, Wehrmeister FC, Ferreira LZ, Vidaletti LP, Hosseinpoor AR, Victora CG. Are the poorest poor being left behind? Estimating global inequalities in reproductive, maternal, newborn and child health. BMJ Glob Health. 2020;5(1):e002229.
6. Akseer N, Wright J, Tasic H, et al. Women, children and adolescents in conflict countries: an assessment of inequalities in intervention coverage and survival. BMJ Glob Health. 2020;5(1):e002214.
7. George AS, Amin A, de Abreu Lopes CM, Ravindran TS. Structural determinants of gender inequality: why they matter for adolescent girls' sexual and reproductive health. BMJ. 2020:368.
8. Shah S, Padhani ZA, Als D, et al. Delivering nutrition interventions to women and children in conflict settings: a systematic review. BMJ Glob Health. 2021;6(4):e004897.
9. Shekar M, Okamura KS, Vilar-Compte M, Dell'Aira C. Investment framework for nutrition 2024. Washington, DC: World Bank; 2024.
10. World Health Organization. Nutrition in universal health coverage; 2019.

MIX
Papier aus verantwortungsvollen Quellen
Paper from responsible sources
FSC® C105338

If you have any concerns about our products,
you can contact us on
ProductSafety@springernature.com

In case Publisher is established outside the EU,
the EU authorized representative is:
**Springer Nature Customer Service Center GmbH
Europaplatz 3, 69115 Heidelberg, Germany**

Printed by Libri Plureos GmbH
in Hamburg, Germany